Pregnancy, Birth and Maternity Care:
feminist perspectives

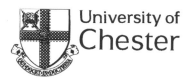
University of
Chester

ARROWE PARK
LIBRARY

This book is to be returned on or before the last date stamped below. Overdue charges will be incurred by the late return of books.

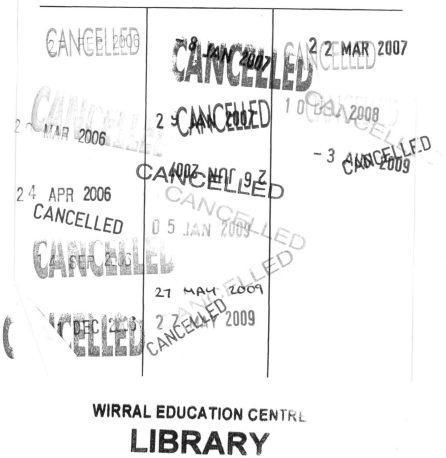

For Books for Midwives:

Senior Commissioning Editor: Mary Seager
Development Editor: Catharine Steers
Project Manager: Pat Miller/Samantha Ross
Designer: George Ajayi

Pregnancy, Birth and Maternity Care: feminist perspectives

Edited by

Mary Stewart RGN RM BSc (Hons) MSc

Senior Lecturer in Midwifery, University of the West of England,
Bristol, UK

Foreword by

Sheila C. Hunt PhD MBA MScEcon RGN RM PGCE

Dean, School of Nursing and Midwifery, University of Dundee, Dundee, UK

BfM Books *for* Midwives

EDINBURGH LONDON NEW YORK OXFORD PHILADELPHIA ST LOUIS SYDNEY TORONTO 2004

Books for Midwives
An imprint of Elsevier Science Limited

First published 2004

ISBN 0 7506 5601 8

British Library Cataloguing in Publication Data
A catalogue record for this book is available from the British Library

Library of Congress Cataloging in Publication Data
A catalog record for this book is available from the Library of Congress

Medical knowledge is constantly changing. Standard safety
precautions must be followed, but as new research and clinical
experience broaden our knowledge, changes in treatment and drug
therapy may become necessary or appropriate. Readers are advised
to check the most current product information provided by the
manufacturer of each drug to be administered to verify the
recommended dose, the method and duration of administration, and
contraindications. It is the responsibility of the practitioner, relying
on experience and knowledge of the patient, to determine dosages and
the best treatment for each individual patient. Neither the Publisher
nor the editor assumes any liability for any injury and/or damage to
persons or property arising from this publication.

The Publisher

**ELSEVIER
SCIENCE** your source for books,
journals and multimedia
in the health sciences

www.elsevierhealth.com

The
Publisher's
policy is to use
**paper manufactured
from sustainable forests**

Printed in China

Contents

Contributors

Carol Bates MA PGCEA ADM RM RN
Education & Professional Development Adviser,
Royal College of Midwives, Past Director
Midwifery Education, University
College Hospital, London

Ann Cronin BSc PhD(Sociology)
Lecturer in Sociology, University of Surrey,
Guildford, UK

Lorna Davies RN RM BSc(Hons) PGCEA MA
Senior Lecturer in Midwifery, Anglia
Polytechnic University, Chelmsford, UK

Sheila C. Hunt PhD MBA MScEcon RGN RM PGC
Dean, School of Nursing and Midwifery,
University of Dundee, Dundee, UK

Tara Kaufmann
Change Facilitator, Barts and the London NHS
Trust, London, UK

Nicky Leap RM MSc
Director of Midwifery Practice, South East
Sydney Area Health Service, and Associate
Professor of Midwifery, University of
Technology, Sydney, Australia

Sally Marchant PhD RM RN DipED
Midwife/Editor, MIDIRS (Midwives Information
& Resource Service) Midwifery Digest,
Visiting Fellow, Bournemouth University, UK

Gabrielle Palmer MSc Human Nutrition
Lecturer, Public Health Nutrition Unit,
London School of Hygiene and Tropical
Medicine, London, UK

Liz Stephens MA BSc(Hons) PGDipEd RM RGN
Consultant Midwife, Surrey, UK

Mary Stewart RGN RM BSc(Hons) MSc
Senior Lecturer in Midwifery, University of the
West of England, Bristol, UK

Ruth Surtees NZRN NZPN RM BA(Hons) PhD
University of Canterbury, Aotearoa,
New Zealand

Jane M. Ussher BA PhD DipClinPsych AFBPS
Professor of Women's Health Psychology,
School of Psychology, University of Western
Sydney, Australia

Denis Walsh RM DPSM PGDipE MA
Independent Midwifery Lecturer and PhD
Student, University of Central Lancashire,
Preston, UK

Sarah Wickham RM MA PGCE(A) BA(Hons)
Senior Lecturer in Midwifery, Anglia Polytechnic
University, Chelmsford, UK

Foreword

I was delighted to be asked to write the foreword for this exciting and imaginative new text. Childbirth is a woman's issue and I have always wondered why anyone could possibly believe that childbirth and midwifery, in particular, could be studied without some reference or even a mention of a feminist framework. Theory, in this case feminist theories, can be described as 'a way of seeing' or the lens through which we see and subsequently construct our explanation of the world. Feminism according to Beasley (1999) is a troublesome term and one of those terms that conveniently defies simple explanation. It is a term which is over-used and often abused and one that has become part of everyday conversation. It is not a single entity but is as the reader of this book will discover, a complex, diverse and still changing concept. It does not belong in academic institutions and to unreadable academic texts but should be available to shine the light on almost every aspect of modern midwifery care.

The authors of this stimulating new text, selected from all regions of the globe, have taken on the task of defining this multifaceted concept with a combination of intellectual rigour, humour, experience and passion. In nearly every chapter the author has defined feminist theories but more importantly has sought to apply these theoretical explanations of the world to aspects of midwifery and to the reality of clinical practice. For the first time, Mary Stewart as editor, has brought together midwifery academics and experienced clinicians to challenge us and to help us to think differently about midwifery care and to shed a new light on many aspects of midwifery care. Questions for reflection challenge the reader to pause and ask 'So what does this mean for midwifery care and for childbearing women and their families'?

The text is also important as a statement of 'So where are we now'? Midwifery as still a relatively new academic discipline is growing rapidly. Its place now firmly established in Higher Education, it still draws on theory and knowledge from other disciplines such as psychology, sociology, and social policy but that which is the essence of midwifery is step-by-step becoming clearer and more expertly defined. This book then is a statement of some of where we are now. We have to know and understand these issues if we are to consciously plan where we would like to be and perhaps more importantly have some sense of how might we get there. As midwives we have to understand all aspects of current clinical practice, but we also have to know and understand the meaning of practice, we have to appreciate the origins of its roots, its beginnings, its attitudes and its beliefs and values. This understanding and depth of thinking is essential if we are to go forward to develop and redefine the fundamentals of our own discipline – its values and its philosophy of care.

This book then will be a jewel in the growing body of midwifery literature, it will become essential reading for every student and qualified midwife. In due course no-one will attempt to define midwifery without acknowledging the feminist 'way of seeing'. Only then we will move confidently to woman-centred care and really mean it.

Sheila C. Hunt

REFERENCE

Beasley C (1999) What is feminism? Sage Publications, London

Preface

Why have a book on feminisms and childbirth? It is a fair question and my first response would be 'well, it seemed like a good idea at the time'. But that is a flippant and untrue response. The reason this book has come into being is because I believe passionately that women matter, and yet we live in a society that, although blessed with many advances and privileges, continues to systematically disadvantage women. Of course, not all women are disadvantaged in the same way. As a white, professional women I am subject to far fewer disadvantages than some of my less-fortunate peers. Nonetheless, we still live in a society that overwhelmingly privileges the male role while undermining the work, both paid and unpaid, of women. I believe this matters immensely, not only to women, but to men too, and that a society where men and women were truly treated as equals would make life better for women *and* for men.

The great majority of those working in the maternity services are women and women are the primary focus of our care and support. For this reason, I think that all those working in the maternity services need an awareness of what feminisms are and how they can be used to underpin both theory and practice. I don't imagine that this book, on its own, will convince a committed sceptic that feminisms are the answer. However, I hope it may begin to sow a seed and to perhaps even persuade you to view the world in a different way.

The book has only reached completion through the immense commitment and enthusiasm of the individual authors of each chapter. Although the chapters follow in a logical format, each is complete in itself so, while you may want to start at the beginning and work your way through to the end of the book, it is equally possible to pick a chapter at random and start with that.

As I write this preface, in July 2003, a study commissioned by the Equal Opportunities Commission has been published which suggests that feminism is 'outmoded and unpopular'. (However I cannot refrain from pointing out that this same study, which grabbed all the headlines, only included the opinions of 35 people.) I hope this book may persuade you otherwise.

Bristol, 2004   Mary Stewart

1

Introducing feminism

Tara Kaufmann

INTRODUCTION

This chapter provides an introduction to feminism: its origins, its theories and its complicated history. It does not attempt to be comprehensive – that would require a whole series of books, not just one chapter. Rather, it focuses on the main themes and concepts of modern feminism and on their implications for women, including midwives. Its message is that feminist thought is a powerful resource for midwifery practice, one that offers a deeper understanding of the forces and feelings that shape women's lives.

Box 1.1

A woman arrives for her booking appointment, delighted to be pregnant after several years delay in starting a family while she worked to establish her career and buy a suitable home. She has read widely on pregnancy, including numerous accounts of women's own experiences, and has decided to choose a home birth.

The next woman to come in is on her third pregnancy. She is accompanied by her husband, a dominating presence who does most of the talking. The woman is pale and tired; there is fresh bruising on her arms and abdomen. Suspecting domestic abuse, the midwife works out a reason for seeing the woman on her own for a few minutes. She gathers together a selection of information on the support services that are available, in case they are needed.

Next, a lesbian couple. This is their first child and they are overjoyed and wanting to share every moment of the pregnancy together. The midwife carefully takes them through the booking form, ensuring that the non-biological mother is recorded as a full partner and co-parent.

These scenarios show how much feminism has changed our social landscape. Just two generations ago, women had restricted access to contraception, making planned parenthood difficult. Their career options were limited, as was the freedom to enjoy sexual relationships outside tightly defined norms. The concept of women's rights over their own bodies, including the right to give birth in the way they chose, was alien to mainstream maternity care. Violence in the home was commonplace but taboo: women were expected to suffer in silence and the caring professions did not consider it their place to intervene.

It is easy to forget the transformations in consciousness wrought by feminism. Many women can recall the exhilaration and freedom they felt the first time they realised that housework was *real* work, that it was OK not to want to be with your children all the time, that it was not hung up to be upset by sexual harassment. Feminism changed women's lives and although it is not now the active movement it once was, its ideas and its influence are still clearly evident. Although only a minority of women call themselves feminists, the vast majority fully endorse equality of opportunity, equal treatment and the belief that women should be accorded their true value. The central tenets of feminism have become 'common sense' and although many of its goals are unrealised, it would now seem impossible to return to the days when sexual inequality was considered normal, natural and desirable – by women as well as by men.

A BRIEF HISTORY

There have always been women who fought for the rights and interests of other women. Mary Wollstonecraft's *Vindication of the Rights of Woman* was published in 1792 and she drew inspiration from the feminist activists of revolutionary France. But the first mass movement in support of women's rights – the 'first wave' of feminism – took place in the early years of the 20th century, with the struggle for enfranchisement. As with the Women's Liberation Movement of some 60 years later, the campaign for suffrage was a coalition of mainstream liberals, radical activists and sympathetic male supporters. When the vote was

finally won, after the end of the First World War, the movement dissolved into fragments. Some continued their work through socialism, social reform or fighting to enter higher education and the 'male' professions, while others simply melted back into their everyday lives.

During both world wars, but most markedly during the second, women were needed to take over men's jobs in order to support the war effort and keep the economy going. This probably did as much to change women's expectations as any amount of formal political activism. The state was forced to support this reserve army of labour by providing childcare and canteen services. Employers found that women could work as swiftly and as skilfully as men, and many women enjoyed their increased financial and social independence. With the return of an army of newly unemployed men, however, women were expected to surrender their jobs and return to domestic labour. The years after the Second World War witnessed an overwhelming backlash against women working outside the home. The cult of the housewife reached its peak, buttressed by new theories about the damage women could do to themselves, their husbands, and above all their children, if they were 'selfish' enough to seek paid work.

'Second-wave' feminism burst onto this stifling ideology like a saltwater wave. It was part of the late 1960s explosion of radical and countercultural activism, and also in part a reaction to how women were treated within that activism. This new feminism was a roar of frustrated rage: rage that formal equality had not dislodged male privilege and rage that the radical social movements of the time – the New Left, black power, CND, gay liberation – still relegated women to tea making and leaflet typing. Although some women found new opportunities for self-expression and leadership in radical politics, others felt exploited and abused – not least because of the loosening codes of sexual behaviour, which expected women to become more sexually available without demanding increased respect for their autonomy and dignity. Radical politics was still male politics and women's experiences were ignored or trivialised.

Many women defected from male-dominated left wing politics in order to apply its analytical framework to their own situation. They borrowed from class politics in order to explore the oppression of women *as* women. Reacting against traditional ways of organising, they formed non-hierarchical, women-only groups which blended campaigning with 'consciousness raising', discussing the detail of their personal lives, uncovering the myriad ways in which sexist ideologies had constrained them from reaching full personhood. It may sound trivial now but for many women this was the first opportunity to talk about how unhappy and restricted they felt in a social code that expected them to find smiling fulfilment living for and through their husbands and children. They began to question all aspects of their lives, even (or especially) those considered normal, natural, trivial or taboo, in order to map out the web of ways in which women were systematically exploited and disadvantaged. 'The personal is political' was ground breaking in its insistence that the battlegrounds of sexism were as much in women's beds and hearts and kitchens and bodies as they were in the public sphere.

Following the lead of earlier feminists like Simone de Beauvoir and newer writers like Germaine Greer, women began to question the very concept of 'woman'. They had been taught all their lives that women were 'naturally' domestic, maternal, sexually submissive, non-intellectual, unambitious and emotionally fragile. Now they wondered why, if women's role was so natural, it had to be so strongly taught and so heavily policed. They unpicked the blanket of messages that teach girls how to be women – messages that are built into language, culture and civilisation – and asserted that the very ubiquity of these messages does not prove that what we call 'femininity' is natural, but that it is propaganda that has to be reinforced for every generation.

Why, for example, does femininity, 'looking like a woman', require so much artifice and hard work? Feminists began to analyse the tremendous pressure put on women, especially young women, to be thin, pretty and sexy. They asked why women spend so much time and money ensuring they look acceptable, by plucking, waxing, bleaching, dyeing, dieting and dressing. It is not that there is anything intrinsically wrong with these activities,

and they bring great pleasure to many women, but equally they are not a freely chosen activity – the penalties for refusing to conform to conventional ideals of beauty are significant. Any woman who has dared to be fat, leave obvious hair on her upper lip or wear short skirts without shaving her legs is aware of how much derision and distaste she will attract. Conversely, there are real and important social rewards for looking beautiful.

Similarly, feminists began to untie the knot of conflicting social expectations around paid work. In the first half of the last century, women were expected to work inside the home, not outside it. Although many women always did take on paid work, not least for economic necessity, this was considered rather shameful and a definite second best to domesticity. When women did work, it was nearly always in a limited set of jobs considered appropriate (like midwifery and nursing) and it was usually an alternative, not a complement, to marriage and children. As increasing numbers of women entered the job market, in the second half of the last century, little was done to reallocate domestic labour more fairly. Women were, and are, expected to combine both. The stress, inconvenience and expense this incurs are considered the responsibility of individual women and are not shared equally with fathers or with wider society. Women find private solutions, usually involving the labour of other women, either poorly paid (au pairs, childminders, nursery workers) or unpaid (grandmothers). If these private solutions fail then that is taken as evidence of the mother's own inadequacy or as a failure of feminism.

The early agenda of second-wave feminism focused on the main obstacles to women's full emancipation: the burdens of housework and childcare, the right to control one's own fertility, equal pay for equal work, access to 'men's jobs'. Later, these were joined by deeper manifestations of socially constructed femininity and male power: cultural representations of women, sexual identity, gender violence. The scope of sexual politics widened, too, embracing global concerns like imperialism, racism and the nuclear threat.

Many of these political concerns seemed alien to the general public. The questioning of heterosexuality and family life, in particular, was received as extremist, anti-men and unnatural. A hostile media portrayed feminists as ugly and shrill and their demands as inimical to the interests of 'ordinary women'. Popular stereotyping of feminists as lesbians (with that considered a bad thing) and as unattractive to men helped drive a wedge between the movement's radical and liberal elements and persuaded many women to stay away altogether. It is notable that the feminist campaigns that attracted the largest public support were those that allowed women to build on, rather than subvert, their traditional role as nurturers of the next generation – as with the peace camp at Greenham Common. This despite the fact that feminism was and is a highly practical movement, with a strong emphasis on the provision of help and support for all women. Very many women have used the rape crisis helplines, women's aid refuges, pregnancy advisory clinics and childcare services provided by feminists, while publicly disavowing the political initiatives in which these services were rooted.

External hostility to feminism weakened its support base, but its potency as a political force was also fissured by its many internal disputes. The very strength and cohesiveness of the original consciousness-raising focus were built, at least in part, on the shared experiences and mutual recognition of 'women like us': the mainly young, white, middle-class women of the Left. Women within the movement who did not fit this model were very much a minority at first, but as the women's movement grew, it encompassed more and more women who rightly demanded that its analysis address the complexities of class, race and sexual preference.

A more hierarchical, disciplined, strongly led movement may have disowned or suppressed these challenges. But feminism was built on a veneration of personal experience as the foundation stone of political awareness and credibility: it had to take on the challenge. Many of its members felt uneasy at the passing of the cosy camaraderie and shared experience that they had hitherto enjoyed; some slipped away, while others despaired over the loss, as they saw it, of the easy solidarity of the political label 'woman'. Those

who stayed entered a difficult period where external struggles faded beside the internal challenge of attempting to build a feminism that could truly speak for all women. Paradoxically, the very structure of feminism (non-hierarchical, leaderless, organic) made it both ideally set up to represent diverse constituent interests and unable to build a coherent political programme that knitted together the solidarity and diversity of women.

Sectarian infighting is a classic feature in the growth of political movements and feminism was not spared. There were times, particularly in the 1980s, when it felt ready to implode under the weight of its own internal battles. 'The personal is political' – that powerful evocation of the strength and insight of feminist analysis – spawned an obsession with identity politics, with women competing to claim 'ownership' of the moral high ground, and of feminism itself, by obsessive self-labelling, glorifying victimisation and putting down others because of their social, sexual or racial identity. This destructive tendency has often been blamed on those women who started questioning the complacent hegemony of white, middle-class, heterosexual feminism, but that was not accurate or fair. Identity politics was used just as much to defend against radical challenge as it was to pose such challenges and in a movement founded on personal experience, it is not surprising that so many used personal experience as their weapon of choice.

Feminism failed to muster the political discipline to sustain a mass movement, but its energy and ideas did not disappear. Even as the Women's Liberation Movement was disintegrating, feminist campaigns and networks were growing. Many feminists moved into the mainstream and worked to influence public services, government and the professions. Others created imaginative and radical campaigning and support groups like Southall Black Sisters, Justice for Women, and the Maternity Alliance. Others worked in international alliances with burgeoning feminist movements across the globe. Meanwhile, a new generation of young feminists emerged with a confident and articulate attack on everything they felt their foremothers had done wrong.

Writers like Naomi Wolf and Katie Roiphe blamed feminism for being puritan and policing and issued a clarion call for independent young women to take forward their own kind of feminism.

The heyday of second-wave feminist activism was over with the dawn of the 1990s. Over the last decade, feminism as a political movement with a mass following has waned in Europe and the USA. Feminist debates continue and have influence but the radical promise of the second wave has not been realised.

Whether you judge feminism a success or a failure depends entirely on your perspective. Given the enormity of its task and the strength of the forces allied against it, its achievements are impressive. It succeeded, in just a couple of decades, in making significant changes to public consciousness about women's place and women's worth. But consciousness itself is not enough to deliver sustained changes to women's lives. There may be greater public awareness of the problem of sexual violence but the sexual violence itself continues unabated. Campaigns against pornography won real support from large numbers of women but the proliferation of misogynist and sexualised images of women – and now children – continues across both mainstream and fringe media. Feminism still has enormous potential to improve women's lives and that potential is yet to be realised.

FEMINIST THEORIES

While it is useful and important to have an understanding of feminism's theoretical roots and analytical frameworks, these must come with a strong health warning. There is no one feminist theory: feminist thought is interdisciplinary and diverse. While it is possible to attempt to divide it into discrete strands (as I have done below) these can only introduce the major wellsprings that fed feminism in its infancy: they do not do justice to the eclectic and permeable nature of feminist thought.

Nor, indeed, do they reflect the intensely personal and practical nature of most women's feminism. Ask any feminist about her feminism and she is likely to tell you about her passion for getting women their fair due, for tackling injustice and creating a more positive world. She is unlikely to identify herself as a socialist or liberal feminist, though she may say she is a radical feminist to indicate the strength of her commitment. Being a feminist is a world perspective and a life journey and that all-encompassing sense of self and purpose defies easy categorisation.

Liberal feminism

Liberal feminism is one of the oldest forms of feminist thought and is still heavily influential in Western Europe. It is rooted in the classic liberal philosophies of Locke, Rousseau, Bentham and Mill and their calls for equal rights, individualism, liberty and justice. The language of liberal feminism is that of equal opportunities and legal rights: in the UK, this was expressed in campaigns for legal reform focused on equal pay and the outlawing of sex discrimination.

The influence of liberal politics is also evident in the style of liberal feminism, notably in the emphases on education, lobbying, rational argument and balancing rights and responsibilities. Liberal feminists believe that once women have been allowed a level playing field, they will demonstrate their equal worth.

But what if women are given an equal crack at the whip and then found wanting? Critics of liberal feminism suggest that although it has strengths in dealing with the public sphere, it has less to offer in the private arena or in explaining how psychology, language, culture, history and identity work to systematically disadvantage women. For example, legal reform on rape has been useful but not highly significant in reducing the incidence of rape. Although reforming the criminal justice system was necessary and desirable, that barely dents the complex social and psychological drivers that make rape happen in the first place. Similarly, gaining access into the world of work has been of undoubted benefit but women would have profited more if their burden of unpaid work had also been addressed. As Rosemarie Tong has said, liberal feminism 'sent women out into the public realm without summoning men into the private domain'.

Socialist feminism

Unlike the individualist orientation of liberalism, socialism emphasises egalitarianism and the collective good. Marxist theory sees class as the ultimate determinant of woman's social and economic status but later socialist feminists have developed more complex analyses that identify the interplay of gender, class and race within an exploitative capitalist system. The profit to be gained from women's disadvantaged position derives from both their lower pay in the workplace and in the unpaid labour they perform at home.

Engels first described how women's unpaid work helps to shore up capitalist exploitation. Not only are women a reserve army of labour who have been called into the workplace when needed (during the Industrial Revolution and during war) and dispensed with when they are not, but women 'service' male workers by taking care of their physiological and psychological needs. Without women's nurturing care, men would be far less tolerant of their exploitation at work. Within the family, women also raise and socialise the next generation of workers.

Socialist feminists have drawn attention to these aspects of capitalist exploitation, so familiar to us that they now seem 'natural'. Why is women's work within the home accorded so much less value than men's work outside the home? Why is it unpaid? Within the job market, why are women concentrated in 'service' jobs – midwifery, nursing, cleaning, cooking, serving – and why then do those jobs attract the lowest rates of pay? How does capitalism manage to pit its victims against each other, getting men and women, black people and white, workers in different economies, thinking that they are in competition when they should be in solidarity?

Critics of socialist feminism argue that it has no adequate conceptual tools to understand specifically sexual oppression. Not everything comes down to class and experience has shown that socialism does not necessarily liberate women. They note that many socialists have been hostile to feminism, seeing it as a bourgeois diversion from the 'real' struggle. Nevertheless, socialist feminism's commitment to detailing the multiplicity of factors determining the lives of poorer women, and its coalition building between different strands of radical activism, have had a powerful impact in this country.

Radical feminism

Radical feminism believes that women are oppressed by a patriarchal system that is so powerful and so pervasive that we have come to see it as the natural order of things. It claims that women are oppressed *as* women (not just as workers) and that men derive direct and significant benefit from their oppression. While it does not hold that all men necessarily want to exploit women, they inevitably do so, individually and collectively. This oppression of women by men (patriarchy) was the original power system, which became the template for all others.

Radical feminists conceptualise gender as a system that classifies people and behaviour in order to find one (the feminine) inferior to the other (masculine). They question the very concept of inborn sex roles and argue that women are taught to be women and men are taught to be men. This teaching is ubiquitous; it is in how we learn to walk, to talk, to be sexual, to expect more or less according to the genitalia we are born with.

If we are to tackle this teaching, we have to 'unlearn' it. Radical feminism aimed to create a revolution in female consciousness by helping women to recognise how sexism shaped every aspect of their lives. Many feminists looked for new ways of living their lives, adopting alternative lifestyles, promoting women's culture (through art, literature, festivals) and creating women-only space. Although separatism gained considerable publicity for its supposed outlandishness, very few women tried to live without men altogether. Many, though, spent more time apart from men, on their own or in the company of other women, as 'time out', a chance to learn what they could be when they were not trying to attract, manipulate or mollify men.

Radical feminists provided much of the energy and passion of the second wave of feminism. It was largely (though not only) radical feminists who pioneered 'reclaim the night' marches, women's aid refuges, rape crisis centres and a strong women's health movement. They argued that women must take back control of their own bodies and set out to educate them on how to do so. The legacy of this campaigning is even now evident in 'woman-centred care' and in a vastly changed provision of women's health services. One of the most exciting and attractive aspects of radical feminism was the voice it gave to the very large numbers of women who had been hurt or exploited through their sexuality. Radical feminism insisted that rape, domestic violence, sexual harassment, child abuse and male-dominated medicine were not unavoidable phenomena. It argued that male violence was a continuum that affected all women, keeping them 'in line' through fear of provoking male violence and never allowing them to feel that their bodies were truly their own. Not all women experience sexual violence (though very few get through life without any unpleasant experiences of harassment or aggression) but *all* women are systematically undermined and taught their 'place' through daily assertions of male power.

Critics of radical feminism have found this approach essentialist and ultimately hopeless. If patriarchy is that pervasive, and all men profit from the daily exploitation of women, then what possibility is there of effective change? They also object to the way the concept of patriarchy was used in an ahistorical and universalising way, implying that gender relations are essentially the same wherever you are in the world and taking insufficient account of issues of race and class. In addition, many women felt policed and judged by radical feminists. If developing consciousness about the social meaning of, for example, high heels means 'enlightened' women ditch the heels, then what does that say about women who enjoy teetering in stilettos? What about women who enjoy pornography or who want caesareans or who cannot reconcile their feminist anger with their love of individual men?

'The personal is political' ate radical feminism in the end. But its influence was out of proportion to its numbers and its impact is evident in all other strains of feminist thought. It has also had a lasting impact on culture, fuelling a new generation of artists, musicians, actors and writers who are not afraid to celebrate and explore women's lives and women's concerns.

A plethora of feminisms

There are not just three feminisms, but many. Lesbian feminism, black feminism, psychoanalytic feminism, eco-feminism, even postfeminism: there are many streams of feminist thought, feeding in and out of each other, coming together at some points and then diverging at others. Most women, in truth, are not that worried about the root cause of sexism; they just want it stopped. So it is that most feminist activism of today is focused around common agendas rather than shared theory.

Black feminism, for example, has developed a strong agenda of concerns that are central to black women in the UK. Many black women were uncomfortable with white-dominated feminist groups and preferred to follow Alice Walker's lead and focus on 'womanism' – working for and with black women and rejecting pressures to choose between solidarity with either black men or white women. White feminists were often casually dismissive of the specificity of black women's experiences, insisting that black men were the enemy or drawing facile analogies between the position of 'women' (presumably white women) and 'blacks' (presumably black men). Their hostility to the family ignored the role that black family life can play as a haven and a focus of resistance to racism. Their condemnation of feminine adornment was predicated on the assumption that all women are expected to be beautiful dolls at all times and was bemused by the insistence of many black women that making oneself beautiful could also be a badge of honour and defiance of the racist perception that black women are ugly and fit only for work. And feminist campaigns for the right to control one's reproduction through access to contraception and abortion failed to take account of black women's experience of coercive fertility control.

Black feminism acted as a powerful wake-up call for the women's movement, forcing it to engage more critically with its own assumptions: to examine how women, too, exploit their privilege over others and to develop imaginative new alliances with women activists across the world.

Lesbian feminism also had a disproportionately powerful impact on feminism. Originally seen as the dirty little secret of 'respectable' feminism, lesbian activists exploded into action in the early 1970s, around the time the Radicalesbians defined a lesbian as 'the rage of all women condensed to the point of explosion'. Lesbian feminists felt that although they faced specific oppression as a subgroup of women, *all* women were effectively kept in place by heterosexual policing of their sexuality. In her groundbreaking essay 'Compulsory Heterosexuality and Lesbian Existence (Rich 1980), Adrienne Rich explored the concept of a 'lesbian continuum' of female relationships. She included on this continuum women's friendships, mother–daughter relationships and all exchanges of love and support between women. While many lesbians felt that this theory denied the specificity (and the sexuality) of their identity, it nonetheless provided a highly influential analysis of the power of female bonding and convinced many feminists of the centrality of homophobia to women's oppression. Until we are all free to choose, none of us is free.

FEMINISM IN PRACTICE

Few women explicitly align themselves with any feminist theory or activism these days, but none of us is untouched by feminism. It has become a commonplace truism that the phrase 'I'm not a feminist but …', so often uttered by so many women, is invariably followed by a central tenet of feminist thought. When women say 'I'm not a feminist', they nearly always mean 'I'm not an extremist', but much feminist thought is now considered mainstream common sense.

Who, after all, would question that women are and should be fully the equal of men in the eyes of the law, in employment and in public policy? Who does not back equal pay for equal work? Who believes that rape in marriage should not be a criminal offence? Who thinks men have a right to beat their wives? Today, these questions sound ridiculous: 30 years ago, they did not. That is a measure of how far we have come.

But what does all this mean for midwives?

Nearly all midwives are women and all midwives work with women at the lifestage that most

powerfully identifies them *as* women, in the eyes of our world. Inescapably, social attitudes to women, and to their reproductive function, have a deep impact on those who make this their life's work. Feminist theory has identified reproduction as both the site of women's worst exploitation and of their power. Early writers, like the radical Shulamith Firestone, argued that women had to escape the destiny their biology gave them and this meant freedom from reproduction. Later thinkers felt that reproduction *was* woman's power, albeit one that was heavily restricted and policed, and that women must fight new attempts to appropriate that power from them (like the new assisted reproductive technologies). Sociologists like Ann Oakley described motherhood as a myth based on the threefold belief that 'all women need to be mothers, all mothers need their children, all children need their mothers'. Many feminists explored the complex web of maternal privilege, maternal power and maternal drudgery. The whole world of maternal joy, love, entrapment, resentment, boredom, exhilaration, exploitation and liberation is a central preoccupation of feminist thought and a major resource for all those who want to understand better the complexity of women's transition into motherhood.

Many feminists practise midwifery as a direct and important way to support and empower women. But feminism is not a precondition of midwifery and midwifery is very far from being a feminist profession. Many women have been drawn into midwifery because of their desire to help other women, but without being a feminist. Many others have been informed and influenced by the women's health movement and by feminist ideas about bodily integrity, empowerment and choice. Whether you sign up to the label or not, there is clearly a lot that all midwives can learn from, and contribute to, feminist thought.

Often, feminism is seen as lending itself more naturally to a particular type of birth experience. It is cited by those who favour a natural birth, 'liberated' from male medicine, in which women are 'in control'. It is also cited by those who claim women's right to be free from pain, to escape their biological destiny, to refuse vaginal birth and breastfeeding if that is their wish. Women are expert at policing each other, especially when they become mothers, and many women complain about being bullied by both sides, guilt-tripped by midwives, doctors and other mothers, because they are being 'selfish', because they are not putting their baby's health before everything else.

Debating which kind of birth is truly feminist may be missing the point of feminism. At this point in time, and in the absence of a cohesive feminist movement, we can surely best understand feminism as a process rather than an endpoint. A feminist Utopia will look very different for different women. We can define it by its absences – of exploitation, coercion, abuse – but not so easily by its presences. The important thing is to understand what women are going through here and now. Women may have more control over their reproductive lives than they ever did before but their autonomy is still heavily affected by ideological forces that prescribe what is 'natural' and desirable for their sex, about how and when they can mother, and about the authority of medical (and midwifery) expertise.

A feminist midwifery profession is one that understands the depth and the power of these forces and engages with each woman to identify what they mean for her and what support she needs to navigate her journey into parenthood. It does not attempt to deny the power of its own authority but uses that power in support of women. It also supports and values the women who work within it, asking them to work in solidarity with each other and with the women in their care in order to help all women have the birth experience they deserve.

Questions for Reflection ?????

A feminist midwife is one who:

- *is committed to supporting women*
- *believes that supporting women's empowered decision making is a positive end in itself, as well as a vital means of ensuring they are provided with high-quality care*

- *understands power and powerlessness and how they shape women's experiences as service users, as well as midwives' experiences as workers*
- *understands the realities of women's lives*
- *aims to maximise women's autonomy and agency, especially those for whom it is hard (teenage mothers, refugees, women who misuse drugs), and sees this as the pinnacle of professional practice*
- *has a vision of good birth but does not impose it or disrespect women's autonomous decision making*
- *understands that by giving women – colleagues as well as clients – agency and respect, she contributes to women's liberation.*

What do you make of this list?

Are there any points you disagree with?

Can you think of any that have been left out?

Key points

- Feminism has had a major impact on women's lives, including women's needs and expectations in pregnancy and childbirth.

- There are a range of feminist theories, with differing analyses of the origins of gender injustice and differing agendas for political action. All these theories have something to teach us about how and why women are disadvantaged.

- Although feminism has failed to sustain a cohesive activist movement in the UK, the main tenets of feminist thought have been mainstreamed and become 'common sense' to most women.

- Understanding and embracing feminism can help midwives to understand the diverse realities of women's lives, and to support and respect the women with whom they work.

FURTHER READING

Faludi S 1992 Backlash: the undeclared war against women. Chatto and Windus, London

Figes K 1995 Because of her sex: the myth of equality for women in Britain. Pan, London

Greer G 1984 Sex and destiny: the politics of human fertility. Picador, London

Hooks B 1982 Ain't I a woman: black women and feminism. Pluto Press, London

Rich A 1980 Compulsory heterosexuality and lesbian existence. Signs 5(4): 631–660

Rowbotham S 1989 The past is before us: feminism in action since the 1960s. Pandora Press, London

Tong R 1992 Feminist thought: a comprehensive introduction. Routledge, London

Vance C (ed) 1992 Pleasure and danger: exploring female sexuality. Pandora Press, London

Walter N 1999 The new feminism. Virago, London

Whelehan I 1995 Modern feminist thought: from the second wave to 'post-feminism'. Edinburgh University Press, Edinburgh

Wilkinson S, Kitzinger C 1993 Heterosexuality: a feminism and psychology reader. Sage, London

Wolf N 1990 The beauty myth. Chatto and Windus, London

2

Gender and sexuality

Ann Cronin

INTRODUCTION

We live in a society, indeed a world, that organises and regulates sexual identities, behaviours and practices. For example, the law in the UK permits people in opposite-sex relationships to marry but denies the same right to people in same-sex relationships. In other countries, for example Sweden and Holland, same-sex couples enjoy the same legal and social status as opposite-sex couples. Similarly, the age of consent varies from country to country; in some it is as young as 12 and in others as old as 21. Additionally, the age of consent depends on whether the relationship is between same-sex or opposite-sex partners. Where there is a difference it is likely to favour a younger age of consent for opposite-sex relationships. In the UK, after years of campaigning by gay rights groups, the age of consent is 16 for all. However, while male homosexual acts between consenting adults were decriminalised in 1967, homosexual behaviour remains illegal in many countries. There has never been any legal age of consent in this country for women who have sex with other women. Co-existing alongside laws that regulate sex, there are more informal rules and norms governing sexual behaviour. For example, there is cultural disapproval of teenage pregnancy, women who have babies on their own through choice, people with disabilities becoming parents and later life pregnancy.

These examples suggest that sexuality is subject to laws and regulations in our society and in others. Furthermore, heterosexual relationships have a higher status than homosexual ones and gender is important for our understanding of sexuality. It is these sorts of issues that will be explored in this chapter and along the way there are questions to help you consider your own views on the material presented. For as Wilton (2000) argues, all too often training for the healthcare professions fails to adequately address issues of human sexual diversity, leaving those delivering healthcare ill equipped and often unsure as to how to deal with people who present with a different sexuality from their own. While there are many relevant issues that could be explored in this chapter, for example teenage pregnancy, I have decided to focus on the experiences of non-heterosexual women because the needs of this group of women are often overlooked.

The chapter begins with a discussion of gender and its impact on our lives before moving on to look at the relationship between gender and sexuality. This is followed by a brief overview of the theoretical explanations for the existence of homosexuality, focusing on the feminist understanding of sexuality. The chapter then examines the attitudes of healthcare workers towards non-heterosexual people and concludes with an assessment of the issues raised in this chapter and the implications they contain for healthcare delivery and practice.

LIVING IN A GENDERED WORLD

The range of feminist theoretical perspectives explored in the last chapter demonstrates that feminism, at both a theoretical and political level, is neither a static or unitary body of thought. Instead it offers alternative accounts for the existence and resolution of personal and institutional inequality between women and men. Despite these differences there is consensus amongst the majority of feminists on the relationship between gender and sex. While sex refers to biological differences between women and men, gender refers to the social construction of male and female roles (Oakley 1982). Although the two are interlinked, sex is regarded by many feminists as a biological given and, for most, unalterable. In contrast, gender, the social meaning of maleness

and femaleness, is socially learnt behaviour and ensures the continuation of a sex/gender system, characterised by some as patriarchy and reliant on male supremacy (Ramazanoglu 1989, Stanley & Wise 1993).

We can use this view of gender to help us understand particular social worlds and histories, for example the division of labour, both inside and outside the home. Work is generally defined as activities carried on outside the home in return for a wage. This dismisses the vast amount of work performed by women, work that receives no remuneration and often no recognition, for example housework and childcare, tasks which are the world over predominantly performed by women. Furthermore, women are not just involved in unpaid work but are an integral and necessary part of the global economy. Seager (1997) estimates that 41% of all women aged 15 or over are economically active; that is, either involved in or actively seeking paid work. Nevertheless, the majority of women are confined to low-paid, low-status work, thus carrying the double burden of paid work and unpaid work. The failure to recognise women's multiple activities contributes to the institutionalisation of unequal relations between women and men.

Therefore, the application of the concept of gender to the division of labour enables us to locate our own individual experiences of being a woman or a man in a wider social context. By this I mean that without the concept of gender we might think that our experiences of living as a woman in this society are unique to us; gender enables us to realise that such experiences are patterned and reproduced through the social organisation of society. This in turn highlights that gender is not just located in individuals but is a social relation where one gender group (men) has more power than another gender group (women). Gender lies at the heart of any society and structures and mediates our daily lives.

However, recognition of the important role gender plays in our lives should not occur at the expense of dismissing other social variables, nor their interaction with gender. Women's experience of work, both paid and unpaid, is mediated by the interaction of gender with other factors such as class, race, geographical location or age. A black woman experiences discrimination at work because she is a black woman; her race and her gender cannot be separated out. Her experience of work will be very different from that of a white woman, yet both of them are affected by gender. Likewise, girls and women in Afghanistan have until recently been denied the right to be educated, been banned from work and have not even been allowed to show their faces in public. While these experiences are so very different from our own that they might be difficult to comprehend, they nevertheless remain gendered experiences, mediated in this case by fundamentalist religious beliefs, which in turn are connected to the global political order. What these examples show us is that the intersection of gender with specific social and cultural factors fractures the notion of a unitary category of woman:

While all women potentially experience oppression on the basis of gender, women are, nevertheless, differentially oppressed by the varied intersections of other arrangements of social inequality.
(Lengermann & Niebrugge-Brantley 2000, p 471)

While recognition of this is important for our understanding of gender in our own culture and others, it may also have an impact at a personal or individual level. This may lead us to question our own norms, values and beliefs about what it means to be a woman in our own society, let alone the rest of the world. One issue that often raises such discussion and debate is sexuality, which of course is the focus of this chapter.

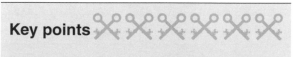

Key points

■ Sex refers to biological differences between women and men while gender refers to the social meaning attached to being female or male.

■ Gender is a social relation where one group has more power than another group.

■ Gender intersects with other social variables to produce different gendered experiences.

Questions for Reflection ?????

How do you think gender has affected your life?

What do you think are the points of similarity and difference between women in this country and women in, for example, South Africa?

GENDER AND SEXUALITY

A few years ago I ran a workshop entitled 'Lesbian Health Matters' for an all-female group of health professionals undertaking postgraduate studies in women's healthcare. Following introductions, I asked the women to reflect on their own attitudes towards women who have same-sex relationships and to consider how this might affect their delivery of healthcare to these women. At this point I did not know their sexual identity, although in the ensuing discussion all the women indicated they were heterosexual. Below are a few comments from that discussion.

Woman 1: I don't like the word 'lesbian'.
Myself: Why not?
Woman 1: Well, I used to get called it when I was little at school because I used to hold my friend's hand ... and no-one would tell me what it meant – not even my mum ...
Myself: Well, I guess if the word has very negative associations for you then you wouldn't like it ...
Woman 1: Now 'gay', that's a nice word – why can't you use that?
Woman 2: Yes, but then again that used to mean happy and joyful, now look what it means ...

'While I would never treat anybody differently because of their sexuality, I have to say that I find what lesbians and gay men get up to sexually absolutely abhorrent.'

'Now, I can understand why men and women want to have sex together because that can lead to reproduction but I just can't understand why two women would want to have sex together.'

'Well, I think that lesbians and gay men bring it all on themselves – why can't they just keep quiet and then people would just assume that they were heterosexual.'

In contrast, below are extracts from the stories of three women who self-identify as lesbian:

I knew from overhearing some of their conversations that there were thoroughly sick people in the world who loved their own sex, men and sometimes women who wanted nothing better than to kiss each other and sleep in the same beds. It was very depressing to hear them speak like that.
(Helen, in NLGS 1992, p 1–2)

I thought I was a lesbian but then I thought it was ridiculous and awful and every book on psychology I ever read … told me that it was immature and that I should really get my act together and reconcile myself to my femininity and find myself a good man and have children. And so I thought, I must simply get on with being a normal woman.
(Diana, in Inventing Ourselves 1989, p 49–50)

The message was the same each time. There was a 'real' lesbian, generally mannish, though not always, and a 'real' woman, who eventually left the lesbian, usually for a man. The lesbian then committed suicide, conveniently. She was always a sad, pathetic figure, or totally despised and unlikeable.
(Steph, in NLGS 1992, p 16)

Both sets of statements – those from the health professionals and those from women who self-identify as lesbian – are instances of a particular way of talking about lesbians. Lesbians are 'sad', 'pathetic', 'mannish' and 'miserable', they are women who perform abhorrent sexual acts with each other. Thus, they represent a particular type of knowledge or way of talking about lesbians. They also say something about the way in which gender and heterosexuality are conceptualised in our society. The invisible nature of relationships between women is based on an underlying assumption that we all are or should be heterosexual. Hence, they say something about who is allowed to have sex and for what purpose. Likewise, they refer to the rules governing gender appropriate behaviour. Finally, by highlighting the negativity associated with the word 'lesbian', they valorise heterosexuality. In short, there is a relationship between what we know about 'the lesbian' and what we know about gender and heterosexuality.

Many of us consider our sexual identity, desires and practices are a private matter and of no concern to anyone else and at one level they are, in as much as being sexual is in general an activity that takes place in private with one other person. However, both the examples cited at the beginning of this chapter and the subsequent discussion suggest that sexuality, just like gender, is subject to cultural norms, values and belief; while there is variation, all societies have laws and regulations that govern sexuality. Obviously we might feel that some of these laws are right and fitting, for example laws against sexual abuse or paedophilia, while others we might question. Nevertheless, it is for these sorts of reasons that we can talk about the social organisation of sexuality. Furthermore, as the statements by both the healthcare workers and women who identify as lesbian suggest, there is a close relationship between gender and sexuality, which constrains all of us regardless of our sexual identity or preferences. For example, many heterosexual women feel it is unfair that women who have multiple sexual partners receive derogatory labels while men have similar behaviour condoned or even supported.

Key points

- There is a relationship between sexuality and gender.
- Sexuality is socially organised and regulated in all societies.
- There are different theoretical approaches to understanding sexuality.

Questions for Reflection ?????

What are your own views on the statements made by the health professionals? Do you agree or disagree with them, and why?

Can you think of examples of the way in which this society or any other society organises and regulates sexuality? What are your views on this?

THEORISING SEXUALITY

Accepting that sexuality may not necessarily be a strictly private affair leads us to ask why it is that societies and cultures sanction some forms of sexual behaviour or relationships and condemn or prohibit others? In particular, why do societies support opposite-sex relationships while often condemning, either informally or formally (and often both), same-sex relationships? Again, theory can help us answer this question although, as with feminist theory, there is not a single monolithic explanation for sexuality but instead different explanations, some of which will hold more validity for you than others.

A full account of the different theoretical approaches to sexuality is beyond the remit of this chapter, therefore what follows is a brief overview of the main theoretical approaches, with most attention being given to the feminist analysis of sexuality. I will talk about theories that can be categorised as 'essentialist' and theories that can be categorised as 'social constructionist'. While in practice there may be some overlap, for convenience I have separated them out here. Essentialism assumes that sexuality is an instinct or a drive and that our sexuality identity, whether we identify as heterosexual, homosexual or bisexual, is representative of our true inner self. Therefore, there is a focus on the biology of the individual. In contrast, there is the view that sexuality is socially constructed; that is, we are not born with any particular sexuality or sexual identity but rather it is formed through our social experiences and the particular society we live in.

Essentialist explanations of sexuality

Gay liberation in the 1970s, alongside the re-emergence of the women's movement, signalled a new form of political action aimed at challenging the hegemonic control and power of heterosexual and male-dominated society. It demanded change in the political, judicial and social treatment of lesbian and gay men and signalled the birth of a modern lesbian and gay culture that has continued to grow and extend over the last 30 years. The last 30 years of political activism have

had a beneficial impact on the lives of those that do not identify or live as heterosexual. Nevertheless, such improvements should be viewed with caution given that the dominant institutional and cultural framework continues to promote heterosexuality as the only truly valid way of life (Cronin 2000). However, what has often been forgotten in the flurry of activity over the last three decades is that the terms 'homosexual' and 'heterosexual' to denote different sexual identities have only been in existence for some 130 years (Foucault 1979, Weeks 1985).

The development of sexology as a discipline in the latter half of the 19th century can be regarded as the starting point of contemporary scientific and medical investigation into the aetiology of homosexuality and indeed, the invention of discrete sexual identities. Such investigations are united by the underlying assumption that homosexuality has an individual biological basis or that any investigation into the causality of homosexuality should include a consideration of the biological make-up of the individual. While united by this assumption, the moral judgements placed on it differ considerably. For example, Le Vay (1993), whose research findings support a genetic or biological basis for male homosexuality, has used this to argue for social reform on the basis that individuals are not responsible for their sexual identity and therefore should not be condemned for it. Others have argued that homosexuality's biological basis should be regarded as a pathology or disease and thus research should focus on a 'cure'.

While the sexologists of the late 19th century favoured a biological explanation for homosexuality, it was Freud's psychoanalytic theory of psychosexual development that led to the psychological construction of the homosexual in the first half of the 20th century. However, as we shall see, underlying Freud's model is an assumption of the normalcy of the biologically constructed heterosexual. Freud's model is a sequential systematic model, in which an individual progresses from an initial polymorphous sexuality in early childhood through to the development of a mature sexuality; that is, the achievement of a stable heterosexual identity. Within this model, homosexuality is viewed as a temporary stage of development (usually occurring during adolescence) on the path towards heterosexuality. This implies that those who identify as homosexual in adulthood are 'fixated' on an early and hence immature phase of sexual development. Alternatively, they have due to psychological disturbance 'regressed' back to this early phase of sexual development. Either way, homosexuality is located within a discourse of deviance, psychopathology and illness.

Evidence for this can be found in the understanding and treatment of homosexuality: until 1973 the American Psychiatric Association classified homosexuality as a mental disorder requiring psychiatric treatment. Following a long and protracted debate amongst members of the APA, the trustees ruled in 1973 that homosexuality should be reclassified as a sexual orientation disturbance (White 1979). Of this category the APA writes:

This category is for individuals whose sexual interests are directed primarily towards people of the same sex who are disturbed by, in conflict with, or wish to change their sexual orientation. This diagnostic category is distinguished from homosexuality, which by itself does not necessarily constitute a psychiatric disorder. (APA 1975, p 1)

Despite this ruling there remains a diverse range of opinion amongst the APA and others working in the mental health services, with many practitioners continuing to regard homosexuality per se as a mental disorder. For example, research suggests that non-heterosexual clients who present with identical symptoms to their heterosexual counterparts are viewed with greater negativity (Levy 1978). Likewise, other studies (for example, Garfinkle & Morin 1978, White 1979) suggest that an awareness of a lesbian identity can affect clinical assessment, diagnosis and subsequent treatment.

The social construction of sexuality

In contrast to the long history of scientific and medical investigation, the sociological study of homosexuality is a relatively new phenomenon. The Kinsey Reports (Kinsey et al 1948, 1953) and the development of the labelling perspective in the 1960s provided the catalyst for sociologically informed studies on homosexual identity, communities and culture.

Kinsey's large-scale study of human sexual behaviour highlighted the discrepancy between the number of people who either had or continued to engage in same-sex behaviour and the number who identified as homosexual. This led Kinsey to develop a six-point sexual continuum, designed to encompass a variety of sexual behaviours and thoughts, ranging from exclusively heterosexual (1) to exclusively homosexual (6). In between was a range of thoughts and behaviours that cannot be categorised as exclusively heterosexual or homosexual, with bisexuality, a desire for both sexes, somewhere in the middle. Based on extensive research, Kinsey argued that men and women often move between categories during their lifetimes. This led to doubts being expressed about the validity of dividing people into homosexual and heterosexual, a division which has dominated the modern discourse of sexuality as witnessed by the laws and rules governing sexual behaviour. Based on empirical evidence, Kinsey reasoned that the category 'homosexual' should be dismissed because there are only individuals, some of whom have had more homosexual experiences than heterosexual ones. Indeed, we could extend this to the category 'heterosexual' as well. For Kinsey the development of an exclusive homosexual identity was the outcome of society's rejection of homosexual behaviour.

Labelling perspective focuses on the social construction of deviance and deviant labels so it is not surprising that it gained favour with an emerging sociology of homosexuality. It provided a theoretical basis for those sociologists who wanted to move away from causal explanations for homosexuality with their essentialist notions of what constitutes normal and natural sexual behaviour. In contrast, labelling theory offered a new way of looking at homosexuality. Based on the premise that all sexual behaviour is socially constructed, people who engage in homosexual behaviour are labelled deviant due to the reactions of a hostile society, hence, there is nothing intrinsically deviant about a homosexual identity. The aim of such a stance is to expose the effect of stigma and social ostracism on the homosexual. The move away from causal explanations enabled research to focus on how: 'Historically produced stigmatising conceptions surrounding same-sex experience have had dramatic consequences for those experiences' (Plummer 1981, p 17).

For example, McIntosh (1968), critical of the ahistorical universalism of the medical model, argues that homosexuality, as we currently experience it in the Western world, did not exist until the 17th century. That is, while people may have engaged in homosexual behaviour, they were not necessarily labelled homosexual. Therefore, a specific homosexual role is socially and historically constructed.

Thus the sociological understanding of sexuality, and in particular homosexuality, moves away from essentialist understandings of human sexuality, to examine the social construction of sexuality. Depending on your own personal perspective, you might regard this as a good or bad thing. Many welcomed this fresh approach to understanding sexuality, particularly as it provided arguments for the destigmatisation of non-heterosexual people, yet it has not been without criticism. Feminist researchers (for example, Dworkin 1981, Faraday 1981, Kitzinger 1987, MacKinnon 1979, Rich 1980, Richardson 1981, Wilton 1995) and, more recently, queer theorists (for example, Duggen 1992, Epstein 1994, Gamson 1995, Namaste 1994, Seidman 1994, Warner 1993) have added their voices to the theoretical debate concerning sexuality. While supporting the social constructionist implications of labelling theory, both sets of theorists have identified specific problems in relation to the way in which it is used to theorise sexuality: first, that gender and heterosexuality are inadequately theorised and second, that insufficient attention has been paid to historical and social factors. These points are further expanded on below in my discussion of the feminist understanding of sexuality.

While a radical feminist perspective is by no means the only feminist perspective to address the issue of sexuality, it has nevertheless served as a starting point for later understandings of sexuality and therefore is worthy of consideration here. Space does not permit me to examine queer theory here but if you are interested in

following up this perspective, then the edited collection by Seidman (1996) is an excellent starting point.

Feminist understanding of sexuality

As discussed in the last chapter, radical feminism is united by a number of assumptions about human nature and social reality, in particular a belief in the universal domination of women by men, which is the primary form of social control practised through a system of patriarchy. While explanations for this may differ, radical feminists regard biology or, to be specific, the different roles that women and men play in reproduction as the basis of this patriarchal oppression of women. For example, Firestone (1970) explores male control of reproduction, while Brownmiller (1976) and Dworkin (1981) focus on the use of pornography to control women's sexuality. Thus radical feminism offers a radical critique of male power so it is not surprising that it focuses on the relationship between gender and sexuality, which is regarded as a key feature in the analysis of society (Walby 1990). This has led to a feminist analysis of both lesbianism and heterosexuality as political institutions aimed at regulating and controlling women's sexuality, which helps to ensure the continuation of unequal relations between the sexes.

We can shed light on this claim through examining Faderman's (1985) feminist account of the social construction of lesbianism, which she links to the rise of feminism in the 19th century, with its demands for equality for women in a variety of different areas including education, marriage, work and the enfranchisement of women. According to Faderman, before the rise of feminism 'romantic friendships' between women were viewed as a normal part of social relations. They had been neither labelled nor discouraged; indeed, they were often regarded as preparation for marriage. However, Faderman documents the harsh treatment of women who transgressed gender roles by cross-dressing as men in order to lead independent lives, which may or may not have included sexual relationships with women. Likewise, Robson (1992) discusses the punishment, including death, administered to those women who in having relationships with other women challenged the nature of gender relations prevalent in society at that time. It could be surmised that relationships between women, which were seen to challenge the hegemonic male control of women, were punished, while those relationships deemed as innocent and non-threatening were overlooked.

Nevertheless the emergence of an organised feminist movement in the 19th century brought with it the possibility of economic independence for women. This resulted in those relationships previously characterised as 'romantic friendships' being recategorised and labelled abnormal. Feminist demands, which were in general met with hostility, were contested through the utilisation of developing scientific/medical knowledge, which warned of the harmful effects of equality on women's health. Behind this lay a fear that gender distinctions, on which the social structure was dependent, would become blurred or indistinct, leading to subsequent social disorder and chaos. Such fears led speakers of the day such as Horace Bushnell to speak out against women attaining the vote on the grounds that women were a separate species and that the vote would lead women to become like men (Faderman 1985). Contained in this fear was the belief that women's fight for equality, which implicitly challenged women's traditional dependence on men, would lead to a situation where women, having gained economic independence, would elect not to get married. This fear fed into existing 19th-century concerns about the falling birth rate and the eugenics movement, which was concerned about the power and strength of the British Empire (Weeks 1985). If the economic imperative to get married disappeared then women would have little use for marriage and would turn to women, not for 'romantic friendships' before or during marriage but as a replacement for it. For the first time 'love between women became threatening to the social structure' (Faderman 1985, p 238).

Such fears were given legitimacy through the scientific and medical construction of the lesbian. Based on essentialist notions of women, sexologists claimed women's desire for independence (equated with desire for relationships with other women) was unnatural. Therefore, those women

who demanded it were not 'real women', because 'real women' accepted their natural dependence on men. Westphal, one of the early sexologists, writing in 1869, used the term 'congenital invert' to argue that these women were abnormal due to hereditary degeneration and neurosis (Faderman 1985). Westphal's work led to a proliferation of literature on this subject, suggesting that women who wanted equality were either 'unsexed' or 'semi-women'. Faderman argues that this theoretical stance reflects the need to secure women's compliance to their traditional role through acceptance that a desire for independence from men was unnatural. Hence the category 'invert' was developed and applied to those women who rejected their natural role. This meant they were sexually active rather than passive, desired to be in the public world of education and work instead of the private world of the home and family and their primary allegiance lay with women, not men. These women ceased to be real women but instead became members of a 'third sex'. The demands of feminism, which offered the possibility of freedom for all women, became associated with pathological inversion.

Feminists have argued that these early sexology theories weakened the first wave of feminism because women were stifled by a powerful ideology that labelled them as 'non-women' if they fought for women's rights (Faderman 1985, Kitzinger 1987). For example, Kraft-Ebing (1965) and Havelock Ellis (1897), who wrote extensively at the end of the 19th century about the pathological nature of the 'female invert', influenced 20th-century notions of lesbianism, notions which still persist today to some extent. Ellis warning against the dangers of feminism and distinguished between the 'true invert' and the woman drawn into same-sex sexual activity during adolescence or due to situational reasons. Ellis identified three defining factors of the true invert: childhood crushes on another female; the adoption of masculine physical and social characteristics; the adoption of male attire. Assuming that any 'normal woman', given the chance, would choose to have relationships with men, he warned that feminism could lead women to have contact with true inverts and thus occasion 'spurious imitation', the implication of his argument being that 'normal women' should stay away from feminism and, moreover, feminists. Ellis directed his concerns towards professional or middle-class women whom he believed to be particularly at risk from inversion. Arguably, these women were well positioned to argue for women's equality.

While this section has focused on inversion theories in relation to women, these were also applied to men. Nevertheless, given the existence of gender, it is important to distinguish between women and men when assessing the impact of such theories. While it was expedient for both male and female homosexuals to accept the scientific explanations of congenital defects, their reasons for doing so differed. Due to stringent anti-homosexual laws aimed at men and based on the notion of chosen depravity, it was expedient for men to accept such explanations (Faderman 1985, Weeks 1985). However, for women, while congenital defective explanations granted legitimacy to women who wanted to pursue an independent life, they discouraged the majority of women from becoming involved in feminism. Viewed from this perspective, it could be argued that the social construction of lesbianism had little to do with women loving other women and more to do with isolating women who desired greater independence in life. The labelling of lesbianism as an abnormality prevented the majority of women viewing it as a viable option, thereby enabling a separate group of women 'inverts' to develop. While not all feminists were (or are) lesbians, the link between feminism and lesbianism has become firmly entrenched and acts as an effective control against feminism. In turn, this weakens the threat of a social system dependent on equal relationships between women and men. For some feminists this constitutes heterosexuality as a compulsory institution, hence contributing to women's subordination by men (Rich 1980). Rich argues that the compulsory nature of heterosexuality ensures that men retain their physical, economical and emotional control over women. For Rich, as for Faderman, the institution of heterosexuality is dependent upon ensuring that the experiences of lesbians either remain invisible or are associated with disease and illness.

To summarise, examination of the social construction of lesbianism in the 19th century exposes the close relationship that exists between gender and sexuality and hence the implications it has for all women regardless of sexual identity. Furthermore, we can see the way in which the development of scientific theory was used to maintain existing gender relations and deny women's access to the public world. While Faderman and Rich adopt a broadly radical feminist perspective, other feminists have contributed to our understanding of sexuality. In particular, recent work has focused on the institution of heterosexuality and the implications of this for women who continue to have relationships with men. For anyone wishing to explore this further I recommend the edited collection by Richardson (1996) or the book by Wilkinson & Kitzinger (1993) which contains the autobiographical stories of heterosexual women.

Key points

- Essentialist explanations suggest that investigations into the causes of homosexuality should begin with the biology of the individual concerned.

- Social constructionist explanations are less concerned with the biology of the individual but more concerned with the social organisation of sexuality and the stigmatisation of non-heterosexual identities.

- A feminist understanding of sexuality prioritises the relationship between gender and heterosexuality and examines the contribution that the institution of heterosexuality makes to the social control of all women.

Questions for Reflection

Where would you place yourself on Kinsey's six-point continuum?

What do you think makes someone heterosexual or homosexual?

Do you think homosexuality is biologically natural or a biological deviation?

What do you think about the feminist explanation for the social construction of lesbianism?

SEXUALITY AND HEALTHCARE

The last section explored different theoretical explanations for sexual identity, in particular a homosexual identity, although in reflecting upon homosexuality such theories also reflect on heterosexuality. Theory does not just exist at an abstract level but has an impact on how we think, feel and behave, as illustrated by the statements made by the health professionals. You might reasonably argue that these statements are anecdotal and cannot be generalised to all health workers. In order to put these comments in a wider context this section examines first, the findings from research on the attitudes of healthcare workers to lesbians and second, the experiences of lesbians seeking healthcare. While the majority of this research is American in origin, this does not imply that the issue is not relevant elsewhere. As Rose (1993) argues in her UK study of nurses' attitudes towards lesbian colleagues and patients, homophobic attitudes are not only commonplace amongst nursing staff but affect working relations and patient care.

Before proceeding it is worth saying something about the term 'homophobia'. Homophobia is regarded as an individualised pathological trait, characterised as 'an irrational fear of homosexuals' (Rose 1993, p 500). Although this definition is valid, it does not take sufficient account of the social origins of homophobia, namely heterosexism or, as it has been called more recently, heteronormativity. Such terms refer to the assumption that the only true and valid relationship is that between a man and a woman, leading to the social organisation of society for the benefit of people who define as heterosexual. This should be borne in mind when reading this section, for in the following discussion I am not suggesting that healthcare workers are more prejudiced than any other group in society although, given that their

task is one of providing healthcare to individuals, such attitudes may have particular implications. As Douglas et al (1985) argue, levels of homophobia are similar to the general population, while Randall (1989) illustrates that there is little evidence to suggest that homophobic attitudes are actively challenged during medical training.

The attitudes of healthcare workers

The research in this area (for example, Douglas et al 1985, Matthews et al 1986, Young 1988) suggests that significant numbers of healthcare workers hold homophobic attitudes towards lesbians and gay men. For example, Matthews et al's (1986) study of medical doctors categorised 23% of the sample as severely homophobic, with the most homophobic attitudes being expressed by surgeons, gynaecologists and family practice doctors. Forty percent expressed discomfort at treating lesbians and gays, and 30% were opposed to lesbians and gay men being admitted to medical schools. Forty percent would not refer their clients to known lesbian or gay colleagues. These findings have implications for the healthcare of non-heterosexual women, particularly when those expressing the most severe homophobic attitudes are to be found in those specialties that women are most likely to come in contact with: gynaecologists and family practice doctors. Similar homophobic attitudes were expressed in Young's (1988) study of registered nurses, with negative attitudes ranging from pity, disgust, repulsion and unease to embarrassment, fear and sorrow. Furthermore, many nurses who expressed such feelings stated they had no desire to change, leading Young to contend that such strong attitudes are likely to affect the level of care that lesbian and gay patients receive. In addition to this, Randall (1989) and Eliason & Randall (1991) show that there exists a high degree of ignorance about lesbianism in general, for example the popular belief that lesbians constitute a high-risk category in relation to the transmission of HIV infection. In assessing the implications of such hostility, it could be argued that research indicates that knowledge of a lesbian identity can detrimentally affect assessment, diagnosis and treatment.

This is supported by Rose's (1993) study of UK nurses' attitudes towards lesbian colleagues and patients, where data were collected from lesbian identified nurses. The majority of the 44 nurses who took part in the research were 'out' at work although half of this group felt that 'coming out' had been a difficult process and had detrimentally affected the nature of their relationships with colleagues. Younger lesbian nurses who were not out feared that disclosing their sexual identity could have an adverse effect on future career plans. The majority of the nurses reported witnessing homophobic behaviour directed at patients. This included colleagues refusing to care for a homosexual patient, hearing lesbianism being referred to as an illness, deviant or sinful, or patients being the butt of prejudicial jokes. Faced with such behaviour, all the nurses reported self-censorship in social conversation. In conclusion, Rose suggests that her findings imply that there are nurses whose uniqueness and dignity are not being respected. This in turn is indicative of a gap between equal opportunity policy and practice which, until it is addressed, will continue to affect individual self-esteem and career progression.

Such research indicates that a significant number of healthcare workers hold homophobic attitudes, which are often based on ignorance. While acknowledging that the relationship between attitude and behaviour is a contentious one, this research does raise the question about the effect such prejudicial attitudes have on clinical practice. This issue is addressed in the next section, which explores the findings from research on the healthcare experiences of women who identify as lesbian.

Accessing healthcare

Research (for example, Cochran & Mays 1988, Dardick & Grady 1980, McGhee & Owen 1980, Reagon 1981) suggests that lesbian women seeking healthcare are concerned that disclosing their sexual identity may result in negative reaction, ranging from hostility and ignorance through to inadequate care or at worst being denied access to treatment. For some women these fears are well founded and based on previous experience.

Reagon (1981) reports negative reactions to a disclosure including anxiety, hostility, less likelihood of touch, mental health referral, excessive curiosity and demeaning jokes. Similarly studies of lesbian mothers support many of the findings already mentioned (Harvey et al 1989, Olesker & Walsh 1984). Many women had not disclosed their sexual identity when seeking prenatal care and assumptions of heterosexuality had often led to the exclusion of a lesbian partner. Stewart's (1999) research with lesbian parents highlights the consequences of women facing hostility and a lack of understanding from health visitors, which can result in a reluctance to seek support when necessary for fear that the child might be taken away. A position paper published by the Royal College of Midwives (2000) documents the difficulties faced by lesbian mothers when seeking healthcare and is worth reading.

Women who have decided not to disclose their sexual identity report that health workers often make an assumption of heterosexuality, which may lead to inappropriate advice being given, for example contraceptive advice. Such assumptions are evidence of the close relationship between homophobia and sexism; regardless of a woman's sexual identity, doctors often assume that women are in need of contraceptive advice, thus illuminating the hidden assumptions held by the medical world in general concerning the inability of women to make appropriate independent decisions concerning their own fertility.

Taken collectively, such findings suggest that lesbian women may feel alienated from the healthcare process, which may result in them not seeking treatment, even for routine screening for breast or cervical cancer. Saunders et al's (1988) study indicates that many lesbians prefer to seek out informal healthcare via friends or, when forced to seek out traditional healthcare, base their choice of healthcare worker on the advice and experience of friends. In conclusion, they argue that lesbian networks are very influential in decision-making processes concerning healthcare behaviour, the implication of this being that socially or geographically isolated women will not have access to networks or support when making healthcare decisions.

Despite these negative experiences it is equally important to acknowledge the positive experiences of disclosure, as it is possible to learn from these and take them forward into healthcare practice. For example, Dardick & Grady (1980) and Olesker & Walsh (1984) report that lesbians who receive a positive reaction to their sexuality feel able to develop an open and trusting relationship with their healthcare provider, leading them to believe they are receiving a better level of healthcare. However, such women are in a minority and until women feel they are in a safe and supportive environment they will delay coming out to healthcare workers.

What are your attitudes to non-heterosexual women? How do you think these attitudes might affect your delivery of healthcare?

How would you deal with a woman in your care who disclosed her lesbian status? (You might want to draw on an actual experience to answer this question or simply consider how you might react.) Do you envisage any problem with this?

What issues might you need to take into account when working with (a) all women, (b) women who have identified as lesbian, bisexual or non-heterosexual to you?

Key points

■ A significant number of healthcare workers hold homophobic beliefs which may be expressed in a variety of ways towards non-heterosexual colleagues and patients.

■ Women who do identify as lesbian have experience of or fear they may experience a negative reaction if they disclose their sexuality to a healthcare worker, leaving them feeling alienated from the healthcare process.

■ Some women have experienced positive reactions to disclosure, enabling them to build an open and trusting relationship with their healthcare worker.

Questions for Reflection

What do you think about the research findings presented in this section?

CONCLUSION

This chapter has taken a brief look at the social organisation of gender and sexuality and the relationship between the two. In doing so, I discussed the different theoretical explanations for homosexuality and in particular lesbianism. While the primary focus in this chapter has been on lesbian identity I have tried to demonstrate the close relationship that exists between heterosexual and non-heterosexual identities. I did this to make the point that all women, regardless of sexual identity, are constrained by culturally varied expectations regarding gender and sexuality. How you feel about the material presented is of course your own choice and it is not for me to persuade you of the merits of one perspective over another. However, as the last section suggested, there is a close relationship between attitude and behaviour. Given the commitment of healthcare practitioners to provide the best possible service for those who come under their care, the purpose of this chapter has been to invite you to examine your own attitudes and practices to women who may not have the same sexual identity as you and to consider ways in which this may be improved upon.

REFERENCES

American Psychiatric Association 1975 Press release. American Psychiatric Association, Washington DC
Brownmiller S 1976 Against our will: men, women and rape. Penguin, Harmondsworth

Cochran SD, Mays VM 1988 Disclosure of sexual preferences to physicians by black lesbians and bisexual women. Western Journal of Medicine 149: 616–619

Cronin A 2000 Deconstructing the sociological closet: the queering of lesbian identity. University of Surrey, Guildford

Dardick L, Grady KE 1980 Openness between gay persons and health professionals. Annals of Internal Medicine 93: 115–119

Douglas CJ, Kalman CM, Kalman TP 1985 Homophobia among physicians and nurses: an empirical study. Hospital and Community Psychiatry 36(12): 1309–1311

Duggen L 1992 Making it perfectly queer. Socialist Review 22: 11–32

Dworkin A 1981 Pornography: men possessing women. Women's Press, London

Eliason MJ, Randall CE 1991 Lesbian phobia in nursing students. Western Journal of Nursing Research 13: 363–374

Ellis H 1897 Studies in the psychology of sex: sexual inversion (reprinted 1911). FA Davis, Philadelphia

Epstein S 1994 A queer encounter: sociology and the study of sexuality. Sociological Theory 12: 188–202

Faderman L 1985 Surpassing the love of women. Women's Press, London

Faraday A 1981 Liberating lesbian research. In: Plummer K (ed) The making of the modern homosexual. Hutchinson, London

Firestone S 1970 The Dialectic of sex: the case for feminist revolution. William Morrow, New York

Foucault M 1979 The history of sexuality: an introduction (trans. R Hurley). Penguin, London

Gamson J 1995 Must identity movements self-destruct? A queer dilemma. Social Problems 42(3): 390–407

Garfinkle EM, Morin SF 1978 Psychologists' attitudes towards homosexual psychotherapy clients. Journal of Social Issues 34(3): 101–112

Hall Carpenter Archives 1989 Inventing ourselves: lesbian life stories. Routledge, London

Harvey SM, Carr C, Berheine S 1989 Lesbian mothers: health care experiences. Journal of Nurse-Midwifery 34(3): 115–119

Kinsey AC, Pomeroy WB, Martin CE 1948 Sexual behaviour in the human male. WB Saunders, Philadelphia

Kinsey AC, Gebhard P, Pomeroy WB, Martin CE 1953 Sexual behaviour in the human female. WB Saunders, Philadelphia

Kitzinger C 1987 The social construction of lesbianism. Sage, London

Kraft-Ebing 1965 Psychopathia sexualis: a medico-economic study (trans. ME Wedeck). Putnam, New York

Lengermann PM, Niebrugge-Brantley J 2000 Contemporary feminist theory. In: Ritzer G. (ed) Sociological theory. McGraw-Hill, London

Le Vay S 1993 The sexual brain. MIT Press, Boston

Levy T 1978 The lesbian: as perceived by mental health workers. Unpublished doctoral dissertation, California School of Professional Psychology, San Diego, CA

McGhee RD, Owen WF 1980 Medical aspects of homosexuality. New England Journal of Medicine 303: 50–51

McIntosh M 1968 The homosexual role. Social Problems 16(2): 182–192

MacKinnon C 1979 The sexual harassment of working women: a case of sex discrimination. Yale University Press, New Haven, CT

Matthews WC, Booth MW, Turner JD, Kessler L 1986 Physicians' attitudes toward homosexuality: survey of a California country medical society. Western Journal of Medicine 144: 106–110

Namaste K 1994 The politics of inside/out: queer theory, poststructuralism, and a sociological approach to sexuality. Sociological Theory 12: 220–231

NLGS 1992 What a lesbian looks like. Routledge, London

Oakley A 1982 Subject women. Fontana, Glasgow

Olesker E, Walsh LV 1984 Childbearing amongst lesbians: are we meeting their needs? Journal of Nurse-Midwifery 29(5): 322–329

Plummer K (ed) 1981 The making of the modern homosexual. Hutchinson, London

Ramazanoglu C 1989 Feminism and the contradictions of oppression. Routledge, London

Randall CE 1989 Lesbian phobia among BSN educators: a survey. Journal of Nursing Education 28: 302–306

Reagon P 1981 The interaction of health professionals and their lesbian clients. Patient Counselling and Health Education 3(1): 21–25

Rich A 1980 Compulsory heterosexuality and lesbian existence. Signs 5(4): 631–660

Richardson D 1981 Lesbian identities. In: Hart J, Richardson D (eds) The theory and practice of homosexuality. Routledge and Kegan Paul, London

Richardson D (ed) 1996 Theorizing heterosexuality. Open University Press, Buckingham

Robson R 1992 Legal lesbicide. In: Radford J, Russell DEH (eds) Femicide: the politics of women killing. Open University Press, Buckingham

Rose P 1993 Out in the open. Nursing Times 89(30): 50–52

Royal College of Midwives 2000 Position paper no 22: maternity care for lesbian mothers. Royal College of Midwives Journal 3(4): 118–120

Saunders JM, Tupac JD, MacCulloch B 1988 A lesbian profile: a survey of 1000 lesbians. Southern California Women for Understanding, West Hollywood, CA

Seager J 1997 The women in the world atlas. Penguin, Harmondsworth

Seidman S 1994 Symposium: queer theory/sociology: a dialogue. Sociological Theory 12: 166–177

Seidman S (ed) 1996 Queer theory/sociology. Blackwell, Oxford

Stanley L, Wise S 1993 Breaking out again. Routledge, London

Stewart M 1999 Lesbian parents talk about their birth experiences. British Journal of Midwifery 7(2): 96–101

Walby S 1990 Theorising patriarchy. Blackwell, Oxford

Warner M (ed) 1993 Fear of a queer planet: queer politics and social theory. University of Minnesota Press, Minneapolis

Weeks J 1985 Sexuality and its discontents. Routledge and Kegan Paul, London

White TA 1979 Attitudes of psychiatric nurses towards same sex orientation. Nursing Research 28(5): 276–281

Wilkinson S, Kitzinger C (eds) 1993 Heterosexuality: a feminism and psychology reader. Sage, London

Wilton T 1995 Lesbian studies: setting an agenda. Routledge, London

Wilton T 2000 Sexualities in health and social care: a textbook. Open University Press, Buckingham

Young EW 1988 Nurses' attitudes towards homosexuality: analysis of change in AIDS workshops. Journal of Continuing Education in Nursing 19(1): 9–12

3

Feminisms and the body

Mary Stewart

The body is pregnant with symbolic meanings, deep, intensely charged and often highly contradictory. (Porter 2002, p 53)

INTRODUCTION

One of the many fascinating aspects of the body is that it is so often used as a metaphor for other aspects of life. In general terms, the head represents intellect and power: for example, 'head of the organisation', 'head start', 'head hunted'. The heart represents emotion: 'cold-hearted', 'heartache', 'heart of gold'. The genitalia and bodily functions are used as insults: ' he's a pain in the bum', 'kiss my ass'. Even sides of the body have powerful meanings, with the right side representing goodness and competence – 'he's my right-hand man', and the left side representing misfortune or incompetence – 'she's got two left feet'. Indeed, the word 'sinister' comes from the Latin, meaning 'on the left hand'. As the quote at the start of this chapter illustrates, the pregnant body creates further metaphors. This is only a tiny sample of the innumerable examples that exist but it demonstrates that the body informs our language and reinforces cultural beliefs about whether different parts of the body are good or bad.

The body, as a subject for sociological debate, has been under scrutiny for several decades. Many eminent academics have based their careers on developing an understanding of the body and of how and why it is represented, used and displayed. The purpose of this chapter is not to try and summarise all those debates, as that would be

25

an impossible task. Instead, my intention is to give a brief overview of some of the key sociological debates, highlighting how and why the subject of the body is of particular interest to feminists. I will go on to look at the debates about the body in relation to medicine and healthcare in general and then move on to discuss how these theories can be used to inform our understanding of the way in which pregnancy and childbirth may be experienced and viewed in contemporary Western society. I have given a reading list at the end of the chapter and hope that if you find something of interest in this chapter you can use it as a springboard for reading about the subject in greater depth. However, the subjects I have highlighted only touch on some of the debates that I find particularly interesting: inevitably this is a personal choice and you may disagree vehemently with the stance I have taken. If so, I will be delighted – my intention is not to convince you that I am right but to provoke debate.

We are inhabitors of our own bodies and other people view us and may make judgements on those bodies; we are also viewers of bodies (our friends, our lovers, the man on the street, the soap star on television) and, as midwives, we have privileged access to bodies. The subject of bodies generally triggers a reaction: sometimes irrational, sometimes appreciative, but rarely disinterested. I hope this chapter will explain some of those reactions and, at the same time, make clear why I believe the subject to be both endlessly fascinating and of supreme importance.

Exercise 3.1

It may be helpful to begin by contemplating how you feel about your own body. Look at yourself in a mirror, full length if possible. Imagine, at the same time, that you have a fairy godmother, benevolent genie or someone similar who can grant all your wishes, however wild and improbable. Now make a list with two columns. In the left-hand column, make a note of those physical attributes you would like to change. In the right-hand column, list all the physical attributes you would keep.

Now compare the two. My guess is that the list on the left is longer than the list on the right. When I did this

exercise myself, the column on the left had 10 items I wanted to change (and could have had more) whereas the column on the right had two. Why? I am a fairly average-looking woman, in good health and with no obvious physical impediments. Why would I want to change any of those things that my ancestors have bequeathed me? The answers to these questions are far from straightforward. However, I suggest that you now put the list on one side and, having read the chapter, revisit it in the hope that you will then have a clearer understanding as to why so many of us have complex and often unsatisfactory relationships with our bodies and how this can be explained in feminist terms.

A HISTORICAL OVERVIEW

The sociology of the body came about, in part, as a reaction to the work of the 17th-century philosopher Descartes, who conceived of the body and mind as distinct entities, giving rise to the expression Cartesian dualism (Annandale 1998) and a philosophy, common within science, that biochemical changes within the body were unrelated to mental, spiritual or emotional events (Abercrombie et al 2000). Sociological interest in the body reflects the challenge to this notion (Russell 2000).

Whilst beliefs about separatism persist, particularly, as we shall see later, in medicine and healthcare, sociologists argue that the body and mind are inseparable. Thus, as Hughes (2000) points out, there is a significant difference between the medical body, which is often referred to as a machine and may be perceived as simply a collection of body parts, and the sociological body, which constructs the body from a holistic perspective, subject to the constant interaction of psychological, physical and cultural phenomena (Abercrombie et al 2000). Between the sexes, Cartesian dualism led to a belief that men could be represented by the mind, whereas women are represented by their bodies (Kent 2000). Thus, men have traditionally been portrayed as rational and in control (and, until very recently, were presumed to be the 'head of the household') whereas women are perceived to be at the mercy of their wild and unpredictable bodies.

The study of the sociology of the body is of considerable importance because the exercise of social power includes power over bodies (Wilton 2000) and sociologists are interested in how regulation of the body is necessary for the regulation of society. This may be exercised at the highest levels through 'bio-power'; that is, the structural mechanisms used to manage populations and discipline individuals (Foucault 1977). Such power has far-reaching effects, influencing as it does the ways in which individuals manage and monitor their own bodies. Bio-power can usefully be applied to consider the ways in which society constructs and controls bodily ideals.

Ideas about the body are socially constructed and are influenced both by the individual's own culture and by social structures, such as the person's position in the workplace, as well as age, ethnicity and social class (Freund & McGuire 1995). So, for example, an 80-year-old white woman living in London is likely to have a different notion of how the body should be used and dressed from an 18-year-old black man living in the same city. Each of these believes their ideas to be normal but while ideas of normality are strongly held within each culture and society, they may differ markedly from one society to another. Think, too, of Queen Elizabeth, who most people in Britain would consider to be a normal size and shape, and contrast this with the King of Tonga, who is perceived to be equally normal by his subjects. Where do these ideas of normality come from and whose interest do they serve?

Contemporary society is based upon domination of the representational self (Turner 1987). In other words, the way we represent ourselves and the way others are represented, both in words and images, are key features of Western culture. Whilst in previous generations religion held ultimate control over people's bodies, with a focus on management of the soul, or the 'interior body', modern-day consumerism places emphasis on organisation and management of the exterior body. Foucault, a French philosopher, has been a key influence for sociologists. He was particularly interested in the ways in which the body was disciplined and much of his research focused on the power and authority exerted in both prisons and hospitals. However, he also highlighted the extent to which governmental organisations control the human body, through what he described as panopticism – systems of rational, detailed and bureaucratic surveillance.

I will return to Foucault's work later. For the moment, though, I want to focus on some aspects of what Helman (2000) describes as the 'body politic'; that is, control of the body, including its shape, size, clothing, diet, posture, behaviour and activities.

It seems self-evident to point out that we all have a body. However, it is not simply a physical entity that we each inhabit; it is ambiguous and problematic in human cultures (Turner 1987). Traditionally, the body has been 'managed' by three institutions: religion, law and medicine. Religion disciplines and controls the body through a process of confession, penance and forgiveness. The legal system exerts its power through a system of allegation, punishment and rehabilitation. Medical control of transgression involves diagnosis and therapy (Freund & McGuire 1995). However, while medicine and the law are still very powerful systems of control, in our largely secular society, religion wields less influence. Whereas for previous generations, the person's soul was the object of their salvation and this was monitored and controlled by the Church, the soul has now been replaced by the body (Baudrillard 1970) and this is monitored by society. Therefore, while in previous generations, moral worth was judged by a person's behaviour, in 21st-century Britain it is arguably more likely to be measured by the perception that an individual maintains control of their body and conforms to norms of fitness and weight (Urla & Swedlund 1995). However, these norms are highly gendered. For example, muscle definition, denoting strength, is highly valued in men but is perceived to be less attractive in women.

Bodily control, however it is achieved, can be seen as a powerful form of social control and attitudes towards the body act as a mirror, reflecting the social concerns of a group or culture (Freund & McGuire 1995). In contemporary British society there is a focus on the size and outward presentation of the body. Body image is an important aspect of the presentation of self: thinness is perceived to be a norm of beauty (Chernin 1981, Turner 1987) and moral judgements may be made about those who do not conform to this norm, with obesity frequently viewed as a lack of personal control (Abercrombie et al 2000, Freund & McGuire 1995). For example, in an ethnographic study Hunt & Symonds (1995) observed that midwives caring for obese women believed them to be out of control and totally responsible for their size.

Whilst our cultural obsession with dieting and fitness is often presented as a good thing, reflecting concerns with health and well-being, it also demonstrates the extent to which self-control and physical appearance are valued. While bodily control is expected of both men and women, in a patriarchal society it is women's appearance that is subject to greater social scrutiny. It is this discrepancy that is of particular interest to feminists.

WOMEN'S BODIES: FEMINIST THEORIES

Just as norms regarding the body are variable, so the 'ideal' woman's body varies across cultures, generations and societies but at the same time appears fixed and natural (Kent 2000). The ideal, with which most of us are now bombarded, is one of a slim, fit, youthful, white and able-bodied woman. Fashion has become increasingly influential in creating those norms, implying that women must be very thin in order to be socially acceptable (Bordo 1993, Eckermann 1997). A good example of how strongly this ideal is upheld is the model Sophie Dahl who, when she first began a career in modelling, was a size 16. Reams of newsprint were given over to discuss the extraordinary fact that a model who was the same size as many women in this country should be used to advertise clothes aimed, presumably, at those very same women.

Fashion is not only used to dictate the ideal size; it may also be used to alter body shape and to control physical activity. For example, high heels not only change the wearer's centre of gravity but it is impossible to move as freely in stilettos as it is in trainers. So, clothing which is marketed as being a highly desirable fashion accessory can also be seen as a way of controlling women's movement and behaviour, ensuring that they remain relatively passive and slow.

It is interesting to note how the perceived ideal has changed subtly, but significantly, even in relatively recent times. As Arthurs & Grimshaw (1999) point out, in the 1960s and 1970s, women were 'simply' expected to be slim. In recent years the requirement of a toned and fit body has also been added to the equation. Every image we are exposed to, whether visual or in the written word, underlines this notion of normality and desirability. Advertisements, 'celebrity' magazines, television programmes all portray successful individuals who have in common a specific body shape. And, despite our increasingly multicultural society, Caucasian standards of beauty still dominate: despite the suggestion that through exercise and diet, everyone can achieve the 'body they want', it is equally clear from all the visual images that surround us in the media that only a certain type of body will do (Bordo 1993).

Despite the evidence that women's bodies are the site of control, through systems of surveillance and oppression, it is also worth pointing out that individual women resist and subvert these efforts to control them in a multitude of different ways (Davis 1997, Kent 2000). For example, some authors argue that both anorexia and overeating can be seen as a means of asserting personal control and resisting social norms (Freund & McGuire 1995, Orbach 1986).

Of course, physical attraction is not the exclusive concern of women but it is nonetheless *more* of an issue than it is for men. For example, while women in Western society are likely to be judged solely on their appearance, men are far more likely to be judged by their performance, whether occupational, athletic or sexual (Freund & McGuire 1995). Similarly, the meaning given in contemporary society to growing older demonstrates that this is perceived to be more of a problem for women than men (Featherstone & Hepworth 1991). Ageing is perceived as particularly problematic chiefly because women's physical attractiveness is valued so highly (Abbott & Wallace 1997). You only have to look at the ways in which women's cosmetics are marketed. The emphasis is on creams and potions that 'minimise fine lines', that promise to 'reduce wrinkles' or that even guarantee to 'slow the signs of ageing'. The clear underlying message is that if women want to be perceived as attractive they have to look youthful, whatever their age.

Women's bodies have also been the subject of what Berger (1972) describes as the 'male gaze'; that is, men have a privileged gaze, allowing them to look at women critically or lustfully. Not only are women expected to be the passive recipients of this, they are also expected to modulate their appearance to please the gaze (King 1992). Many aspects of our consumer culture still depend on erotic sexuality, and this privileged gaze, to market goods for men (Turner 1991). For example, in a recent radio discussion, editors and publishers involved in the production of men's magazines acknowledged that the partly clothed women pictured on each front cover are used intentionally to 'sell' the magazine (The Message 2003). I am not referring here to *Playboy* or to pornographic magazines that are placed on the top shelf of the newsagents but to very mainstream publications, such as *FHM* and *Loaded*. While men's magazines depend on this objectification of the female body, women's magazines are sold on the basis of promising alternatives, whether it is a younger body, one that is more beautiful or, indeed, a body modelled on someone else entirely. I recently saw a magazine on the supermarket shelf called *Celebrity Bodies* carrying the subtitle 'You can have one too'.

While men view women's bodies as a source of titillation and gratification, women are bombarded with the message that they have a duty to maintain and beautify their body. It is this sharp contrast, between the observer and the observed, that has been the focus of feminist interest in the body.

Women need the power that comes from being at ease within their bodies. (Counihan 1999, p 195)

Counihan's quote puts forward one of the key issues for feminists with regard to the body: that women will only be equal with men when their bodies are accepted in the same way as men's bodies; when the observed and the observer are equal.

As Kent (2000) notes, feminist thought has been instrumental in creating and shaping debates around the body. So, while social theorists have recognised for some time that bodies are affected by social and psychological as well as physical elements, feminists have pointed to the ways in which women's bodies in particular are situated, used and portrayed. Feminist theories focus on how patriarchy determines social attitudes towards women and how women's bodies can be seen as the site of inequality, domination and oppression (Williams & Bendelow 1998).

As other authors within this book demonstrate, 'feminism' is not one single, simple perspective. In contrast, feminists may hold widely differing views on how and why women are oppressed within society and how and why this should be changed. Similarly, they may be at odds when discussing how and why the body is and should be represented within contemporary society. However, feminists agree that women are *generally* disadvantaged and that the patriarchal society in which we live benefits men more than women.

The subject of women's bodies is of particular interest and concern because, as we have seen, it is an effective site for controlling women's behaviour. Many young women today would argue that they have no need of feminism, that they have the same opportunities as their male peers. Putting aside the incontrovertible evidence that women still earn less than men, while being expected to work both within and outside the home, there is also evidence that women are spending more time on the management and discipline of their bodies than they have for many generations (Bordo 1993, Roberts 2002).

At this point it is worth briefly visiting some of the specific feminist critiques of the body. However, this is really only scratching the surface, to highlight the differences that exist. You should not feel that you have to ally yourself absolutely with one stance, although you may feel strongly that you want to do this. All feminists share common objectives of identifying ways in which patriarchy (i.e. the system, not necessarily men, either as individuals or a group) undermines women's health, but there are significant and highly political differences between them (Annandale 1998). However, many feminists are now less insistent on an unswerving loyalty to any single theoretical framework (Jaggar & Rothenberg 1993).

Liberal feminisim

Liberal feminists recognise that the body is the site of control of women but argue that women need to work alongside men in changing this, for example by rejecting or reshaping the beauty and fashion industries (Wolf 1991, 1994). This is based on a core belief of liberal feminism, that while men and women are equal in potential, the differences that exist result from social expectation, including the differing ways in which boys and girls are treated from infancy onwards, as well as from discriminatory legislation (Abbott & Wallace 1997). Particular interest has been paid to the social construction of gender roles and the argument that women are taught, from an early age, how to use and dress their bodies. However, the suggestion by liberal feminists that this oppression and control can be countered by a process of re-education, in which divisive gender roles are replaced by more equitable behaviour, has been criticised for being overly simplistic and for ignoring the fact that financial, social or educational barriers exist among and between women (Annandale 1998, Gatens 1983, Turner 1987).

Radical feminism

Radical feminists argue that patriarchy is the primary cause of women's oppression and that this is specifically experienced through male control of female bodies (Abbott & Wallace 1997, Annandale 1998). For example, radical feminists are highly critical of male control over women's fertility, exemplified by the new reproductive technologies, arguing that this is an example of patriarchal medicine brutalising women's bodies, without analysing how infertility can be prevented (Rowland & Klein 1996). Similarly, some radical feminists argue that pregnant women should reject technological birth and reclaim 'natural' birth. However, this is problematic for several reasons. As current debates clearly demonstrate, there is no consensus on what natural birth actually is (Hanson 2002). Moreover, to focus on natural birth as the ideal devalues those women and babies who actually benefit from medical intervention.

Central to radical feminism is the belief that what women have in common is greater than the factors that divide them (Abbott & Wallace 1997). Its proponents believe that women share a common experience of oppression built around male control over women's bodies and, in contrast to liberal feminists, seek to celebrate the female body as superior to rather than equal with the male body. Critiques of radical feminism argue that this stance denies differences between women, such as those of 'race' or class, and that it pits women against men by holding up a female 'counterculture' based on a premise of women's biological superiority (Annandale 1998).

Poststructural feminism

Poststructural feminists have been heavily influenced by the work of Foucault and have developed this to focus on two key issues, the first being the ways in which discourse constructs our understandings of the body. Therefore, the way in which we understand words such as 'body', 'sex' or 'gender' is not accidental: the meanings have been created purposefully and the words are used as labels, defining what is and is not normal (Kent 2000). Similarly, poststructuralists argue against the use of binary concepts, such as male/female or masculine/feminine, which generally privilege the former to the detriment of the latter. They contest the assumption of difference based on sex or gender, arguing that our understanding of this difference has been created by the omnipresent discourse of patriarchy (Annandale 1998). For example, most people believe that men are 'naturally' stronger than women and, often enough, this proves to be true. However, poststructuralists would argue that, far from being a biological given, this results from centuries of discourse which has valued male members of society over women, with more time and money invested in their education, their diet and their well-being. Inevitably, the men will develop more healthily than women but we cannot assume that this is because Y chromosomes are somehow healthier than their X counterparts.

Secondly, poststructuralists criticise liberal and radical feminisms for focusing on the viewpoints of white, middle-class, North American and Western European women. In contrast, poststructuralists are specifically concerned with the diversity of women's experiences, emphasising difference and plurality and arguing that there is never one, universal account and, moreover, that men can also be the victims of patriarchy (Annandale 1998). So, while current discourse generally devalues women's bodies, an affluent white woman will experience this very differently from a young black lesbian and a woman with cerebral palsy, each of them experiencing pregnancy for the first time. Concerns have been expressed that poststructuralism will dilute feminist critiques of patriarchy and that this relativism, and the focus on individual accounts, will challenge the universal thrust of feminists' opposition to male dominance (Riley 1988).

THE BODY IN MEDICINE AND HEALTHCARE

As we have seen, society in general exerts considerable control over the body but bodies have now also become the site of health surveillance (Howson 1998). Once again, Foucault has been one of the most influential thinkers in this field. He described what he referred to as the 'medical gaze', a new way of seeing the body whereby it has become the focus of surveillance and control by the medical profession (Annandale 1998). The medical gaze also represents the universalisation of medical discourse which regards all bodies as essentially the same, which is in turn based upon specific definitions of normality about the ways in which bodies look and work (Kent 2000).

The medical gaze has also led to the rise of biomedicine; that is, modern scientific medicine, which regards the 'body as a machine and ... the doctor's task as the repair of that machine' (Engel 1977, p 131). The body is perceived as a series of parts, each of which, if effectively managed and controlled, can be expected to function in a certain, specific way. This focus on parts of the body, rather than considering the whole person, led to what Porter (2002, p 55) calls a myopic reductionism, ignoring as it does the fact that social and psychological conditions may both contribute to the

illness or promote healing (Freund & McGuire 1995). Randomised controlled trials (RCTs) are a supreme example of the universalisation and myopic reductionism endemic within biomedicine. While RCTs can demonstrate a causal link between an intervention and an outcome, the findings cannot be automatically applied to individuals, as human behaviour is 'irredeemably contextual and idiosyncratic' (Greenhalgh 1999, p 324).

As I discussed earlier in the chapter, whereas in previous generations religious institutions largely shaped world views, in our increasingly secular society it is now health which acts as a moral model of the universe (Helman 2000). So, the notion of an unhealthy lifestyle resulting in ill health has replaced earlier religious concepts of sinful behaviour leading to divine retribution. Biomedicine then becomes something of an arbiter of social values, holding the individual responsible for their malady, while absolving society of responsibility and, at the same time, acting as a forceful agent of control. Witness current debates about whether alcoholics should be 'allowed' to have liver transplants or whether smokers should have to pay for treatment for lung cancer. These arguments place blame solely on the individual and do not allow for any discussion of *why* the individual started to smoke or drink heavily in the first place, nor whether society may have had a hand in this.

I do not want to suggest here that individuals bear no responsibility for their actions. However, it is far too simplistic to suggest that they bear sole responsibility: this, as Williams (2002) suggests, lets society off the hook without requiring any self-questioning, any contemplation that collectively we may bear some responsibility for the actions of individuals within that society.

Current public health messages make clear that individuals have a responsibility to monitor their own health, through diet and exercise, whilst also subjecting their bodies to external control and surveillance, for example through regular visits to the dentist. The growth of preventive medicine relies on an internalisation of powerful discourses of health and fitness. I do not want to suggest that preventive medicine is, by definition, bad, nor that a balanced diet and exercise have no place in our lives. Rather, I simply want to make the point that public health messages, both the overt ('Eat five pieces of fruit or vegetables a day') and the subliminal (fat people are undeserving), are a powerful and effective way of controlling bodies. As Turner (1987) argues, though, the seeming virtues of preventive healthcare may be far more interventionist than more conventional, 'curative' medicine as it involves more intrusive management of lifestyles and bodies.

Public health messages demonstrate the extent to which the medical gaze has become a seemingly acceptable means of monitoring lifestyles. Arguably, the National Health Service, with its underlying principle of providing a free service at the point of care, which is an undeniable privilege, also acts as a powerful system of control over people's health. While the system remains free at the point of delivery, it is reasonable to demand that individuals who wish to use and benefit from the system have a responsibility to maintain their own health. As well as demanding responsibility, biomedicine may also require a person to accommodate themselves to an unsatisfactory role, rather than suggesting that the role could be changed (Freund & McGuire 1995). So, for example, a worker with backache on a factory production line will be expected to take painkillers, rather than being given the tools to challenge their working conditions. (In Chapter 8, Jane Ussher considers the ways in which women are expected to accommodate themselves to the often unsatisfactory expectations of mothers in society.)

While modern medicine is increasingly used as an agent of social control, this is especially true for women, making them dependent on the medical profession. This can be vividly seen in the levels of surveillance to which women are subjected during their reproductive lives. The female reproductive system is seen as problematic in contrast with the male reproductive system which, apparently unaffected by age, is seen as largely efficient. Physiological processes, from menarche to the menopause, have come under medical control to the extent that this is accepted as normal (Freund & McGuire 1995). As Annandale & Clark (1996) point out, the removal of sexual organs is never recommended in the same way for men as it is for women which implies that women's reproductive organs are not only problematic, but that they are dispensable. This suggests that we have not moved far beyond the Victorian notion that women's emotional instability arose from the uterus and could be cured by a hysterectomy. (The word 'hysteria' comes from the Greek word for womb, since it was originally believed to be a disorder of the uterus and therefore a disorder unique to women.)

Women are perceived to be the victims of their hormones, resulting in a belief that the whole of women's reproductive lives can, and indeed needs to be, controlled (Abbott & Wallace 1997), whether this involves antidepressants to 'treat' premenstrual tension, the pill to 'regulate' the menstrual cycle or hormone replacement therapy (HRT) to 'relieve' women of problems associated with the menopause. (It is also worth pointing out here that one of the marketing strategies used to promote HRT is that it preserves women's youthful appearance, emphasising the ideology that the only attractive female body is a young one.) It seems perverse, though, that while many 'women's problems' are perceived to be hormonal in origin, the treatment, too, involves the use of hormones. This suggests that biomedicine feels threatened by the natural physiological processes which mediate women's reproductive lives and that therapy and interventions, prompted by the medical gaze, are a technique for governing these processes.

Even modern contraception, such as the development of the Pill with its promise of sexual liberation, has been problematic for feminists (Kent 2000, Thomas 1998). While on the one hand it gives women far more independence and control over their reproductive lives, nevertheless it also extends medical and social control over women's bodies (Abbott & Wallace 1997). 'Liberation' and sexual freedom come with enforced surveillance and control. Moreover, most contraceptives carry small but significant health risks for women's bodies, the only exception being natural family planning that depends on temperature and mucus assessment.

Regulation of women's bodies, through each stage of their reproductive lives, can be seen as an effective way of reminding women of their powerlessness in the face of patriarchy (Helman 2000). Perhaps this is nowhere more clear than in the control exerted over women's bodies during pregnancy and childbirth.

WOMEN'S BODIES DURING PREGNANCY AND CHILDBIRTH

Childbirth experienced

Childbirth is, or at least should be, primarily about women's experiences. These experiences are intensely personal and will be influenced by a multitude of factors. In this section I want to consider what we know of those experiences, in particular exploring experiences that relate to the body. Clearly, all women experience a change in body shape but their body also becomes more public: it becomes a site of interest to friends, family and complete strangers. Moreover, women's bodies are likely to be touched more during and immediately after pregnancy than at any other time.

A universal experience of pregnancy is the accompanying change in body shape. Some women luxuriate in the change, with a sense of womanly fulfilment. Equally, others dislike the change, whether because of the loss of the shape that they enjoyed and/or the sense of being invaded by the fetus.

I love pregnant bodies, and I love the way pregnant women look. I would stand in front of the mirror and look at myself and touch my belly. I just like the way I look pregnant. I like the way pregnant women look; I think they're beautiful. I had no problems with my body image; I really loved it. (Counihan 1999, p 201)

I do have to say I felt a lot less attractive pregnant. I felt more matronly, I guess, is the word instead of sexy. When you're pregnant, you're used to that being your goal. You want to look attractive to the opposite sex. (Counihan 1999, p 201)

While some women revel in their changing shape, others find it quite appalling. For the latter, this dislike arises, in large part, as a reaction to societal expectations that the only worthwhile woman is a young, sexy, slim one. Interestingly, though, as women get physically larger, many of them express a feeling that they, as a person, are disappearing.

Just as all pregnant women experience a change in body shape, so too most women in more developed countries also experience antenatal care. One aspect of that care, which most midwives regard as routine, is abdominal palpation. There seems little doubt that this is one of several useful tools for assessing the growth and development of the fetus. In my own practice, I have always enjoyed doing palpations and marvelling at that close contact with the baby before it is born. I had always presumed that women enjoyed this experience too and was taken aback when I read that this is not always the case (Olsen 1999). Similarly, women can feel cheated when the midwife or doctor listens to the fetal heart.

The first time we heard the heartbeat I wasn't as excited as my husband, and I couldn't figure out why I wasn't excited, and then I realized that the reason I wasn't is because my doctor gave me the heartbeat. It's like he took it away from me … Maybe I'm a real independent person or something, but I felt funny that I had to rely on him. I wanted to do it myself. (Martin 1987, p 72)

Women may experience antenatal care as devaluing their own lived experience and knowledge of their own body and their growing fetus. Conversely, of course, some women rely on technology to provide them with confirmation of their pregnancy.

[With ultrasound] you have an idea of what you have inside you. I became conscious that it was a person. I hadn't felt it as much before, I had to see it first. (Georges 1997, p 98)

Clearly, pregnant women may experience the development of technology in either positive or negative terms. However, these two contrasting stories are also stark examples of power and control. The first woman expresses her frustration when the doctor takes control and 'allows' the woman to hear her baby's heartbeat. In the second account, the woman defers to medical power and authority: she has lost belief in her own ability to know her own body and looks to health professionals to provide this for her. It is too simple to suggest that the medical profession is solely responsible for this. We live in an increasingly technocratic society, where computerised microchips are the medium for the provision of more and more information. As a result, women will experience more and more of their pregnancy 'second-hand', whether through the use of ultrasound imaging, Doptone to monitor the fetal heart or serum screening to assess the well-being of the woman and her fetus. However, I refuse to believe that the most sophisticated technology in the world can replicate the endlessly subtle and ongoing interaction of a pregnant woman and her baby. Equally importantly, it is vital to recognise the infinite number of ways in which professional power can undermine and devalue women's own unique experiences of pregnancy and childbirth.

Women's experiences of breastfeeding provide a fascinating insight into their perceptions of body image. In a study of lived experiences of the let-down reflex associated with lactation, two women express sharply contrasting views.

I don't think leaking ever bothered me though, I think if I've had a patch I've just thought 'Oh sod it' sort of thing, I think I've got to the stage where I think well, this is natural and if other people don't like it they can lump it. (Britton 1998, p 72)

[Leaking] is not very nice, it's sort of like wetting yourself really. You don't want stains round your clothes, especially if you've got a blouse on or something on when it can really show up ... You wouldn't want to see wet knickers in public, so you don't want people to see this either. (Britton 1998, p 75)

Women's perceptions of breastfeeding may be shaped by a dominant perception within society that the female body is leaky, messy and troublesome, that it offends public sensibilities and requires containment (Hughes & Witz 1997, Shildrick 1997). This message is so powerful and all-pervasive that it is no surprise that breastfeeding rates are low in Westernised societies as few women have the confidence to ignore the instruction to cover up their leakiness, as the woman in the first interview did.

There are many more issues that are obviously relevant to women's experiences of pregnancy and childbirth, such as their experiences of touch during labour and, in particular, during vaginal examination, but space does not allow me to elaborate here. However, from the examples of women's experiences of pregnancy and birth discussed in this section, two key issues emerge.

One is the issue of knowledge, and whose knowledge counts. The second issue is the way in which society and the medical profession shape women's experiences, appropriation and ownership of women's bodies.

Questions for Reflection ?????

In what ways do you think your practice could affect women's experiences of pregnancy and birth? Think about where you look when you are doing an abdominal palpation or vaginal examination.

What do you say when you listen to the fetal heart, whether with a Pinard or a Doptone?

Do you comment on the woman's changing shape or other parts of her body (such as stretch marks)?

Pregnancy and childbirth portrayed

This section will consider how women's childbearing bodies are represented, whether during pregnancy, labour or the postnatal period. Representation refers to the ways in which a topic is written or spoken about and the visual imagery associated with it, and is of great importance to feminists (Wilton 2000).

When women's child-bearing bodies are photographed, painted, sculpted or even described in words, when their images are displayed, whether in the pages of *Hello!* magazine or an obstetric textbook, what we see is more than a simple visual or verbal image. Such depictions both produce meaning and construct women's pregnant or child-bearing bodies in specific ways. Every image is 'read' and interpreted by the observer. Our understanding of the image is affected by the context in which it is presented, by our own cultural beliefs and personal experiences, as well as by the personal experiences and cultural beliefs of those who created the image.

As we saw earlier in this chapter, women are commonly seen and portrayed through the 'male gaze'. This is equally true during pregnancy and early motherhood where women are commonly portrayed in Madonna-like contemplation, whether gazing at their pregnant belly or new baby, suggesting that these are natural and wholly happy experiences, creating a sense of womanly fulfilment (Kent 2000). This image has been remarkably resilient to change over the centuries. If you compare a medieval painting of the Madonna and child with a front cover photograph on a contemporary parenting magazine, you will see that although clothing has changed, little else has altered in the ways in which women are portrayed.

However the pregnancy has been conceived, whether it is being experienced by a single woman, a heterosexual couple or a couple in a lesbian relationship, pregnancy is the most overt sign of a woman's sexual activity and yet, until very recently, visual images rarely portrayed pregnant women in a sexual or sexy way. The photograph of Demi Moore, nude and pregnant, which made the front cover of *Vanity Fair* in 1992 caused considerable debate because it confounded socially constructed notions of the ways in which pregnant women should display their bodies. Arguably, this photograph was hugely influential as it is hard now to avoid images of pregnant celebrities, displaying their bodies with pride and in a manner that would have been unheard of even 20 years ago. However, it is also worth pointing out that those same bodies are, without exception, sleek, toned, slim and healthy.

I also imagine it will be many years before a woman's postnatal body is celebrated in the same positive way: for the most part, they remain clothed and hidden. One striking contradiction to this norm is a series of three photographs by the Dutch artist Rineke Dijkstra on permanent display at Tate Modern in London,* each of which shows a naked woman and her baby gazing directly at the camera. I loved these photographs when I saw them and find them profoundly moving – to me they are a wonderful testimony to the strength, as well as vulnerability of child-bearing women.

They demonstrate that childbirth changes women's bodies – there is no hiding from the reality of the photos, there is no soft focus to romanticise the images. However, these frank portrayals of women's bodies clearly can make people uncomfortable, as was apparent by the behaviour of some of the visitors when I visited the gallery where the photos were displayed. People saw them and glanced quickly away, perhaps ashamed, embarrassed or disgusted by what they saw. These photographs seem to me to be an attempt to reframe cultural notions of normality and acceptability, to put forward an alternative viewpoint where, rather than creating a romanticised and false ideal, childbirth is portrayed as hard work and yet is a source of power and strength for women.

It is illuminating to reflect on how women are portrayed in midwifery and medical textbooks. In one study, the authors examined the ways in which women are portrayed in 17 editions of *Williams' Obstetrics*, an obstetrical textbook, over a period of more than 90 years (Smith & Condit 2000). The authors describe three key findings. First, within the textbooks, depictions of healthy or 'normal' pregnant bodies were virtually absent. Second, images portraying women's full bodies, rather than simply parts of their anatomy, were dominated by images of white women. Third, the authors concluded that the images communicated to readers a clear message of the pathology of pregnancy and the belief that women can be seen simply as a series of body parts. This leads to objectification, where the body is seen as an object of analysis rather than as a sentient, sensitive person, which in turn ensures subordination of women (Counihan 1999, Kent 2000). It would be reassuring to think that this was only true of medical textbooks. However, a quick glance through any standard midwifery textbook suggests that this is far from true. Just as in Smith & Condit's study, most focus on pictures of pathology rather than physiology, with a predominance of Caucasian women. Most notably, pictures which celebrate the joy of birth and the strength and beauty of women's bodies during pregnancy and childbirth are virtually absent.

So it is clear that portrayals of pregnancy and early motherhood, whether in the media or in

---

* (www.tate.org.uk/servlet/AWork?id=26250

professional texts and journals, are often far removed from women's lived experiences. However, despite the disparity between representation and reality, it is the former which becomes the instrument of control, articulating societal norms which in turn dictate the ways in which women are expected to dress and behave and the ways in which others see them during pregnancy and after the birth of their baby.

Questions for Reflection ?????

Look through some medical textbooks and note the way bodies have been portrayed over time. What do you see?

Is this intentional?

Childbirth surveyed

As any woman who has been pregnant will testify, the pregnant body becomes the site of public interest and discussion. Not only do people comment on women's changing size in a way that would be undreamt of in the non-pregnant state, but rights of access to the woman's body also change. Pregnant woman often comment, whether in shock, amazement or amusement, that friends and even strangers feel free to comment on the woman's changing bodily shape and to touch and stroke their bodies (Bailey 2001). While much of this public interest seems harmless, if impertinent, women may find that their behaviour is monitored, demonstrating that motherhood is commonly associated with a loss of privacy (Richardson 1993). During pregnancy and motherhood, women will find that other people are always telling them how to behave and what to do (Oakley 1993). This is true of friends and strangers, who may tell the woman anything from the seemingly sensible, such as 'You should get more rest', to the frankly bizarre. One woman I know was told by her mother-in-law never to stretch higher than her shoulder, as this would strangle the baby. As the woman in question stood less than

5 feet tall, following this advice would have made her life extremely problematic.

Pregnant women's behaviour is of particular interest to health professionals. As we saw earlier, women's bodies have been, and continue to be, sites of medical surveillance, with the medical gaze defining both the 'normal' and the 'abnormal' (Foucault 1973). The underlying perception that women's bodies are problematic extends into pregnancy (Kent 2000) and, of course, pregnancy and childbirth are unique as there are now two or more bodies that become the subject of detailed scrutiny simultaneously. Indeed, while attention is ostensibly being paid to the pregnant woman, often she is merely a vessel, container and incubator, while the fetus is the primary focus of attention (Bordo 1993).

Professional knowledge and the legitimisation of science have led to pregnant women being subjected to the medical gaze through regular antenatal appointments and screening programmes. This can be seen as an extension of preventive healthcare that was explored earlier in this chapter and is an important tool in the surveillance of women (Oakley 1986). While antenatal care may be 'sold' as entirely altruistic, and promoting the health and well-being of both mother and baby, it can also be seen as a strategy for ensuring medical control over the female body. For example, there is an assumption that women will participate in antenatal care, whether clinic attendance or ultrasound screening, not only to secure their own health but also because the woman is perceived to have a duty of care to the fetus (Bordo 1993, Howson 1998).

Similarly, while there is a growing emphasis on informed choice, prompted in part by *Changing Childbirth* (Department of Health 1993), there is still an expectation that women will make the 'right' choice, within unwritten limits of acceptability. So, women may choose not to have serum screening for Down's syndrome and no-one is likely to make a fuss, but the woman who chooses not to have any antenatal care is deemed unnatural or irresponsible. A woman may be offered the choice of a home birth but only if she meets certain criteria: if she opts to have a home birth of twins or a baby in the breech presentation she is likely to become the subject of unwonted attention. Women who do not comply with this surveillance or are seen to make the wrong choices may be charged with irresponsibility, selfishness and even insanity. Consider the women who have refused a caesarean section and have subsequently been sectioned under the Mental Health Act (Cahill 1999). Women clearly do not have absolute control over their bodies. As Stapleton et al (2002) point out, the reality, in fact, is one of informed compliance, with the expectation that women will agree to the package of care they are offered.

Questions for Reflection ?????

How do you feel when a woman comes to your labour ward having not had any antenatal care?

What words do you or your colleagues use to describe this woman?

Is there an alternative version to this story?

I made the point earlier that within medicine, the body is often seen as a machine made up of separate parts. This metaphor is particularly true with relation to childbirth, where labour itself comes to be seen as analogous with factory production, a 'hierarchical system of centralized control organized for the purpose of efficient production and speed' (Martin 1987, p 66). Within this factory, the woman's body becomes an object that is managed and acted upon by the health professional, whether midwife or obstetrician. Again, it is worth reflecting on the content of standard midwifery textbooks, which often have chapters and subheadings focusing on the *management* of antenatal, intrapartum and postnatal care, suggesting that women's bodies need to be controlled. This management is based, in turn, on a premise that health professionals *know* certain truths about the body. Sara Wickham discusses feminist approaches to knowledge in Chapter 11. However, it is worth reflecting here how current understanding affects surveillance of women's bodies during labour.

Think, for example, of some of the 'facts' we are taught as midwives, such as that labour can be divided into three stages, each of which can be clearly defined and measured. However, this concept is specific to a certain culture and time. While we may think it is of crucial importance to time and measure the three stages of labour, it seems clear that our ancestors interpreted labour as a single event, that was not divided into arbitrary stages. Similarly, it is not impossible, perhaps it is even likely, that midwives in the 24th century may divide labour into four stages. For example, they may argue that what we now think of as being the latent stage is, in fact the first stage of labour, followed by the second stage (more regular contractions), third stage (birth of the baby) and fourth stage (delivery of the placenta and membranes). Conversely, these stages may be abandoned altogether. I do not want to suggest that one alternative is better than another. I simply want to point out that what we think of as being 'truths' about the body, whether pregnant or not, are always influenced by cultural and societal norms which shift over time but which have a profound effect on medical surveillance.

The growth of a technocratic society where now the interior as well as the exterior of people's bodies can be scrutinised means that a body viewed on a screen, whether via X-ray, MRI scan or CAT scan, may become more real than the physical body (Annandale 1998). This is amply demonstrated in the use of technology in pregnancy and childbirth. You only have to consider how, during ultrasound scan, the focus of everyone in the room is on the image of the fetus on screen, rather than on the ways in which the woman can describe her changing body and her knowledge of the baby's behaviour. (I use the term 'baby' here intentionally as I believe this is the word that almost all women use, at whatever stage of their pregnancy, rather than 'embryo' or 'fetus'.)

Increasing medical intervention in childbirth demonstrates how the unpredictable nature of the female body needs to be disciplined by medicine (Britton 1998). From her first appointment early in pregnancy, where the woman will be offered blood tests to assess her own state of health, through ultrasound scan, birth and thereafter, technology is at hand, ostensibly to make pregnancy and birth both safer and less traumatic to mother and baby. The most vivid example of this is the assumption by most midwives and doctors that women should be offered pain relief in labour. The prevailing belief is that the pain of birth is extreme and unacceptable for most sophisticated, modern women but that they can be saved from this distress by technology. While a wish to help others avoid pain appears laudable, it also puts forward the ideology that women are not capable of doing this alone and must rely on health professionals who, as result, remain in control of the birth. Compare this with a contrasting philosophy, as described by Nicky Leap (2000), of being with women in pain and resisting the urge to take away that pain. Being truly 'with woman' through a long and arduous labour, in which she remains in control of what happens to her and when, is one of the best examples of feminism in practice.

CONCLUSION

Feminists are interested in the ways in which women are disadvantaged within society. The body is a prime example of such disadvantage and, as I hope this chapter has demonstrated, women's bodies are subject to close scrutiny, both overt and covert, which informs women about the ways in which they are expected to clothe, use and display their bodies. This scrutiny is extraordinarily powerful and pervasive and is particularly evident in the ways in which women's bodies are observed and controlled during pregnancy, labour and birth. Heightened levels of interest vary from the seemingly innocuous, such as a pat on a woman's growing belly, to the extreme, for example, labelling as insane a woman who does not comply with treatment.

I made the point earlier that, as midwives, we have privileged access to women's bodies. While the subject of the body has been of great interest to sociologists and feminists for several decades, it rarely features on the midwifery curriculum. However, the ways in which we relate to our own bodies, and the bodies of those around us, are likely to have a profound effect on the women we support through pregnancy, birth and beyond. For this reason, I think we have an obligation to engage with current debates and theories, using them to inform our practice.

Bodies matter. The bodies we inhabit as individuals, the bodies we see on our television screens, the bodies of pregnant women and their babies: all these contribute to and are shaped by our understanding of the world around us. The subject of the body is both complex and ever changing and this short chapter cannot hope to do justice to all the many differing debates. However, I hope that it has whetted your appetite to know more.

Key points

- The body is the subject of extensive debate amongst feminists.

- The body is the site of both social and medical control.

- In healthcare, the body is often seen as a series of parts rather than an inseparable whole.

- Women's bodies are the subject of increasing scrutiny during pregnancy and childbirth.

- Our relationships with bodies, whether our own or others, are often intense, complex and contradictory.

REFERENCES

Abbott P & Wallace C 1997 An introduction to sociology: feminist perspectives. Routledge, London

Abercrombie N, Hill S, Turner BS 2000 The Penguin dictionary of sociology. Penguin, London

Annandale E 1998 The sociology of health and medicine: a critical introduction. Polity Press, Cambridge

Annandale E, Clark J 1996 What is gender? Feminist theory and the sociology of human reproduction. Sociology of Health and Illness 18(1): 17–44

Arthurs J, Grimshaw J 1999 Introduction. In: Arthurs J, Grimshaw J (eds) Women's bodies: discipline and transgression. Cassell, London

Bailey L 2001 Gender shows: first-time mothers and embodied selves. Gender and Society 15(1): 110–129

Baudrillard J 1970 La societé de consommation. Cited in Berthelot JM 1991 Sociological discourse and the body. In: Featherstone M, Hepworth M, Turner BS (eds) The body: social process and cultural theory. Sage, London

Berger J 1972 Ways of seeing. BBC Books, London

Bordo S 1993 Unbearable weight: feminism, Western culture and the body. University of California Press, Berkeley, CA

Britton C 1998 'Feeling letdown': an exploration of an embodied sensation associated with breastfeeding. In: Nettleton S, Watson J (eds) The body in everyday life. Routledge, London

Cahill H 1999 An Orwellian scenario: court ordered caesarean section and women's autonomy. Nursing Ethics 6(6): 494–505

Chernin K 1981 The obsession: reflections on the tyranny of slenderness. Harper and Row, New York

Counihan CM 1999 The anthropology of food and body: gender, meaning and power. Routledge, New York

Davis K (ed) 1997 Embodied practices: feminist perspectives on the body. Sage, London

Department of Health 1993 Changing childbirth part 1: Report of the Expert Maternity Group. HMSO, London

Eckermann L 1997 Foucault, embodiment and gender subjectivities: the case of voluntary self-starvation. In: Petersen A, Bunton R (eds) Foucault, health and medicine. Routledge, London

Engel G 1977 The need for a new model: a challenge for biomedicine. Science 196(129): 164–171

Featherstone M, Hepworth M 1991 The mask of ageing. In: Featherstone M, Hepworth M, Turner BS (eds) The body: social process and cultural theory. Sage, London

Foucault M 1973 The birth of the clinic: an archaeology of medical perception. Tavistock, London

Foucault M 1977 Discipline and punish: the birth of the prison (trans. A Sheridan). Penguin, Harmondsworth

Freund PES, McGuire MB 1995 Health, illness and the social body. Prentice Hall, Englewood Cliffs, NJ

Gatens M 1983 A critique of the sex/gender distinction. In: Allen J, Patton P (eds) Beyond Marxism. Intervention Publishing, Leichhardt

Georges E 1997 Fetal ultrasound imaging and the production of authoritative knowledge in Greece. In: Davis-Floyd RE, Sargent CF (eds) Childbirth and authoritative knowledge: cross-cultural perspectives. University of California Press, Berkeley, CA

Greenhalgh T 1999 Narrative based medicine in an evidence based world. British Medical Journal 318: 323–325

Hanson S 2002 Definitions of normality. Midwifery Matters 95(winter): 3–4

Helman CG 2000 Culture, health and illness. Butterworth Heinemann, Oxford

Howson A 1998 Embodied obligation: the female body and health surveillance. In: Nettleton S, Watson J (eds) The body in everyday life. Routledge, London

Hughes A, Witz A 1997 Feminism and the matter of bodies: from de Beauvoir to Butler. Body and Society 3(1): 47–60

Hughes B 2000 Medicalized bodies. In: Hancock P, Hughes B, Jagger E et al (eds) The body, culture and society: an introduction. Open University Press, Buckingham

Hunt S, Symonds A 1995 The social meaning of midwifery. Macmillan, Basingstoke

Jaggar A, Rothenberg P 1993 Feminist frameworks: alternative theoretical accounts of the relations between men and women. McGraw-Hill, New York

Kent J 2000 Social perspectives on pregnancy and childbirth for midwives, nurses and the caring professions. Open University Press, Buckingham

King C 1992 The politics of representation: a democracy of the gaze. In: Bonner F, Goodman L, Allen R, Janes L, King C (eds) Imagining women: cultural representations and gender. Polity Press, Cambridge

Leap N 2000 'The less we do, the more we give'. In: Kirkham M (ed) The midwife–mother relationship. Macmillan, Basingstoke

Martin E 1987 The woman in the body: a cultural analysis of reproduction. Open University Press, Milton Keynes

Oakley A 1986 The captured womb: a history of the medical care of pregnant women. Basil Blackwell, Oxford

Oakley A 1993 Essays on women, medicine and health. Edinburgh University Press, Edinburgh

Olsen K 1999 'Now just pop up here, dear…': revisiting the art of abdominal palpation. Practising Midwife 2(9): 13–15

Orbach S 1986 Hunger strike: the anorexic's struggle as a metaphor for our age. WW Norton, New York

Porter R 2002 Blood and guts: a short history of medicine. Allen Lane, London

Richardson D 1993 Women, motherhood and childrearing. Macmillan, London

Riley D 1988 Am I that name? Feminism and the category of 'women' in history. Macmillan, Basingstoke

Roberts T-A 2002 The woman in the body. Feminism and Psychology 12(3): 324–329

Rowland R, Klein R 1996 Radical feminism: history, politics, action. In: Bell D, Klein R (eds) Radically speaking: feminism reclaimed. Zed Books, London

Russell R 2000 Ethical bodies. In: Hancock P, Hughes B, Jagger E et al (eds) The body, culture and society: an introduction. Open University Press, Buckingham

Shildrick M 1997 Leaky bodies and boundaries: feminism, postmodernism and (bio)ethics. Routledge, London

Smith SA, Condit DM 2000 Marginalizing women: images of pregnancy in Williams' Obstetrics. Journal of Perinatal Education 9 (2): 14–26

Stapleton H, Kirkham M, Thomas G 2002 Qualitative study of evidence based leaflets in maternity care. British Medical Journal 324 (7338): 639–643

The Message 2003 Broadcast on BBC Radio 4, 3 January

Thomas H 1998 Reproductive health needs across the lifespan. In: Doyal L (ed) Women and health services: an agenda for change. Open University Press, Buckingham

Turner BS 1987 Medical power and social knowledge. Sage, London

Turner BS 1991 Recent developments in the theory of the body. In: Featherstone M, Hepworth M, Turner BS (eds) The body: social process and cultural theory. Sage, London

Urla J, Swedlund AC 1995 The anthropometry of Barbie: unsettling ideals of the feminine body in popular culture. In: Terry J, Urla J (eds) Deviant bodies. Indiana University Press, Bloomington

Williams R 2002 Writing in the dust: reflections on 11th September and its aftermath. Hodder and Stoughton, London

Williams SJ, Bendelow G 1998 The lived body: sociological themes, embodied issues. Routledge, London

Wilton T 2000 Sexualities in health and social care: a textbook. Open University Press, Buckingham

Wolf N 1991 The beauty myth. Vintage Books, London

Wolf N 1994 Fire with fire. Vintage Books, London

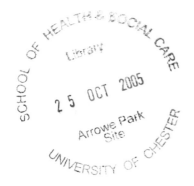

4

Pregnancy

Liz Stephens

INTRODUCTION

Birth is a women's issue: birth is a power issue; therefore birth is a feminist issue. (Buckley 1997)

Pregnancy and childbirth is claimed to be a rite of passage and one of the most important achievements in a woman's life. Yet reproduction and mothering are central to theories of patriarchy and women's unequal position within Western society. Women's bodies have been medicalised by the definition of normal body functions, such as childbirth, as medical problems with medical solutions, so that they have become sites of medical knowledge (Jackson et al 1993). Having a baby is a biological and cultural act; a woman reproduces the species yet childbirth is shaped by culture (Oakley 1980).

Feminists have since the 1970s questioned the reasons for women's oppression, identifying marriage, child bearing, child rearing and capitalism as basic causes; central to all these is biological reproduction (Hanmer 1993). Childbirth paradoxically can be seen as both a cause of woman's subordinate position in society and as a means of empowerment. By the expectation that women will stay at home to carry out child rearing, they are placed in a subordinate unpaid role in a society that values material possessions above all else. Yet success in childbirth can be empowering for women. In my research into midwives' lived experience of being 'with woman' (Stephens 1998) this is expressed by one of the midwives interviewed.

At the end of it if they feel like they've got through a difficult labour, they feel they can conquer the world, and so I do think that's empowering, yes, I do think that any woman that gets through a natural birth feels yeah, I can do it. (Lisa)

Within the maternity services the two main professions of obstetrics and midwifery are gendered, with obstetrics being gendered male and midwifery gendered female (Oakley 1993, Witz 1992). How midwives help women to achieve successful and empowering birth experiences must therefore be a subject of interest to feminists.

The 20th century saw enormous changes in the ways in which pregnancy and childbirth were viewed and managed. The century started with the Midwives Act of 1902, which ensured the future of midwives and midwifery but at a cost of putting them in a disadvantaged position amongst professions. The Act secured occupational demarcation, dividing maternity into normal and abnormal, a deskilling strategy by 'medical men' (Witz 1992). Midwives have since perpetuated this demarcation. It was also a time of great change for women and the women's movement.

This chapter will look at how these are linked and their impact on the way women experience antenatal care. A feminism for midwifery will be offered that will explore how midwives and women can work in partnership in order to help women achieve safe, satisfying and empowering birth experiences.

FEMINIST THEORY: THE BIG THREE PERSPECTIVES

Feminist theory has attempted to offer critical explanations of women's unequal position in society, in order to identify why women have less power than men. Feminists have produced competing theories of women's subordination in order to analyse, understand and challenge it (Reynolds 1993). Second-wave feminism originating in the 1960s and 1970s placed the emphasis on women's 'biological fate' (Humm 1990), minimising the differences between women and theorising feminism into the big three perspectives of liberal, radical and socialist feminism (Banks 1981).

Radical feminism puts sexuality at the heart of male domination; it is seen as the way in which men control and maintain power over women (Mackinnon 1982). Socialist or Marxist feminism does not regard sexuality as the fundamental cause of women's oppression (Richardson 1993), but believes that women are the underclass in a society that depends on the working classes and that elimination of a class society is the priority. Liberal feminism aimed to achieve equal rights for women within the framework of society, by political lobbying and equal rights legislation (Eisenstein 1993).

These three 'big perspectives' dominated feminist theory until the early 1980s. However, from the mid 1980s feminist theory began to be criticised by lesbians (Rich 1980) and black women (Carby 1982), amongst others, for its white heterosexual ethnocentric focus, which did not address the problems of women in these groups. Maynard (1995) argues that a further difficulty with classifying feminism in this way is that it implies that there is some kind of unity of approach and intention between writers placed in each category, with the implication that there is sufficient similarity between those allocated to each group to warrant a claim of coherence within the group.

It is interesting to note that whilst feminists were challenging the male domination of our society, the Peel Report (Department of Health and Social Security 1970) advocated hospital birth on the grounds of safety, ensuring that childbirth took place in hospitals that were medically dominated. This notion of the safety of hospital birth has been a feature of the medically dominated maternity service, despite increasing evidence that it is simply not the case for all women. Paradoxically, at a time when male power was being challenged in the public domain, women were losing power over the essential experience of being a woman, that of childbirth. The ideal of safety in childbirth has become central and is valued over women's satisfaction, although these are not competing ideologies and are not mutually exclusive. Oakley (1993) questions why so much is heard about patient satisfaction and so little done about it, whilst little is heard about doctors' satisfaction when it is a powerful but invisible influence on obstetric care.

Feminism until the 1980s conceptualised women as one distinct oppressed group and that was white middle-class women (Spelman 1990). However, women are of all classes, races, ages and religions so there is in effect no 'category woman', as there is no category of 'pregnant woman'. Spelman (1990) suggests that it is important to acknowledge the 'difference' so that feminism can include the voice of all women, emphasising the complexity of the ways in which the meaning of sexual difference is learned within a patriarchal culture, as femininity is never defined but unconsciously programmed, which causes women to keep seeking acceptance of their femininity. Joan Scott (1988) suggests that we need a theory that can analyse the workings of patriarchy in all its manifestations, ideological, institutional, organisational and subjective, and that allows for pluralities in the classification of women rather than unities and universals. Postmodern feminism, however, rejects any concept that claims to identify the basis of women's unequal position; the concept of women's subordination implies an objective, fixed state, suggesting that women are oppressed in essentially the same ways. Postmodern feminism allows for many different feminisms to enable individuality in aims and experience.

PATRIARCHY

Central to all theories of feminism is the concept of patriarchy. We live in a system that must be acknowledged as patriarchy and this system is mirrored in the structure and functions of the National Health Service (NHS). The term 'patriarchy' was first used to describe the power of the father as head of the household. More recently, it has been used within feminism to describe the systematic organisation of society that allows male supremacy and female subordination (Humm 1989). Kate Millett (1970) argued that male domination within Western society is so widespread that it is invisible and accepted as natural. This subliminal patriarchy could be compared with the subliminal medicalisation of the maternity service described by Gould (2002), in which medicalisation has become so widespread and accepted that we fail to recognise it. Within the

maternity services the effect of this is that the woman as cared for or carer is less valued within the male-dominated system.

Walby (1990) suggests that patriarchy has moved from the private to the public domain. This public patriarchy is based within structures such as employment and the state. Within this model the NHS can be seen as a typical patriarchal institution which may be viewed as a pyramidal structure. The highly paid, highly valued, predominantly male senior managers and consultants are at the apex of the pyramid whilst paradoxically, despite the NHS being ostensibly about caring, the low-status, low-paid work is carried out by a predominantly female workforce. Watson (1990) argues that the present healthcare system operates within a larger patriarchal structure that does not value caring, which is viewed as women's work. Within this system normal life processes are treated as illness and stereotypes of the intellectual physician (male) and the nurturing non-intellectual nurse/midwife (female) persist (Muff 1982).

Questions for Reflection ?????

Write down some examples of patriarchy that you have experienced in your own social and working life.

How did these make you feel?

What was it that allowed those situations to arise?

THEORY AND PRACTICE

The link between feminist theory and midwifery practice may be hard to see, especially as in recent years feminist theory has become more academic and there seems to be a feeling that the war has been won. This is simply not true; women still earn significantly less than men, have difficulty reaching the most senior posts within organisations and are expected to carry out child rearing and home keeping in addition to paid work outside the home. Postmodern feminism has given us smaller groups of women working towards a common goal with groups such as black feminists and eco-feminists.

I suggest, then, a midwifery feminism, the essence of which is a 'with woman' philosophy. Sarah Buckley (1997) argues that 'birth is a women's issue: birth is a power issue; therefore birth is a feminist issue'. As midwives and women, we need to work with the woman we care for to ensure that our maternity services are woman focused. There can be no doubt that birth is a power issue; male dominance within our society has led to male dominance within the health service and professional dominance within the maternity services. In my own research into midwives' experience of being 'with woman' (Stephens 1998), it was issues around power and hierarchies that prevented midwives practising in the way they wanted to. These power issues are echoed within Mavis Kirkham's recent work (Kirkham 1999). These hierarchies are both inter- and intraprofessional but always result in women, as both service users and midwives, being the most disadvantaged people within the hierarchy.

MIDWIFERY FEMINISM

Peggy Foster (1995) believes that women's healthcare is determined by the interests of the providers of that healthcare rather than the needs of the women themselves. Foster (1989) identifies five key principles which underpin a feminist model of healthcare delivery, all of which could be incorporated into woman-centred systems of care. The first of these principles is that all medical knowledge should be shared with the woman in a way that will give her greater control. Second, Foster suggests healthcare providers should work in open egalitarian and democratic ways, which will enable the sharing of knowledge, expertise and other types of medical power. Third, feminist healthcare should be holistic, treating the woman as an individual and listening to her needs. Foster's fourth principle is that healthcare providers should share themselves as well as their expertise, empathising with women rather than taking a professional stance. The fifth principle is that healthcare must

be equally accessible to all women regardless of class, race or sexual orientation (Foster 1989).

As midwives we must position ourselves 'with women', ensuring they have the choice, continuity and control advocated in *Changing Childbirth* (Department of Health 1993). This concept has been used by factions within our society to offer women choices such as caesarean section on demand, choices that are not necessarily in their best interest. The essential point is the link between the three Cs (choice, continuity and control) which starts with antenatal care; to make the choices that suit them, women need to be given the information. Good information based on the best evidence enables women to take control; however, all too frequently information is used as a form of social control. We tell women what not to eat based on little evidence and without telling them what the risks are they are told to stop smoking and drinking alcohol and treated as social pariahs if they do not conform. A midwife up to date with the evidence and able to work in partnership with women should provide this information in an informative and non-judgemental way, so that the woman can make decisions for herself and her baby that suit her needs and circumstances. The way we give this information is important; a recent letter in the midwifery press described how women were getting rid of their cats due to unfounded fears about toxoplasmosis. This partnership with women should be based on equality, with the woman as the driving force as this is about her body, her pregnancy and her birth experience.

Pivotal to midwifery feminism is the concept of continuity and support; we know that continuity of care schemes confer considerable benefits on women, psychologically and physically (Allen et al 1997, Hutchings & Henty 2002, Page 1995, Reid 2002). Women, however, in many areas are still subjected to systems of care that mean they meet many maternity care workers in the antenatal period. This midwifery feminism could be likened to the social model of care as suggested by Walsh & Newburn (2002) (Box 4.1).

Within such a model women's voices become legitimate voices within the system, they work in partnership with midwives to achieve safe,

> **Box 4.1** Medical model vs social (midwifery) model (Walsh & Newburn 2002, with permission)
>
> | Medical model | Social model |
> |---|---|
> | Medical event | Life event |
> | Safe place (hospital) | Safe place (home) |
> | Professional care | Support from friends |
> | Technology | Nature |
> | Control | 'Let go' |
> | Analyse/solve | Mystery/respect |

satisfying birth experiences in the place of their choice. There are schemes that work in this way, such as the Albany Practice in South East London, the Weston Shore Group Practice in Southampton, Queen Charlotte's One to One initiative and my own team at St George's. These teams meet the woman early in her pregnancy, using the first meeting as the basis for a relationship of trust in which the midwives guide the woman through the service to ensure she has the birth she wants. The birth will be the basis of a lifelong relationship with her baby. This model ensures that the woman makes those choices based on information provided by the midwife; such personal decision making can be the start of a lifelong empowerment.

A further key feature of this feminist midwifery model of care will be its community base; the philosophy will be one of following women rather than staffing the institution. Anna Bosanquet (2002) states that if midwives continue to train and work within the hospital they will not be able to free themselves from its political and ideological forces. Yet we still have a system that socialises student midwives into the hospital way of birth and insists on a consolidation period on qualification. Midwife training needs to be community based, rooted in normality and based in one-to-one schemes. When working within the hospital environment midwives feel pressured to conform to hospital times, norms and guidelines, with covert policing by peers, managers and other professional groups (Bosanquet 2002, Kirkham 1999). By moving the emphasis to the community, the hospital way of technological birth will become less dominant and midwives and women able to work in ways that meet the needs of women.

This model provides good outcomes. The Albany Practice has a home birth rate of 43%, with 89% being looked after by their primary midwife. This group also reports a higher vaginal delivery rate, lower rates for induction, caesarean section, episiotomy and use of analgesia (Reid 2002). The Weston Shore Group Practice has a home birth rate of 34% and a normal birth rate of 85% (Hutchings & Henty 2002). My own team, although just starting up, has similarly high rates. This is achieved by offering the woman true choice, a choice frequently made in labour, when the woman decides she does not want to travel into hospital. Home birth is currently often viewed as the choice of middle-class women, yet these schemes have concentrated on women living in social deprivation. The Albany Practice is sited in a poor area in South East London and the Weston Shore Group Practice is sited in a SureStart area in Southampton, an area of acknowledged deprivation. My own team has started out by taking on women who are not finding what they want within the service, but our intention is to target asylum seekers and women living in bed and breakfast accommodation. By working in this way we are targeting our best service at those women in most need.

Hart (1971) described the inverse care law, whereby those most in need of healthcare provision have the least access to services. Although we are now 30 years on, Kirkham et al (2002) show that the inverse care law is alive and well and functioning within maternity care. They describe how time pressures favour educated middle-class women and that young and socially deprived women were treated differently from articulate, economically secure women. This is a function of the way we provide maternity care within the medical model. Where medical dominance has promoted the taking of blood pressure and testing urine over all else, midwives are caught in the middle, expected to carry out these rituals of antenatal care with all the time pressures of the modern maternity system which leaves them unable to move beyond this, frustrated at offering a service that does not meet women's needs. Midwives either learn to fit in or, increasingly it seems, the frustration is such that many leave the profession (Kirkham et al 2002).

Questions for Reflection ?????

What would be the advantages for women and midwives of a midwifery model of care in your own place of work?

Would there be any disadvantages?

What could you do to try and develop a midwifery model of care at work?

ADVOCACY

Within such a model of partnership and continuity the midwife and woman get to know each other and the midwife learns what the woman wants from this childbirth experience. If the woman chooses a birth experience outside the norm approved by institutional obstetrics, such as vaginal birth after caesarean section in a birth pool or vaginal breech birth, the midwife's role is to work with that woman, ensuring she has information that is evidence based without being alarmist. It is a sad fact of recent evidence-based practice that the evidence is often used to coerce women into making choices that they do not believe are right for them, as described by Anderson (2002). This use of evidence can only be described as 'institutional bullying'. The randomised controlled trial gives us information about what is the best treatment for the majority of subjects within that trial; it is unable to tell us which people are in that majority, so for individual woman there are no answers. Trials such as the breech trial (Hannah et al 2000) are being used to ensure women choose caesarean section, yet we know that many women will have perfectly safe vaginal breech births when facilitated by a practitioner experienced in that type of birth.

A midwife who has built up a good relationship with a woman during the antenatal period will want to help her achieve the birth she wants and will support that woman in achieving it, rather than acting as the mouthpiece of the institution, which demands conformity to protocols. This midwife will then act as the woman's advocate within the maternity services, positioning herself 'with woman' rather than 'with institution'. As midwives, we need to be prepared to support women and support each other. Mavis Kirkham (1999) shows how midwives fail to support each other and are left in the position of doing good by stealth but such concealment makes concerted action impossible. The way midwives treat each other is fundamental in defining and maintaining the culture of midwifery (Kirkham 1999). It must be a central tenet of the midwifery feminist model that midwives support each other and through supporting each other, support woman.

ANTENATAL CARE

When a woman was having a baby, nobody seemed to be interested in her until she was seven months pregnant. Nobody thought about antenatal care then. There were no antenatal beds. (Reflections of Ellen O'Brien read at a service for the Royal College of Midwives to celebrate 100 years of professional midwifery, May 31st 2002)

Antenatal care was not a feature of maternity care until the 20th century. Fetal heart sounds had first been recognised by Vicomte de Kergaredec in the early 19th century, abdominal palpation had been described in the late 19th century, but there appears to have been no systematic use of these techniques until the 20th century. In 1901 William Ballantyne published 'A Plea for a Pro-Maternity Hospital' (cited in Rhodes 1995). In the early decades of the century midwives tended to visit a woman early in the pregnancy to make arrangements for the birth, but would then only see her if problems arose (Leap & Hunter 1993).

Ballantyne described a number of fetal and maternal conditions about which little was known and put the case for a hospital that would provide antenatal beds. Ballantyne also established a domiciliary outpatient clinic in Edinburgh. In 1918 the Maternity and Child Welfare Act gave powers to local authorities to set up antenatal clinics. In 1923 Ballantyne wrote the aims of antenatal care which were:

• to remove dread
• to reduce discomfort

- to treat syphilis and pre-eclamptic toxaemia early
- to increase the numbers of normal pregnancies and labours
- to reduce the stillbirth rate
- to reduce maternal mortality (cited in Rhodes 1995).

Ballantyne recognised the importance of psychological aspects of pregnancy in a way that is not recognised by today's medical establishment. The primary focus of current antenatal care is on the recognition and treatment of physical manifestations. It is possible that this is a feature of medical dominance within maternity care, with biological disease seen as more important than psychological and emotional outcomes. In *The ABC of Antenatal Care* (Chamberlain 1997) the aims of antenatal care are given as:

1. management of maternal symptomatic problems
2. management of fetal symptomatic problems
3. screening and prevention of fetal problems
4. preparation of the couple for childbirth
5. preparation of the couple for child rearing.

These aims are much more focused on pregnancy as a problem to be managed, by a paternalistic service that believes it knows what is best for you. Yet a holistic woman-centred model of care should value all aspects of care equally. Within the midwifery model of care the psychological, social, emotional and physical aspects of antenatal care are valued, with the woman being able to express what is important to her at that time. To date, we have still not achieved Ballantyne's aims and indeed, instead of removing dread, women are often so scared of normal childbirth they choose to have major abdominal surgery instead and the numbers of normal pregnancies and labours are decreasing year on year. Intervention has become so widespread we no longer know how to define normal labour and birth.

The foundation of the NHS in 1946 led to an increase in the availability of beds for childbirth and this trend towards hospitalisation was underpinned by the Peel Report (1970) which advocated 100% hospital birth on the grounds of safety. This claim of greater safety was based on little or no evidence yet the trend for hospital birth has led to treating pregnancy as an illness that requires attendance at clinics, necessitating long waits in busy waiting rooms, leading to subsequent submissive behaviour.

Jean Chapple (2000) makes no attempt to state the aims of antenatal care but suggests needs assessment, identifying which women are at risk of pregnancy complications, which babies are at risk and what social factors may cause problems. This is an individualised model of care designed in partnership with women rather than a 'we know best' or patriarchal model of care that tells women what to do.

A decade on, we still have maternity care based on assumptions of the safety of the medical model, assumptions that remain unproven. The pattern of care has been established, challenged, individualised and yet we have no real evidence to show what is an ideal pattern of care. Enkin et al (2000, p 18) state that 'The content of antenatal care visits are more ritualistic than rational. The frequency … and the interval between visits has not been tested'. The evidence we do have is inconclusive, showing that it is probably safe to reduce the number of antenatal visits, yet this will lead to some women being disappointed (Villar & Khan Neelofur 1999). Yet as midwives we carry on without challenging a system that has been imposed and which may have no purpose for that woman at that time. We change one schedule of visits for another yet we know that women are individuals with individual needs so the midwife responsible for planning and implementing care needs to discuss the woman's individual needs and plan her care to meet those needs. Sanders (2000) suggests a gentle and flexible approach in which the woman decides the number and timing of visits. I would suggest if you add venue to these choices this would fit a midwifery feminist model of care. The woman will be aware of the reasons for antenatal care and will feel able to contact the midwife if she feels there is any change in her circumstances.

Within the last few decades more screening tests have been introduced and the use of technology has been increased with little evaluation of its benefits for women and their babies. This is a triumph for the technocratic model of care as described by Davis-Floyd (1992), which values technology above nature and male-oriented scientific knowledge over the soft science of caring and emotion. This is a result of male domination in society, which has led to male domination in the health service and medical dominance within the maternity services. Most recently we have seen the rise and rise of the fetal medicine units which use resources such as technological equipment and personnel but as yet have provided very little evidence in terms of improved outcomes but have increased maternal anxiety that could have a disastrous effect on the relationship that a woman has with her baby (Chapple 2000, Whelton 1993).

The nature of antenatal care

For most women the antenatal visit is their socialisation into the maternity service. This visit usually lasts for 10 minutes and takes place in a hospital outpatient clinic, a general practitioner's (GP) surgery or a community clinic. The emphasis during the visit is on the physical aspects of the pregnancy; blood pressure is taken, urine tested and the abdomen palpated, all of which have a place in antenatal care but are currently promoted over the other aspects. This emphasis on the provision of physical care is, I would suggest, a feature driven by medical dominance. We do need to ensure physical well-being yet in a 10-minute interview this is all we are able to monitor.

Within a midwifery feminist model of care, the majority of care would take place in the woman's home, ensuring she has control over the length, content and social aspects of the visit. This type of visit often has a social side, with tea or coffee being offered, enabling the woman to set the agenda and discuss how she feels and what is important to her. There has been no disempowering wait in a busy clinic waiting area, clutching a bottle filled with urine; such a wait encourages submissiveness, preparing the woman for the controlling nature of the encounter. The woman and midwife are able to build a relationship of trust, getting to know each other in a way that is not possible in a busy antenatal clinic.

The first encounter

The first encounter is often referred to as a booking visit and is arguably the most important visit for the woman and the midwife. For the woman it is usually her first encounter with the maternity services and should therefore be aimed at meeting her needs and informing her about the choices available to her. Within a midwifery model of care this visit should take place in the woman's home, if that is her wish, and should be with the midwife who will be responsible for planning and implementing her care. This encounter should focus on the social aspects and building a rapport, finding out what is important to that woman and her family. A trend I have observed in recent years has been to leave this initial interview until later in the pregnancy in case the woman has a miscarriage; I believe we need to re-examine this trend. Many areas provide early scanning at 12 weeks, for dating and nuchal fold screening. If this occurs before booking, the woman's first contact with the maternity services is one of medical science, possibly with her not being fully informed of the implications and consequences of this test. If the woman does have an early miscarriage it may have been helpful to her to have this pregnancy acknowledged and legitimised by contact with the midwife. Early contact may have given her information that will be of help with future pregnancies, such as advice on folic acid supplementation and smoking cessation.

In Sanders' (2000) study, women attached importance to obtaining information early in pregnancy, recognising that it is a vulnerable time in fetal development, and highlighted the need for antenatal care to start before the time of traditional booking by a midwife. Within the current model resources for the extra time needed to do these bookings may be diverted to other aspects seen as more important. However, the giving of information regarding diet and lifestyle issues may have implications reaching beyond this pregnancy.

If the booking visit is conducted in the woman's home, she will feel comfortable and in control, and able to ensure her own privacy; a small number of women prefer an alternative place and that choice should be facilitated.

Lesley Page (2000) suggests the five steps of evidence-based midwifery, which should form the basis of booking. The first step is finding out what is important to the woman and her family, and understanding her hopes, anxieties and fears by using open-ended questions such as 'Tell me how you feel about being pregnant'. By finding out this type of information early on, the midwife providing continuity can work with the woman to achieve what is important to her and her family. Step 2 is using information from the clinical examination and asking the mother about her lifestyle, nutritional status, personal and family medical history (Box 4.2). Using this information, the midwife can work with the woman to make any necessary changes and give good evidence-based feedback on any areas of risk. Each woman will have specific issues and the midwife must give time and space for her to voice these. There will also be a certain amount of 'form filling' for administrative purposes and the midwife needs to ensure this does not ruin the social interaction necessary to enable the woman to be in control.

Step 3 looks at the evidence informing decisions the woman may wish to make. The final stages are talking it through with the woman and her family (step 4) and reflecting on outcomes, feelings and consequences (step 5). These steps provide a good basis for planning and implementing care at booking, ensuring the woman can be as much a part of the decision-making process as she wishes. The midwife who has carried out the booking has gained an insight into that woman's wishes and lifestyle and is ideally placed to be her prime carer for the pregnancy and birth.

Questions for Reflection ?????

What kind of antenatal care have you witnessed in practice or been taught as a midwife?

Have you ever experienced antenatal care as a pregnant woman?

In your experience, how much time is spent on a physical check?

What other aspects of care are included?

The concept of risk

We have become very used to the concept of risk in recent decades, classifying women as high or low risk. Enkin et al (2000) state that one of the primary objectives of antenatal care is to identify factors that could put the mother or baby at increased risk of adverse outcomes. High-risk classification then puts a woman in a group where she receives a higher level of care designed to prevent these adverse outcomes. There is no universally agreed and tested risk-scoring process that has been shown to be of proven value (Enkin et al 2000). The benefits of risk-scoring systems are to identify those women at risk, treat them appropriately and ensure the safe delivery of a healthy baby to a healthy mother. The disadvantages are socialisation into the medical model, control of women (Oakley 1992), unnecessary interventions and a great deal of stress and anxiety for the woman and her family. Saxell (2000) makes the point that childbirth in Western society is safer than it has ever been, yet the concept of risk has been expanded to unprecedented levels.

Box 4.2 Information to be obtained on a booking visit (adapted from Page 2000)

Personal history
  General health
  Nutritional status
  Smoking history
  Recreational drug and alcohol use
  Any relevant history of illness
  Social support
  Previous pregnancies

Hopes and fears about the pregnancy
  Clinical information
  Blood pressure and urine
  Fetal well-being, growth and movement if appropriate
  Are the height and weight within normal limits?

Family history
  Is there any relevant family history?
  Diabetes
  Cardiac problems
  Inherited illness

Holistic risk-screening systems, which include assessment of social and psychological factors, appear to have more success in identifying 'high-risk' pregnancies. Such systems give consideration to a woman's social circumstances and support systems (Oakley 1992, Sosa et al 1980), nutritional status, and alcohol and drug taking behaviours (Saxell 2000). A midwifery model of care will be a holistic model that incorporates information about a woman's social and psychological as well as biological adaptation to her pregnancy. The continuity of caregiver means that as the relationship develops, many women who felt unable to impart sensitive information at the outset might divulge this information. This may include drug or alcohol use, domestic violence or childhood sexual abuse. The midwife's role in such circumstances is to foster trust and be non-judgemental, offering appropriate help and support according to the woman's wishes. There can be a problem for midwives and women in that such discussions will need to be documented and the midwife has no control over the attitudes and prejudices of other caregivers so she will need to discuss this with the woman.

The *Confidential Enquiry into Maternal Deaths* (CEMD 2001) recommends that a risk and needs assessment should take place at booking to ensure that every woman has a flexible care plan adapted to her needs and this plan should be regularly reviewed. The CEMD includes social as well as physical risk factors, recommending routine enquiry around domestic violence and experience of postnatal depression amongst other things. Midwives need to be aware of how to manage this sensitively and appropriate referral systems need to be in place.

The prevention of eclampsia has long been a stated aim of antenatal care. This condition has important implications for both mother and baby, therefore monitoring of blood pressure throughout pregnancy is important. It is not the intention of this chapter to discuss the aetiology or treatment of this disorder of pregnancy. Midwives do need to be aware, however, of risk factors for individual women and be able to give them relevant information. Pregnancy-induced hypertension is a disorder of first pregnancies that appears during the course of the pregnancy and is reversed

by birth; it rarely occurs before 28 weeks (Enkin et al 2000). This is the most common disorder of blood pressure in pregnancy and for most of these women will only require more frequent checking of blood pressure by a midwife at home. When associated with proteinuria, however, this becomes pre-eclampsia. Proteinuria associated with raised blood pressure is associated with poor fetal outcome and needs referral to an obstetrician.

Oedema is a more difficult sign to interpret and is often a feature of normal pregnancy. Oedema does, however, affect approximately 85% of women with pre-eclampsia (Enkin et al 2000), but cannot be used as a defining sign of pre-eclampsia due to its association with normality. The midwifery feminist model of care will include the taking of blood pressure and testing urine as part of a holistic visit tailored to the needs of the woman.

Urine is also tested for glycosuria, a possible indicator of diabetes in pregnancy. There is no evidence to support the practice of routine blood tests to diagnose gestational diabetes. We need then to question why it is carried out with such frequency. Is this paternalism in action? Women may be shown how to test their own urine if that is their preference. There is no evidence to support the routine weighing of women in pregnancy (Dawes & Grudzinkas 1991, Green 1989). A midwife practising within the midwifery feminist model needs to be aware of the social implications of weighing women; culturally a woman's self-esteem is frequently inextricably linked with her weight.

Abdominal palpation is an integral part of current midwifery care but there is arguably an over-reliance on this procedure early in pregnancy. One reason stated for carrying out this procedure is to assess fetal growth; this should be undertaken alongside a dialogue with the woman about growth as she will know whether she is getting bigger and this should be acknowledged. Assessment of fetal growth is more reliable when carried out by the same person. It is suggested that measuring fundal height may improve identification of small-for-gestational-age babies but a study in Denmark did not bear this out (Lindhart et al 1990). The Cochrane database supports this finding (Neilson 1997) yet recommends continuing the practice, an interesting recommendation when the practice is not in widespread use.

As the pregnancy progresses we perhaps need to question why we undertake abdominal palpation on a routine basis. Does it have a meaning in terms of outcomes? Near to term we do need to be aware of fetal position and engagement of the presenting part. If the palpation is undertaken it needs to be in partnership with the woman, encouraging her to feel fetal parts and informing her of the findings; this will help promote maternal – fetal attachment. Auscultation of the fetal heartbeat is also undertaken, a practice that confers few benefits, as if the baby is moving we are assured of fetal well-being. However, women enjoy it and it has become an essential part of the social meaning of the antenatal visit.

Antenatal screening

Screening for fetal abnormalities has been an area of massive growth in recent years, with the majority of parents taking up antenatal screening tests. It is not possible in this section to look at the full range of screening tests but we will cover some contentious issues and the midwifery feminist's role in screening.

Ultrasound scanning has become an integral part of the childbirth experience, with expectant parents proudly showing the picture of their baby in utero as early as 12 weeks. It would seem that the first scan has become a rite of passage in itself and has meanings for the woman outside merely screening. The majority of women can expect to have at least one scan in their pregnancy and this has increasingly become two, with many centres offering a 12-week nuchal fold scan and a 20-week anomaly scan. Yet medicine has not established definitively the safety of scanning. Enkin et al (2000) state: 'Whether ultrasound imaging should be used routinely for prenatal screening or only used for specific indications has not, as yet, been firmly established'. It can be argued that there are many people walking around now who were scanned as fetuses, yet over the last decades the number of scans a woman has have increased, the intensity of the ultrasound used has increased and the use of transvaginal

scanning has increased. Transvaginal scanning uses a vaginal probe that may not be acceptable to many women, especially survivors of sexual abuse and certain ethnic minorities. By using the vaginal route the ultrasound is emitted closer to the baby and with less tissue to absorb the ultrasound. Beech & Robinson (1996) suggest that this rise in the number of scans increases the amount of ultrasound and we have no data on the safety of this increased dosage.

Many units offer serum screening for Down's syndrome and women need to be aware that many of these tests are for conditions for which there is no cure and the expected treatment will be termination of pregnancy. Samwill (2002) found that midwives were not confident in counselling women about this test and that many had a poor level of knowledge about the test, whilst women have expressed dissatisfaction with the way results are reported (Abramsky & Chapple 1997). The blood test for Down's syndrome serum screening is usually carried out with a range of other blood tests and women often do not think through the consequences until they are being told about the risks of miscarriage associated with amniocentesis or, worse, being informed that abortion is the 'cure' on offer. Deacon (2002) states that midwives should be offering sound advice based on contemporary information, enabling every expectant parent to be able to make informed choices. Unfortunately it is not as simple as this and decisions around aborting less than perfect fetuses are necessarily value laden within our society. The evidence is not always easy to understand, as indeed individual tests are not easy to report, with little understanding regarding false positives and negatives.

The National Screening Committee (NSC) was established in order to provide guidance on screening programmes but to date there are few antenatal guidelines. The current NSC proposal is for second-trimester serum screening, offering amniocentesis to women with a risk factor higher than 1:250. A programme with high levels of both false positives and negatives and regional variations (Wellesley et al 2002) is offered in the second trimester, with all the anxieties and fears that involves for women.

The role of the midwifery feminist in offering antenatal screening tests, whatever their nature, is to ensure women have information appropriate to their area and that they are aware of the reasons and the consequences of the tests. The midwifery feminist will enable that woman to have the best outcome for her. As midwives we need to give women and their partners the time to talk through these decisions, finding out what is important to them, presenting the evidence as best we can and supporting them in whatever decision they make.

Antenatal education

There are some excellent books and workshops on providing antenatal care through a model of empowerment (Priest & Schott 1991, Robertson 1997). This section does not intend covering that area but looks specifically at the midwifery feminist role.

Antenatal classes aimed at preparing women and their partners for their birth experience are provided by most units. More often than not, these classes are held for large groups due to pressure on the service. In my experience they are usually attended by middle-class parents who have already gained most of the information from books, magazines and the Internet. Although there is nothing wrong with this, it seems that those in most need do not attend. The main purpose for many of these parents is to meet people in the same situation. Hospital classes often appear to be aimed at teaching birth 'the way we do it here' and promoting compliance with routines and procedures (Priest & Schott 1991). Midwives should be aware of the needs of women and their partners concerning antenatal education, providing education appropriate to those needs. It may be appropriate to provide this on an individual basis for those who do not wish to go to classes. If the main purpose is to meet others in the same situation, we should make this overt, encouraging them to set their own agenda. Within the midwifery feminist model the midwife would discover what the woman and her partner want and find a way to facilitate that.

THE MIDWIFERY FEMINIST MODEL OF CARE

The midwifery feminist model of care incorporates the ideal of holistic woman-centred care, working in partnership with the woman and her family, with the woman as the driving force in this partnership. This care is best provided within a community-based one-to-one setting but this does not prevent hospital-based midwives working within a midwifery feminist paradigm. The midwife within this model is a facilitator of the woman's choices, positioned 'with woman', providing her with information based on best evidence and supporting the choices she makes based on that evidence. If the woman makes choices that are not approved of by the institution, the midwife supports her and acts as an advocate for her as there will be many people who will try and persuade her against those choices.

This model extends to the intrapartum and postnatal periods, ensuring that women are in control of their experience, so that the woman who has had an emergency caesarean section feels that she has been part of the decision-making process and has not been disempowered by the experience. Although continuity is interlinked with midwifery feminism, the midwife who is not able to work in continuity of care schemes can share a midwifery feminist philosophy, supporting these midwives and giving holistic woman-centred care within the hospital setting. Such a model of care need not be exclusive to midwives. Indeed, it is hoped that many obstetricians will embrace a midwifery feminist model of care within their area of work.

Suggestions for Reflection ?????

Use the midwifery feminist model of care (above) to sketch out your own ideas for woman-centred antenatal care. Consider how you might put some of these ideas into action. Identify colleagues, friends, managers and others who might help you achieve this goal. Revisit this aim in 6 months time and make a note of what you have achieved.

Table 4.1 The midwifery feminist model of care

Features of the model	Rationale
Early first encounter	Social interaction Establish rapport Assess the needs of that woman and her family Information giving Midwife shares self and expertise
Individualised care	Pattern of care to suit the woman and her family Encompasses social, emotional, psychological and physical care Enables women to be in control of their body and decisions concerning the pregnancy and birth Care is offered to all regardless of race, colour, sexual orientation or creed
Informal, equal relationship	Relationship based on mutual trust, ensuring the woman has trust that the midwife will meet her needs, and shares beliefs with her
'With woman'	Acts as advocate for women, protecting them from unnecessary intervention and 'institutional bullying' Midwife is empathic and shares self with woman
Evidence-based practice	Informs women without treating knowledge as power Acts as professional friend
Continuity	Ideally continuity of carer, recognising the uniqueness of the woman–midwife relationship. If this is not possible continuity of care based on a 'with woman' philosophy
'With midwife'	Supports other midwives, encouraging a non-blame culture, enabling them to practise within the midwifery feminist model

CONCLUSION

This chapter has looked at feminist concepts and how they relate to midwifery and in particular to antenatal care. The way we provide antenatal care has been rooted in professional dominance by the male-gendered profession of obstetrics. This has led to antenatal care that is medically driven and focused on screening for physical problems, emphasising physical safety. More recently, there has been an emphasis on the health and safety of the fetus, sometimes appearing to promote the needs of the fetus over those of the mother. Yet for women, birth is a rite of passage that has meanings far beyond safety. By treating women individually and acknowledging the psychological, cultural and emotional aspects of childbirth, midwives can work with women, aiming for not only a safe birth but a fulfilling and empowering birth experience that is the beginning of a lifelong relationship with their babies. As midwives we are uniquely privileged to share this momentous occasion with women and such privilege must involve responsibility. Responsibility for safety because of course, midwives too are concerned with safety, but safety and satisfaction are not mutually exclusive.

I have looked at the role of midwives in most aspects of antenatal care and suggested a midwifery feminist model of care that positions us 'with woman' socially, psychologically and emotionally as well as physically. The majority of midwives are women but I would not want to exclude men from this model, either as midwives or obstetricians. This is about a feminist 'with woman' frame of mind and is inclusive to all those sharing this philosophy.

Key points

■ Antenatal care that is based in the community enables midwives to work in ways that meet the needs of women. This model of care has been shown to provide better outcomes for both mothers and babies.

◼ The inverse care law has shown that those in least need of healthcare provision have the best access to services. In contrast, best practice should be targeted at those groups who are most in need.

◼ Models of care that promote partnership and continuity enable the midwife and woman to get to know each other, so that the midwife learns what the woman wants from this

childbirth experience and can act as her advocate.

◼ Antenatal care has traditionally focused on pregnancy as a problem to be managed, by a paternalistic service. Within the midwifery model of care the psychological, social, emotional and physical aspects of antenatal care are valued, with the woman being able to vocalise what is important to her at that time.

REFERENCES

Abramsky L, Chapple J 1997 47XXY (Kleinfelter syndrome) and 47XYY: estimated rates and indication for postnatal diagnosis with implications for prenatal counseling. Prenatal Diagnosis 14(4): 363–368

Allen I, Dowling SB, Williams S 1997 A leading role for midwives? Evaluation of midwifery group practice development projects. Policy Studies Institute, London

Anderson T 2002 The misleading myth of choice: the continuing oppression of women in childbirth. MIDIRS Midwifery Digest 12(3): 405–407

Banks O 1981 Faces of feminism. Martin Robertson, Oxford

Beech B, Robinson J 1996 Ultrasound? Unsound. AIMS, London

Bosanquet A 2002 'Stones can make people docile': reflections of a student midwife on how the hospital environment makes 'good girls'. MIDIRS Midwifery Digest 12(3): 301–305

Buckley S 1997 Is birth a feminist issue? AIMS Quarterly Journal 5(1): 14–15

Carby H 1982 White woman listen: black feminism and the boundaries of sisterhood. In: The empire strikes back: race and racism in 70's Britain. Centre for Contemporary Studies Hutchinson, London

CEMD 2001 Why mothers die 1997–1999. The confidential enquiry into maternal deaths. RCOG Press, London

Chamberlain G 1997 ABC of antenatal care. BMJ Publishing Group, London

Chapple J 2000 A public health view of the maternity services. In: Page L (ed) The new midwifery: science and sensitivity in practice. Churchill Livingstone, London

Davis-Floyd R 1992. Birth as an American rite of passage. University of California Press, Berkeley, CA

Dawes MG, Grudzinskas JG 1991 Repeated measurement of maternal weight during pregnancy. Is this a useful practice? British Journal of Obstetrics and Gynaecology 98: 189–194

Deacon E 2002 A midwife's role in prenatal screening. British Journal of Midwifery 10(8): 485–488

Department of Health 1993 Changing childbirth: Report of the Expert Committee. HMSO, London

Department of Health and Social Security 1970 Domiciliary midwifery and maternity bed needs (Peel Report). HMSO, London

Eisenstein Z 1993 The radical future of liberal feminism. Northeastern University Press, Pennsylvania

Enkin M, Keirse MJNC, Neison J et al 2000 A guide to effective care in pregnancy and childbirth. Oxford University Press, Oxford

Foster P 1989 Improving the doctor/patient relationship: a feminist perspective. Journal of Social Politics 18(3): 337–361

Foster P 1995 Women and the healthcare industry: an unhealthy relationship? Open University Press, Buckingham

Gould D 2002 Subliminal medicalisation. British Journal of Midwifery 10(9): 418

Green J 1989 Diet and the prevention of pre-eclampsia. In: Chalmers I, Enkin M, Keirse MJNC (eds) Effective care in pregnancy and childbirth. Oxford University Press, Oxford

Hanmer J 1993 Women and reproduction. In: Richardson D, Robinson V (eds) Introducing women's studies. Macmillan, London

Hannah ME, Hannah WJ, Hewson SA et al 2000 Planned caesarean section versus planned vaginal birth for breech presentation at term, a randomised multicentre trial. Lancet 356(9239): 1375–1383

Hart TL 1971 The inverse care law. British Medical Journal 520: 18–19

Humm M 1989 The dictionary of feminist theory. Harvester Wheatsheaf, Hemel Hempstead

Humm M 1990 Feminisms: a reader. Harvester Wheatsheaf, Hemel Hempstead

Hutchings J, Henty D 2002 Caseload midwifery practice in partnership with SureStart: changing the culture of birth. MIDIRS Midwifery Digest 12(1, suppl 1): S38–S40

Jackson S, Prince J, Young P 1993 Science, medicine and reproductive technology. In: Jackson S (ed) Women's studies: a reader. Harvester Wheatsheaf, Hemel Hempstead

Kirkham M 1999 The culture of midwifery in the National Health Service in England. Journal of Advanced Nursing 30(3): 732–739

Kirkham M, Stapleton H, Curtis P, Thomas G 2002 The inverse care law in antenatal care. British Journal of Midwifery 19(8): 509–513

Leap N, Hunter B 1993 The midwife's tale: an oral history from handywoman to professional midwife. Scarlet Press, London

Lindhart A, Neilson LA, Mouritsen LA et al 1990 The implications of introducing the symphyseal-fundal height measurement: a prospective randomized controlled trial. British Journal of Obstetrics and Gynaecology 97(8): 657–680

Mackinnon C 1982 Feminism, Marxism, method and the state: an agenda for theory. Signs 7(3): 515–544

Maynard M 1995 Beyond the 'Big Three': the development of feminist theory in the 1990's. Women's History Review 4(3)

Millett K 1970 Sexual politics. Virago Press, London

Muff J 1982 Handmaiden, battle-axe, whore: an exploration into the fantasies, myths and stereotypes about nursing. In: Socialisation, sexism and stereotyping: women's issues in nursing. Mosby, St Louis, MO

Neilson JP 1997 Symphysis-fundal height measurement in pregnancy (Cochrane Review). Cochrane Library, Issue 3. Update Software, Oxford

Oakley C 1980 Women confined: towards a sociology of childbirth. Martin Robertson, Oxford

Oakley A 1992 Social support and motherhood: the natural history of a research project. Blackwell, Oxford

Oakley A 1993 The doctor's problem. In: Essays on women, medicine and health. Edinburgh University Press, Edinburgh

Page L 1995 Effective group practice in midwifery: working with women. Blackwell, Oxford

Page L, 2000 Putting science and sensitivity into practice. In: The new midwifery: science and sensitivity in practice. Churchill Livingstone, London

Priest J, Schott J 1991 Leading antenatal classes. Butterworth Heinemann, Oxford

Reid B 2002 The Albany midwifery practice. MIDIRS Midwifery Digest 12(1): 118–121

Reynolds R 1993 Feminist theory and strategy in social work. In: Walmsley J, Reynolds J, Shakespeare P, Woolfe R (eds) Health, welfare and practice. Sage, London

Rhodes P 1995 A short history of midwifery. Books for Midwives Press, Cheshire

Rich A 1980 Compulsory heterosexuality and lesbian existence. In: Humm M (ed) Feminisms: a reader. Harvester Wheatsheaf, Hemel Hempstead

Richardson D 1993 Sexuality and male dominance. In: Richardson D, Robinson V (eds) Introducing women's studies. Macmillan, London

Robertson A 1997 Empowering women: teaching active birth. Ace Graphics, Australia

Sanders J 2000 Let's start at the very beginning … women's comments on early pregnancy care. MIDIRS Midwifery Digest 10(2): 169–173

Samwill L 2002 Midwives' knowledge of Down's syndrome screening. British Journal of Midwifery 10(4): 247–250

Saxell L 2000 Risk: theoretical or actual. In: Page L (ed) The new midwifery. Churchill Livingstone, London

Scott J 1988 Deconstructing equality-versus-difference: or the uses of poststructuralism for feminist theory. Feminist Studies 14(1): 33–50

Sosa R, Kennell J, Klaus M, Robertson S, Urrutia J 1980 The effect of a supportive companion on perinatal problems, length of labor and mother infant interaction. New England Journal of Medicine 33: 597–600

Spelman E 1990 Inessential woman. The Women's Press, London

Stephens L 1998 The lived experience of midwives being 'with woman': a phenomenological study. Unpublished Masters Dissertation, available from author

Villar J, Khan Neelofur D 1999 Patterns of routine antenatal care for low risk pregnancy (Cochrane Review). Cochrane Library, Issue 4. Update Software, Oxford

Walby S 1990 Theorising patriarchy. Blackwell, Oxford

Walsh D, Newburn M 2002 Towards a social model of childbirth: part one. British Journal of Midwifery 10(8): 476–481

Watson J 1990 The moral failure of the patriarchy. Nursing Outlook 36(2): 106–112

Wellesley D, Boyle T, Barber J et al 2002 Retrospective audit of different antenatal screening policies for Down's syndrome in eight district general hospitals in one health region. British Medical Journal 325(7354): 15–17

Whelton J 1993 Fetal medicine. In: Alexander J, Levy V, Roch S (eds) Midwifery practice: a research-based approach. Macmillan, Basingstoke

Witz A 1992 Professions and patriarchy. Routledge, London

5

Feminism and intrapartum care: a quest for holistic birth

Denis Walsh

INTRODUCTION

Feminist reflection on labour and birth has much to teach us on a breadth of issues – from historical critique tracing childbirth from the Middle Ages to the present (Donnison 1988) to contemporary feminist research of childbirth complications like preterm labour (Williams & Mackey 1999). It champions the still small voice of women amongst the deafening roar of the childbirth professionals who, through a plethora of journals and books and their appropriated role as the maternity care strategists, continue to extend their power and control in this area.

This chapter summarises the legacy of the recent history of childbirth in the UK and attempts to sketch some contrasting dimensions within current labour and birth approaches that have been termed the biomedical, technocratic model versus the midwifery, woman-centred model (Davis-Floyd & Davis 1997). The latter is predicated on what could broadly be called feminist values and beliefs. These contrasting approaches will then be 'fleshed out' with examples from current labour and birth practices.

Finally, some suggestions will be made as to how feminist ideals could be applied to intrapartum care to humanise it and potentially transform women's experience and the care offered by the childbirth practitioners.

Questions for Reflection ??????

In what contexts have you heard the word 'love' associated with childbirth care or experience?

In what ways have you seen spiritual dimensions of childbirth expressed in the birth environment?

For many midwives, the language of love and the expression of spirituality may be rare events in consultant labour wards today. Yet, if we can strip away our clinical layers to reveal childbirth as an intensely human experience, as feminists have been arguing for decades (Kitzinger 1978, 2000), would not words of love and marks of spirituality be commonplace? What has happened to childbirth in the UK that these aspects of human experience, clearly manifest in other major life events, are rarely observed in this context?

Though feminism is a rich amalgam of different schools of thought – liberal, Marxist, radical in the main (Charles 2000) – all share a desire to make explicit women's experience and women's stories (Kirkham 1997) and to restore women's agency or autonomy (Kent 2000). When the professionals have taken time to listen, they will have heard the plea to reclaim humanness and self-respect from an event that has become sanitised and sterile as a mechanistic, clinical-centred, professional hegemony has held sway. Many feminists would attribute blame for this situation to patriarchy and paternalism as espoused by a male-dominated obstetric profession and there is ample evidence from the recent history of childbirth to support this position (Murphy-Lawless 1998).

HISTORICAL CRITIQUE

It was Tolstoy who wisely counselled that 'those who deem to ignore the mistakes of the past are destined to repeat them in the present'. So the lessons we can glean from the history of childbirth will serve us well as we work to transform the future of the maternity services. Feminist activists have been working on this project for many years. Donnisons' (1988) was one of the first to write this history from a perspective of a struggle to control childbirth, primarily between midwives and doctors, and her work was widely read by midwives. Prior to this time, the midwifery student was exposed mainly to the Maggie Myles version of events through her ubiquitous textbook stretching back some 50 years. As student midwives in the mid 1980s, many of us commented on the paternalistic tone and the almost quaint old-fashionedness of attitudes in the text. Underneath, though, these attitudes masked a stereotyping of gender roles and an uncritical acceptance of obstetric dominance.

Donnison presents an entirely different version of events. She writes so cogently of the systematic, largely successful attempts by the medical profession to discredit lay midwives, to resist the licensing of midwifery practice and to control it when registration became inevitable. In these activities, they were aided and abetted by the advent of science and the scientific method which the medical profession embraced with vigour, rightly judging that it would progress their own professional self-interest. They 'discovered' and embraced new childbirth techniques like the forceps delivery and new drugs that anaesthetised and sedated women in labour. These new, exclusively male practitioners of midwifery, the forerunners of modern-day obstetricians, at first targeted wealthy clients and were content to leave the poor in the hands of the traditional lay midwives. In the 20th century, public health issues began to shape government policy as the development of the welfare state focused attention to all sectors of the population. Therefore access to all client groups was required if this new grouping of obstetricians was to cement total control of maternity care.

An effective strategy for controlling childbirth was to control the place of birth. If this occurred centrally in large hospitals, then both child-bearing women and midwives could be kept under surveillance (Hunt & Symonds 1995) and so the myth of 'childbirth is safer in hospital' was promulgated after the formation of the NHS in 1948. From there, Marjorie Tew (1998) takes up the story to reveal the fallacy of linking falling perinatal mortality with hospital birth. Tew put forward an alternative explanation for falling perinatal mortality rates. She argued convincingly that it was the improvement in public health generally, i.e. better nutrition, better hygiene, that occurred around this time which lowered deaths in childbirth and not the movement of birth from home to hospital.

What can we conclude from this unfolding history that will help us prepare for future change in maternity services? First, that a gender-based analysis of these events emphasises the androcentric or male-dominated dynamic that has operated in recent childbirth history. 'Patriarchy' will constantly seek to dominate an exclusively female client group and a predominantly female professional group which shares the same 'turf'. This is mirrored in other areas of women's health, as Doyal (1998) and Graham (1993) clearly show. Their feminist critique of women's health services also comments on the structured gender discrimination in wider society which manifests endemically at numerous levels, e.g. in the public world of paid employment (women being paid less for the same job and discriminated against in promotion) and the private sphere of domesticity and childcare (much of it is unpaid and invisible). So the feminist analysis of labour and birth reflects wider, ingrained oppression in other areas of women's lives. Any movement for change that does not engage with this reality will flounder. The marginalisation and devaluing of women's and midwives' priorities continue in the present and we need to spot them in their different, subtler guises.

What constitutes feminist ideals and beliefs? It is harder to find the answer to this within feminist literature on childbirth because although extensive critiques do exist, much of it is in a less accessible form. The books and journals containing it are not sold through midwifery networks generally and actually there is a dearth of explicit feminist writing in midwifery journals and books, though much more is implicit in the extensive work of Kirkham (2000), Hunt & Symonds (1995), Downe (2001) and others. It may be that, like nursing, the 'f' word (McLoughlin 1997) causes a range of reactions in practitioners, some of which are distinctly negative and work to discourage publication. Explicit mention in service and educational philosophy is also missing, though some midwifery curricula do source it clearly (Hamilton & McLean 2000). New Zealand midwifery has made it quite central to the profession's philosophy in that country and Guilland & Pairman's (1995) work is an important read for midwives. It may be that the independence of midwifery there was facilitated by this feminist emphasis and that, reciprocally, autonomous, primary care-based practice facilitates the development of feminist thought.

The feminist critique in the arena of childbirth can appear threatening to some and is certainly challenging to men entering the midwifery profession. It rightly asks men to consider very carefully their own gendered behaviours and attitudes and to reflexively resolve the inevitable tensions that impinge on their practice. Anecdotally, male midwives resolve these in a number of ways, some of which can mean leaving the profession but for others the personal adoption of feminist values, coupled with a studied appreciation of the feminist critique (Schacht & Ewing 1997), allows resolution and integration into their practice.

Any attempt to articulate and distil core feminist values and ideals is risky because oversimplification of a complex, dynamic field of thought may reduce it to bland and trite euphemisms. But it is necessary as a starting point when attempting to engage this extremely important critique of current maternity provision that permeates every aspect of care from birth environment and organisation of services to effective labour and birth interventions.

What follows is a summary of key values that underpin feminism.

- The primacy of women's experience. It is a fundamental starting point and ongoing reference.
- Listening to and valuing women's voice and women's version of events.
- Establishing relationships of equality and reciprocity.
- Unmasking of dehumanising and oppressive practices against women.
- Action for empowerment and emancipation (Allan 1993, Webb 1993).

PLACE OF BIRTH

Control of both women's childbirth experience and midwifery practice, two key targets for the colonising intent of obstetric profession, has been neatly dealt with by the brilliant yet simple strategy of moving all childbirth into hospital. Winning this argument after the Peel Report in 1970 (Department of Health and Social Security 1970) has had hugely significant implications for child-bearing women and midwives since. As one anecdote expresses it – how can a midwife have power when the playing field (hospital) is owned by the medics and the choice of game (medicalisation of childbirth) is decided by them? One of their own is the referee (clinical director and other strategy positions) and the rules (policies and protocols) are initiated and regulated by them. Finally, they hold all the players' contracts (acute trust as employer)!

For child-bearing women, the effects are even more profound. As Kirkham (1989) and Hunt & Symonds (1995) so wonderfully describe in their ethnographies of consultant delivery suites, on entering the building, the 'patient' role is waiting to be inscribed at every turn. All the senses – sight, touch, sounds, smell and talk – fashion the patient role in their particular way. Sight reveals a building that couldn't be less like home from the moment it is seen on the horizon, the moment you step into its foyer, the moment you enter its wards. Touch is clinical and sometimes uninvited, not consensual and affectionate, sounds are distinctly foreign and unnerving (alarms, buzzers and constant footsteps of shoes on hard floors). Smells all have a whiff of a cleaning agent, though not one we use at home, talk is esoteric and not necessarily a dialogue and under all of that there are the rules – institutional rules, some of which are clear and some you become aware of the longer you stay.

Now that we know it was improvements in public health which lowered perinatal mortality and not moving the place of birth (Tew 1998), the exploration of alternative birth environments can be embraced with enthusiasm. Helping this cause is a body of quantitative research revealing the unsuitability of consultant delivery suites for normal birth. Numerous randomised controlled trials show less maternal satisfaction and greater number of birth interventions when women give birth in these environments (Hodnett 2002a). There are quite simply no benefits for baby or mother.

Yet the seemingly inexorable trend to centralising birth throughout the UK continues apace. And whenever stand-alone midwifery-led units are mooted as an alternative, a struggle ensues to legitimate this option. Bad decisions continue to be made that fly in the face of evidence. Who makes them? The medical specialties, together with hospital managers, lead on these decisions and it comes as no surprise that they will further their own professional interest and sphere of influence. This is the inherent driving force of patriarchy – the furthering of the androcentric, male-serving interests of men in power over women.

Question for Reflection ?????

List the five senses and place alongside each what women's experience might be in your unit.

Could you initiate small changes where you work to make these sense impressions more home-like?

There is a steadily increasing body of work highlighting the advantages of stand-alone birth centres and midwifery-led facilities, both from quantitative and qualitative research (Campbell 1997, Esposito 1999). Saunders et al's (2000) evaluation of the birth centre model showed low rates of both caesarean section and induction of labour and high levels of maternal satisfaction. Midwifery job satisfaction was also very high. Midwifery interests are rarely researched and there are precious few examples of midwives' views in the significant body of research into childbirth, another example of gender marginalisation. Research from the USA (Rooks et al 1992) and Germany (David et al 1999) supports these findings on birth centres. Coyle et al's papers (2001a,b) reveal to us the significance of relationships and congruence of beliefs between midwives and birthing women. Birth centres facilitate these important quality dimensions of the childbirth experience.

Home birth had always been highly valued by women and in addition to Tew's (1998) work on perinatal mortality, Olsen (1997) has published a meta-analysis of observational studies of home birth revealing the established trend of low birth intervention. Aside from home birth and stand-alone birthing or midwifery-led units, a number of high-quality randomised controlled trials tell us that if neither of these two is available for women, then birthing facilities that are midwifery led within a consultant unit achieve excellent process and outcome figures (Hodnett 2002a).

In conclusion, it is abundantly clear that both improved experiences of birth and a reduction in medicalised birth are achieved in alternative birth environments. As satisfaction with birth is linked to issues of control and agency (Oakley 1984), then women's autonomy is more likely to be respected in these environments as well. This gives midwives a clear imperative to foster change in services along these lines.

STYLE OF CARE

The feminist critique of how birth is done today attacks the very masculine, machine metaphor of parturition (Oakley 1993). This preoccupation with the engineering analogy has been encouraged by a symbiosis between obstetric advancement and the development of birth technologies. Marxist feminism would see this as the inevitable consequence of capitalism where women's bodies are simply reproduction factories and the means of production in generating profits (Crompton & Sanderson 1990). The mutuality of technological and obstetric advance is exemplified by the development and widespread dissemination of electronic fetal monitoring. Some career obstetricians have focused their research on this emerging technology and effectively kick-started its uptake in delivery suites around the world. Their research fails to prove unequivocal benefit as numerous systematic reviews have shown (Thacker et al 2002) yet the technology continues to attract large research grants (RCM 2001). It is almost as if some obstetricians cannot accept its clear limitations and must find a way to make it work.

The growth in the scientific approach to child-birth was part of what philosophers describe as the 'enlightenment age' – an optimistic view that science would solve all the world's problem (Lister 1997). Childbirth became yet another puzzle to solve and therefore control and predict. Latterly, influential writers like Davis-Floyd (2001) and Wagner (1994) have attempted to ascribe a model to these beliefs, coining the phrases 'technocratic' and 'biomedical' to capture the essence of its effects in practice. What is abundantly clear is that the model is blatantly androcentric, reducing child-birth to a neat and tidy succession of anatomical and physiological changes. The language is esoteric and mechanistic – 'powers, passengers and passage' as several standard obstetric textbooks dub them (Llewellyn-Jones 1994, Roth 1998). Feminists have highlighted the adoption of value-laden and victim-blaming terms, like 'failure to progress', 'uterine inertia', 'inadequate pelvis' to name a few, and the effects these have on women (Bastion 1992, Hewison 1993). But they equally criticise the denuding of childbirth of any notions of relationships, emotions and mystery (Bates 1997). Style of care is critical for these dimensions to be given space and expression for style implies an individual's approach and immediately we are referring to persons and the personal.

There is now a vast body of research stressing the primacy of carers in affecting birth experience (Tarkka 1996), intervention rates (Page et al 1999) and birth outcomes (Hodnett 2002b). The findings around birth experience are largely from qualitative designs and cover issues like the impact of midwives' attitudes (McCrea 1993), dimensions of friendship in relationships with carers (Tinkler & Quinney 1998, Walsh 1999), effects on childbirth memories (Simkin 1992) and women's dependence/independence as mediated through carers (Bluff & Holloway 1994, Machin & Scamell 1997). Birth interventions and outcomes linked unambiguously to the presence of professional carers represent one of the most comprehensive bodies of research available in the health field. It unanimously endorses the value of personal ongoing support during labour and birth (one-to-one care) with its profound impact on lowering caesarean sections rates, among a number of other benefits for mothers and babies (Hodnett 2002b).

There's a telling irony here. It concerns one of obstetrics' cherished management protocols for progressing labour, 'the active management of labour' (O'Driscoll & Meager 1986). This package of care represented much that was negative about androcentric and paternalistic approaches (Bates 1997). It presented a very mechanistic model of childbirth (the cervix *will* dilate at 1 centimetre an hour) and was developed by male obstetricians in the main. Paternalism was actioned by 'The Master' (obstetrician in charge) who, in order to keep women's behaviour under control, provided a birth attendant (commonly a student midwife) for each woman. Through research over the past two decades, the protocol has been exposed as ineffective (Thornton 1996), despite widespread adoption in UK delivery suites during the 1970s and 1980s apart from one curious aspect – the provision of the attendant who in effect provided one-to-one care, shown on its own to be very effective as previously mentioned.

The emphasis on relationships in much midwifery research owes a debt to eminent feminists like Oakley et al (1990) in the UK and Jordan (1993) in the USA who wrote tirelessly about the importance of social support and personal agency for child-bearing women. In the UK context this appeared to bear fruit with the publishing of *Changing Childbirth* (Department of Health 1993) which was clearly predicated on the three Cs – choice, control and continuity – the last of which endorses a relational dimension to birth care. Ten year later, the hopes of thousands of women and midwives of building a birth environment and shaping a service founded on those themes have yet to be realised. The very foundational objective of the availability of a professional to provide continuous support to women in labour remains largely unfulfilled.

Questions for Reflection ?????

Who controls resources locally for maternity service provision?

Who makes decisions locally about future maternity care strategy?

Can you think of creative ways in which relational aspects of care, e.g. continuous support in labour, continuity schemes, could be encouraged and implemented where you work?

CHILDBIRTH PRACTICES

Male-led changes in childbirth practices over the 20th century have left a distressing mark, as Graham (1997) eloquently points out in regard to episiotomy. In fact, one wonders if the following litany of interventions – routine repeated rectal or vaginal examinations, routine artificial rupture of membranes, routine episiotomies, pubic shaves, enemas, lying down for birth, restricted mobility, continuous intravenous infusions, instructed pushing, Keillands forceps, withholding food and fluid in labour – would have made it into clinical practice if women were the leading birth practitioners over the time that these interventions came into use. Certainly many of them were linked specifically to practitioner convenience, e.g. lithotomy for forceps deliveries. Mauriceau, a prominent French obstetrician of the 17th century, was one of the first birth practitioners who required his patients to lie down for birth (Dunn 1991). Over 2 centuries later, the shackling of women to beds persists despite growing evidence of its deleterious effects (Gupta & Nilodem 2002). Balaskas (1995), author of *Active Birth*, wrote of the 'stranded beetle' analogy to capture physiological and psychosocial aspects of giving birth in the supine position. The image of a beetle flipped on its back, hopelessly flailing its legs, beautifully illustrates a helplessness and passivity that has parallels with birth on your back. This is reversed by the adoption of an upright posture which communicates an active, 'in control' dimension to care.

Mauriceau's description of the conduct of the second stage of labour in his textbook of 1678 has an uncanny resemblance to what happens in many consultant units across the UK some 230 years later (Dunn 1991). He described the instructed pushing technique that birth attendants need to impart to women so that they can push their babies out more effectively. Research over the last 25 years has shown that this practice is not only dangerous for babies (Caldeyro-Barcia et al 1979) but ineffective as a technique (Knauth & Haloburdo 1986). It is a good example of a practice that reinforces the unequal relationship between childbirth practitioner (person with a repository of specialised information and skills) and women (usually ignorant of this technique), although involuntary and spontaneous pushing behaviours are commonly manifested by women during this phase. It therefore undermines normal physiology and women's trust in their instinctual behaviour.

Normal birth physiology is having something of a renaissance, led by prominent feminists who are midwives (Albers 1999, Bates 1997, Downe 2001) because it is becoming increasingly clear that our inherited wisdom regarding length of labour, among many other physiological parameters, is seriously flawed. It is flawed because it is shot through with androcentric bias, as demonstrated by the early researchers' efforts in describing labour progress. The seminal research on labour progress was done by male obstetricians, in their hospitals, on women who were subjected to intrusive, repeated vaginal examinations while at the same time their labours were being managed and manipulated by drugs (Walsh 2000). Environment, style of care and relational aspects, key confounders in any intrapartum study, were ignored. The research into normal birth physiology needs redoing in situations that are sensitive to a complex and delicate mix of birth hormones, highly susceptible to various stimuli and environmental factors. Research is also required that embraces a holistic approach, valuing the psychosocial as well as the physical.

Chalmers et al (1989) penned wise words when describing the appropriate context for intervention in labour and birth. The two key principles they enunciated were:

1. do not add anything to the physiological process unless it is clear it will bring benefit and improve on nature

2. even when this criterion is met, make certain that side effects of the intervention do not outweigh the potential benefits.

They developed the Cochrane database of childbirth research, a vast repository of randomised controlled trials on many different aspects of pregnancy and birth care, notable though for two other reasons. First, there is a dearth of midwifery-initiated and midwifery-led research and second, an absence of focus on women's experience. The database is full of investigations into potent interventions and procedures yet very few evaluated what women thought or experienced. New research initiatives today should address this at the outset if the mistakes of the past are to be avoided.

Questions for Reflection ?????

Could you appraise your own intrapartum practice in relation to whether interventions you adopt:

1. *are known to be an improvement on natural birth?*
2. *do not have unintended side effects that might outweigh their benefit?*

How much of your care during labour and birth is centred on women's expressed needs?

The almost exclusive reliance on quantitative methods to evaluate women's health has been heavily criticised by feminist authors (Graham 1998, Woodhouse 1998). They rightly champion methods likely to appreciate integration of experience; in other words, a holistic focus. For them, the links between physiology, psychology, emotions and the social are axiomatic. To ignore them is to demean and dehumanise (Inhorn & Whittle 2001). They rail against the objectification of women that this results in (Greer 1999). Yet randomised controlled trials do have their place, as Oakley (1993) explains. If robust drug trials had been undertaken women might have avoided the blight of thalidomide or stilboestrol. In evaluating discrete treatments, e.g. new drugs, and new interventions, e.g. antenatal screening technologies, this design is appropriate but even here it needs to:

- measure outcomes that matter to women
- qualitatively examine women's experience.

Salmon (1999) was one of the first to publish research in a midwifery journal based on an explicit feminist methodology. Her review of perineal care pointed to the contrasting priorities between the professional's and women's concerns. Her own research revealed the importance to women of two areas neglected by midwives and obstetricians – the skills of the practitioner doing perineal repair and the relationship/rapport that she or he has with a woman being sutured. Women spoke of the trauma of insensitive practitioners who either did not ensure that local anaesthetic was working or castigated women for 'moving too much'. Symon's (2000) study of perinatal litigation in Scotland found episiotomy breakdown was a major contributor to litigation related to the perineum, supporting women's concerns about skills in perineal repair.

MIDWIVES AS AN OPPRESSED GROUP

'Doing good by stealth' was how Kirkham (1999) explained repeated behaviour patterns she observed and heard from midwives while investigating midwifery supervision. She also found significant self-blaming language used by midwives. Looking for similarities in other literature to explain these behaviours, she could find no antecedents until she came across writing on oppression. The rationale for 'doing good by stealth' was altruistic, protecting women from unnecessary and potentially harmful intervention. But midwives felt they could not openly express their true beliefs for fear of reprisal within an obstetrically dominated environment. Recent research by Richens (2002) supports this hypothesis. Self-blame patterns are indicative of oppressed groups, as Roberts (2000) explains in her interesting paper on oppression and nursing. 'Doing good by stealth' in her analysis is a form of resistance

to the oppressor that is a passive-aggressive strategy. Her analysis further resonates with much midwifery experience when she explores how the powerlessness of oppression is internalised as low self-worth and then externalised as aggression to colleagues. Leap (1997) has also written of this 'horizontal violence' where the oppressed group oppress their own kind in a perverse outworking of the effects of domination by others.

Oppression is exacerbated by the low status of professions like midwifery and nursing, in part because of their service and caring orientated attributes. Savage (1987) writes how these 'helping' characteristics are popularly ascribed more to women than men and are further reinforced by female dominance in these professions. The devaluing of caring roles in society is evidenced by the non-paid nature of much informal caring within the home, again clearly split along gender lines (Arber 1988).

Underneath the current ideology on multidisciplinary collaboration and team working lurks yet another outworking of the effects of oppression. Though the rhetoric is hard to argue against, anecdotal experience seems to suggest that true equality in team relationships is an elusive goal (Sweet & Norman 1995). Too often committees/groups still defer to the senior medics who will either chair them or control them by exercising the right of veto as decisions are made, often delegating the implementation detail of new initiatives to midwives. One current trend in maternity services, the subspecialisation of obstetricians, for example to fetal medicine or maternal medicine, illustrates this process. The detail associated with setting up specialist antenatal clinics was led by midwives in one maternity unit. Here we had some of the most senior and experienced midwives spending time canvassing for a new name for the clinic, determining how women would access the clinic, how it would be run, etc. But critically important dimensions like referral criteria, the use of appropriate antenatal technologies and screening remained firmly the prerogative of the obstetrician. Similar roles of assistant or secretary to obstetricians can sometimes be seen on delivery suite ward rounds, with the core midwives following the entourage with the clipboard, shepherding and chaperoning male doctors in and out of rooms. As already mentioned, feminists writers have shown up the social ordering of these roles along gender lines, with women socialised as helpers and carers, roles that have little status and power (Savage 1987).

Promotion within this patriarchal and paternalistic system requires highly adaptive behaviours. As a price worth paying to achieve incremental midwifery advancement, midwifery managers may justify compromise and political manipulation. Tactics like 'make them think it is their idea' and ignoring bullying behaviour as a trade-off for support with particular issues occur in practice, as do gender games like mutual flattery and flirtatious behaviours (Porter 1991). Roberts (2000) suggests that individuals with ambition within oppressed groups have to buy into a reward system dispensed by the oppressors in exchange for keeping the status quo, in order to secure promotion.

Advocacy on behalf of women is another dimension to the midwive's role that creates dissonance for many. Although regulatory bodies espouse its importance (UKCC 1996), examples in practice are rare in the literature. Caseload midwifery is an interesting exception (McCourt 1998), where it has been noted that midwives will push the boundaries of normality, e.g. waterbirth following a previous caesarean section, on behalf of women with whom they have built a relationship. More often, midwives act as an appeaser between maternal requests and restrictive institutional policies unless they are comfortable with the inevitable conflict it will engender.

Institutional constraints, the authority of obstetricians within many consultant units and the oppression along gender lines that results are formidable barriers to overcome. Breaking free of this environment by the setting up of geographically separate practices may be the best long-term solution. The severing of links with obstetric and institutional agendas by moving normal birth care to birth units and midwifery-led units does not mean the total cessation of communication with obstetricians. Primary care-based professional groups have been liaising with colleagues in acute services successfully for years, as the

successful birth centres in the UK (Saunders et al 2000) and the USA (Spitzer 1995) demonstrate. Scaremongers opposed to separating obstetric and midwifery services may be demonstrating a more covert fear of losing control of a context they currently dominate.

Questions for Reflection ?????

To what extent is your practice affected by the traditional dominance of obstetricians on labour wards?

Does professional bullying occur where you work and, if so, can you think of ways of addressing it?

Do you think there is any tension between your advocacy role for women and your allegiance to the policies and guidelines of the institution you work within?

GENDER, PSYCHOLOGY AND ETHICS ON THE LABOUR WARD

Discussion so far has sketched the effects of a hegemony that does not serve the interests of child-bearing women and midwives. These reflections have been largely confined to the impact on organisational, clinical and relational dimensions of care. Recent research has also explored alternative feminist thinking in psychology and ethics and the challenges this presents to the current androcentric understandings. LoCicero's (1993) and Harris's (2000) papers will be examined as they have applied their reflections in the context of lowering an excessive caesarean section rate, a hot topic for current labour ward practice.

LoCicero suggests that the intellectual/cognitive framework of obstetrics emanates from a scientific/masculine model that supervalues detached, objective observation in decision making on delivery suites. This model screens out emotional effects which are likely to obscure rational thought so that the obstetrician can respond to referrals for labour complications and make an impartial judgement of the appropriate actions, unencumbered by personal feelings. Jordan and colleagues (1991), by contrast, believe that connectedness and inter-personal relationships are key to making clinical judgements. Empathy, intuition and insight are required to individualise decisions at moments of crisis and these are grounded in active listening, rapport building and sensitive communication with those intimately involved. Connectedness, openness and self-awareness are characteristics of intuition (Davis-Floyd & Davis 1997) and are integral to women's ways of knowing (Belenky et al 1987).

A clear application of these differences occurs daily in intrapartum care. 'Failure to progress' in labour is rooted in physical causation related to the powers, passages or passenger, according to the androcentric biomedical model. The solution is an external birth intervention like artificial rupture of membranes or syntocinon administration. The obstetric decision is not so much what should be done but when it should be initiated and even this parameter is hedged on every side by measurable, verifiable time frames. Simkin & Ancheta's (2000) approach could not be more different. First, the phrase is not used and the biomedical imperative of linking labour and time is broken. They recognise a 'normalising uniqueness' in labour experience, variation in physiology that is special for each women. It only becomes 'prolonged labour' when the woman herself expresses that concern and the language is neutral, not self-denigrating. Then, making the appropriate intuitive judgement of 'how to care' as opposed to 'how to manage' is multifaceted, addressing all the areas that contribute to the 'connective dance of labour' (Davis-Floyd & Davis 1997). Their wonderful book lists a range of supporting strategies that are physiological, psychological, social or spiritual and at the very bottom of the list are the biomedical. Anderson (2000) especially highlights the psychological dimensions of the second stage of labour in her insightful paper, a dimension of care in the second stage completely missing from most standard midwifery textbooks.

Ethics and labour ward decisions have been sharply focused by the forced caesarean section episodes over recent years. Harris (2000) makes a seminal contribution to ethical reflection in this area by challenging the maternal–fetal conflict model which is based on justice, rights and moral obligations. This model holds sway in practice, as the pitting of maternal choice against fetal rights illustrates. She suggests that traditional moral principles of autonomy and beneficence are a particular masculine rendering of ethics from which conflict scenarios inevitably result. She argues for an alternative ethic by applying relational and equality-based moral theories. She writes:

> In this model, clinicians faced with ethical dilemmas should attempt to understand pregnant women and their decisions within their broad social networks and communities, ask how the clinician's personal standpoint influences outcomes judged to be ethical and determine whether their ethical formulations reduce or enhance existing gender, class or racial inequality. (Harris 2000, p 786)

Thus the focus is on the mutual needs of woman and fetus rather than their mutually exclusive needs. Women's decisions are intimately linked with their network of human relationships and the repercussions on these. Bracketing them to one side completely, so that some objective moral imperative becomes the sole arbiter of right or wrong, may result in intolerable dissonance.

The advent of fetal personhood as a separate being in utero is in no small way a consequence of fetal medicine technologies. Bassett et al (2000) call obstetricians focused on this specialty 'fetal champions' and their activities have the effect of raising expectations of the potential to eliminate or treat all fetal abnormalities. This feeds the idea of blaming women if screening and treatments are declined.

Questions for Reflection ?????

Do you value a 'detached disposition' or a 'connectedness disposition' in the approach of obstetricians to labour complications?

What is your view of potential conflict between fetal and maternal rights?

Would it be more helpful from an ethical perspective to view the mother and fetus as an interdependent unit?

SOME IMPLICATIONS OF RECENT DEVELOPMENTS IN FEMINIST THOUGHT

Contemporary feminist thought has added a cautionary note to overemphasising gender differences, whether socially constructed or biologically determined. Many of the critiques of the biomedical model of birth outlined here rest on a socially constructed understanding of gender differences (Kent 2000) but postmodern feminists would urge caution here. Annandale & Clark (1996) are suspicious of grand theories explaining, in this instance, female oppression in the context of maternity care as a consequence of patriarchy. What they refer to as binary thinking and essentialism, i.e. fixed, oppositional categories such as male/female, first condemn us to a kind of gender determinism that is immutable, resistant to alternative explanations, and second, fail to take account of relativist expressions in real life. In other words, there are both obstetricians and midwives who break the mould of socially constructed gender behaviours and attitudes. The postmodernist position sees a fluidity and contingency about knowledge and experience that is more complex, less definable and ever changing (Mitchell 1996).

One of the ways this could be applied in practice is a healthy scepticism about authoritative and absolutist claims, be they from feminists who link all injustice with patriarchy or obstetricians advocating the singular truth of randomised controlled trials. This is not to jettison all traditional feminist analysis, much of which has been outlined in this chapter, but to reflexively evaluate it in the light of one's personal experience and value system. This will lead many to embrace large elements of the feminist critique of maternity care and to continue to integrate professional and personal experience through a feminist lens. Others will adopt other explanations and theories explaining personal and social injustices, though it is hoped that they will seriously engage with what feminism has to say.

CONCLUSION

Returning to an appreciation of values is a satisfying endpoint to these deliberations, for values

---

Box 5.1 Biomedical versus woman-centred models of labour and birth

Biomedical	Woman centred
• Body as machine	• Whole person
• Reductionism – powers, passages, passenger	• Integrate – physiology, psychosocial, spiritual
• Analyse and control	• Respect and empower
• Expertise/objective	• Relational/subjective
• Environment peripheral	• Environment central
• Anticipate pathology	• Anticipate normality
• Technology as partner	• Technology as servant
• Homogenisation	• Celebrate difference
• Evidence	• Intuition
• Safety	• Self-actualisation

---

have the power to unite opposing discourses as well as demarcate them. Box 5.1 is a dichotomous representation of feminist/woman-centred versus androcentric/biomedical perspectives on labour and birth.

But already there is a linkage of shared values/perspectives with the alignment of feminist with woman centred and androcentric with biomedical. Implicit in that alignment are assumptions, some of which have been explored in this chapter. Postmodernism helps us to see that there remain spaces and possibilities between seemingly opposite discourses. One way of exploring these spaces very practically is to involve midwives and obstetricians in 'reverse debates'. In this scenario a proposition is debated, e.g. home birth is intrinsically unsafe, with each professional group arguing against their traditional position on the issue. It is a useful way of exploring each other's often contrasting perspectives.

On the other hand, the recent history of childbirth tells us that spaces can be colonised if one side seeks power over the other. The feminist challenge for all of us is to search out and articulate our own values and beliefs around the life-changing milestone of childbirth, then to examine women's experiences of empowerment and injustice as they undertake this rite of passage to uncover and challenge any gender-mediated effects. This task can be carried out with integrity by midwife or obstetrician, whether male or female.

Questions for Reflection ?????

Do your values and beliefs around labour and birth align more with a patriarchal or feminist model?

What effect might these values have on the care you provide?

In what areas can you see common ground between the two models?

Key points

■ Childbirth broadly follows a biomedical, technocratic model or a midwifery, woman-centred model. The latter is predicated on what could be called feminist values and beliefs.

■ Research has shown that women who give birth in large hospitals experience less satisfaction and a greater number of birth interventions than women who give birth at home or in birth centres.

■ The increase in hospital birth during the 20th century coincided with a mechanistic approach to birth that was increasingly reliant on technology. In contrast, birth at home emphasises the spiritual and emotional elements and a belief in the essential normality of birth.

■ All midwives and obstetricians need to reflect on their own beliefs and values about labour and birth in order to support labouring women more honestly.

REFERENCES

Albers L 1999 The duration of labour in healthy women. Journal of Perinatology 19(2): 114–119

Allan H 1993 Feminism: a concept analysis. Journal of Advanced Nursing 18: 1547–1553

Anderson T 2000 Feeling safe enough to let go: the relationship between the woman and her midwife during the second stage of labour. In: Kirkham M (ed) The midwife–mother relationship. MacMillan, London

Annandale E, Clark J 1996 What is gender? Feminist theory and the sociology of human reproduction. Sociology of Health and Illness 18(1): 17–44

Arber S 1998 Health, aging and older women. In: Doyal L (ed) Women and health services. Open University Press, Buckingham

Balaskas J 1995 New active birth: a concise guide to natural childbirth. Unwin Paperbacks, London

Bassett K, Iyer N, Kazanjian A 2000 Defensive medicine during hospital obstetric care: a by-product of the technological age. Social Science and Medicine 51: 532–537

Bastion H 1992 Confined, managed and delivered: the language of obstetrics. British Journal of Obstetrics and Gynaecology 99: 92–93

Bates C 1997 Care in normal labour: a feminist perspective. In: Alexander J, Levy V, Roth C (eds) Midwifery practice: core topics 2. Macmillan, Basingstoke

Belenky M, Clinchy B, Goldberger N, Tarule J 1987 Women's ways of knowing. Basic Books, New York

Bluff R, Holloway I 1994 'They know best': women's perceptions of midwifery care during labour and birth. Midwifery 10: 157–164

Caldeyro-Barcia R, Giussi G, Storch E et al 1979 The influence of maternal bearing down efforts and their effects on fetal heart rate, oxygenation and acid base balance. Journal of Perinatal Medicine 9: 63–67

Campbell R 1997 Place of birth reconsidered. In: Alexander J, Levy V, Roth C (eds) Midwifery practice: core topics 2. Macmillan, Basingstoke

Chalmers I, Enkin M, Kierse M 1989 A guide to effective care in pregnancy and childbirth. Oxford University Press, Oxford

Charles N 2000 Feminism, the state and social policy. Macmillan Press, Basingstoke

Coyle K, Huack Y, Percival P, Kristjanson L 2001a Ongoing relationship with a personal focus: mother's perception of birth centre versus hospital care. Midwifery 17(3): 171–181

Coyle K, Huack Y, Percival P, Kristjanson L 2001b Normality and collaboration: mother's perception of birth centre versus hospital care. Midwifery 17(3): 182–193

Crompton R, Sanderson K 1990 Gendered jobs and social change. Unwin Hyman, London

David M, von Schwarzenfeld H, Dimer J, Kentenich H 1999 Perinatal outcome in hospital and birth centre obstetric care. International Journal of Gynaecology and Obstetrics 65(2): 149–156

Davis-Floyd R 2001 The technocratic, humanistic and holistic paradigms of childbirth. International Journal of Gynaecology and Obstetrics 75: S5–S23

Davis-Floyd R, Davis E 1997 Intuition as authoritative knowledge in midwifery and homebirth. In: Davis-Floyd R, Sargent C (eds) Childbirth and authoritative knowledge. University of California Press, London

Department of Health 1993 Changing childbirth: report of the Expert Committee on Maternity Care. HMSO, London

Department of Health and Social Security 1970 Domiciliary midwifery and maternity bed needs: the report of the Standing Maternity and Midwifery Advisory Committee (Peel Report). HMSO, London

Donnison J 1988 Midwives and medical men. Historical Publications, London

Downe S 2001 Is there a future for normal birth? Practising Midwife 4(6): 10–12

Doyal L 1998 Conclusions: the way forward. In: Doyal L (ed) Women and health services. Open University Press, Buckingham

Dunn P 1991 Francois Mauriceau (1637–1709) and maternal posture for parturition. MIDIRS 66: 78–79

Esposito N 1999 Marginalised women's comparisons of their hospital and free-standing birth centre experience: a contract of inner city birthing centres. Health Care for Women International 20(2): 111–126

Graham H 1993 Hardship and health in women's lives. Harvester, London

Graham H 1998 Health at risk: poverty and national health strategies. In: Doyal L (ed) Women and health services. Open University Press, Buckingham

Graham I 1997 Episiotomy: challenging obstetric interventions. Blackwell Science, London

Greer G 1999 The whole woman. Doubleday, London

Guilland K, Pairman S 1995 The midwifery partnership: a model for practice. Monograph series 95/1. Department of Nursing and Midwifery, Victoria University of Wellington, New Zealand

Gupta J, Nilodem V 2002 Woman's position during second stage of labour (Cochrane review). Cochrane Library, issue 1. Update Software, Oxford

Hamilton M, McLean M 2000 Pre-registration midwifery degree and diploma curriculum programme document. De Montfort University, Leicester

Harris L 2000 Rethinking maternal–fetal conflict: gender and equality in perinatal ethics. Obstetrics and Gynaecology 96: 786–791

Hewison A 1993 The language of labour: an examination of the discourses of childbirth. Midwifery 9: 225–234

Hodnett ED 2002a Home-like versus conventional birth settings (Cochrane review). Cochrane Library, issue 1. Update Software, Oxford

Hodnett ED 2002b Support from caregivers during childbirth (Cochrane review). Cochrane Library, issue 1. Update Software, Oxford

Hunt S, Symonds A 1995 The social meaning of midwifery. Macmillan, Basingstoke

Inhorn M, Whittle K 2001 Feminism meets the 'new' epidemiologies: towards an appraisal of antifeminist biases in epidemiological research on women's health. Social Science and Medicine 53: 553–567

Jordan B 1993 Birth in four cultures: a cross-cultural investigation of childbirth in Yucatan, Holland, Sweden and the United States. Waveland Press, Prospect Heights

Jordan J, Kaplan A, Miller J, Stiver I, Surrey J 1991 Women's growth in connection. Guilford Press, New York

Kent J 2000 Social perspectives on pregnancy and childbirth for midwives, nurses and the caring professions. Open University Press, Buckingham

Kirkham M 1989 Midwives and information giving during labour. In: Robinson S, Thompson A (eds) Midwives, research and childbirth, vol. 1. Chapman and Hall, London

Kirkham M 1997 Stories and childbirth. In: Kirkham M, Perkins E (eds) Reflections on midwifery. Baillière Tindall, London

Kirkham M 1999 The culture of midwifery in the National Health Service in England. Journal of Advanced Nursing 30(3): 732–739

Kirkham M (ed) 2000 The midwife–mother relationship. Macmillan, London

Kitzinger S 1978 The experience of childbirth. Penguin, London

Kitzinger S 2000 Rediscovering birth. Little, Brown, London

Knauth D, Haloburdo E 1986 Effects of pushing techniques in birthing chair on length of second stage of labour. Nursing Research 35: 49–51

Leap N 1997 Making sense of 'horizontal violence' in midwifery. British Journal of Midwifery 5(11):689

Lister P 1997 The art of nursing in a 'postmodern' context. Journal of Advanced Nursing 25: 38–44

Llewellyn-Jones D 1994 Fundamentals of obstetrics and gynaecology. Mosby, London

LoCicero AK 1993 Explaining excessive rates of caesareans and other childbirth interventions: contributions from contemporary theories of gender and psychosocial development. Social Science and Medicine 37(10): 1261–1269

Machin D, Scamell M 1997 The experience of labour using ethnography to explore the irresistible nature of the bio-medical metaphor during labour. Midwifery 13: 78–84

McCourt C 1998 Update on the future of one-to-one midwifery. MIDIRS 8(1): 7–10

McCrea H 1993 Valuing the midwife's role in the midwife/client relationship. Journal of Clinical Nursing 2: 47–52

McLoughlin A 1997 The 'F' factor: feminism forsaken? Nurse Education Today, 17(2): 111–114

Mitchell D 1996 Postmodernism, health and illness. Journal of Advanced Nursing 23: 201–205

Murphy-Lawless J 1998 Reading birth and death: a history of obstetric thinking. Cork University Press, Cork, Ireland

Oakley A 1984 The captured womb: a history of the medical care of pregnant women. Basil Blackwell, Oxford

Oakley A 1993 Essays on women, medicine and health. Edinburgh University Press, Edinburgh

Oakley A, Rajan L, Grant A 1990 Social support and pregnancy outcome. British Journal of Obstetrics and Gynaecology 97: 155–162

O'Driscoll K, Meager D 1986 Active management of labour. WB Saunders, London

Olsen O 1997 Meta-analysis of the safety of home birth. Birth 24(1): 4–13

Page L, McCourt C, Beake S, Hewison J 1999 Clinical interventions and outcomes of one-to-one midwifery practice. Journal of Public Health Medicine 21(3):243–248

Porter S 1991 A participant observation study of power relations between nurses and doctors in a general hospital. Journal of Advanced Nursing 16: 728–735

Richens Y 2002 Are midwives using research evidence in practice? British Journal of Midwifery 10(1): 11–16

Roberts S 2000 Development of a positive professional identity: liberating oneself from the oppressor within. Advances in Nursing Science 22(4): 71–82

Rooks J, Weatherby N, Ernst E 1992 The National Birth Centre Study. Part II – intrapartum and immediate postpartum and neonatal care. Journal of Nurse Midwifery 37(5): 301–330

Roth C 1998 Reading between the lines: the contribution of obstetric textbooks to professional authority and power. South Bank University, London

Royal College of Midwives 2001 Birth monitoring trial secures £2 million funding. RCM Midwives Journal July: 1

Salmon D 1999 A feminist analysis of women's experience of perineal trauma in the immediate post-delivery period. Midwifery 15(4): 247–256

Saunders D, Boulton M, Chapple J, Ratcliffe J, Levitan J 2000 Evaluation of the Edgware Birth Centre. North Thames Perinatal Public Health, Middlesex

Savage J 1987 Nurses and gender. Open University Press, Milton Keynes

Schacht S, Ewing S 1997 The many paths of feminism: can men travel any of them? Journal of Gender Studies 6(2): 159–176

Simkin P 1992 Just another day in a woman's life? Part 2: nature and consistency of women's long-term memories of their first birth experiences. Birth 19(2): 64–81

Simkin P, Ancheta R 2000 The labour progress handbook. Blackwell Science, Oxford

Spitzer M 1995 Birth centres: economy, safety and empowerment. Journal of Nurse-Midwifery 40(4): 371–375

Sweet S, Norman I 1995 The nurse–doctor relationship: a selective literature review. Journal of Advanced Nursing 22: 165–170

Symon A 1999 Perinatal litigation in Scotland 1980–1995: its incidence, rate and nature. Journal of Obstetrics and Gynaecology 19(9): 239–247

Tarkka M 1996 Social support and its impact on mothers' experience of childbirth. Journal of Advanced Midwifery 23: 70–75

Tew M 1998 Safer childbirth? A critical history of maternity care. Free Association Books, London

Thacker S, Stroup D, Peterson H 2002 Continuous electronic fetal heart monitoring during labour (Cochrane review). Cochrane Library, Issue 1. Update Software, Oxford

Thornton J 1996 Active management of labour. British Medical Journal 313: 378

Tinkler A, Quinney D 1998 Team midwifery: the influence of the midwife–woman relationship on women's experience and perceptions of maternity care. Journal of Advanced Nursing 28(1): 30–35

UKCC 1996 Guidelines for professional practice. UKCC, London

Wagner M 1994 Pursuing the birth machine. ACE Graphics, Sydney

Walsh D 1999 An ethnographic study of women's experience of partnership caseload midwifery practice: the professional as friend. Midwifery 15(3): 165–176

Walsh D 2000 Evidence-based care series 3: assessing progress in labour. British Journal of Midwifery 8(7): 449–457

Walsh D 2001 Birthwrite: continuity and caseload midwifery. British Journal of Midwifery 9(11): 671

Webb C 1993 Feminist research: definitions, methodology, methods and evaluation. Journal of Advanced Nursing 18: 416–423

Williams S, Mackey M 1999 Women's experience of preterm labour – a feminist critique. Health Care for Women International 20: 29–48

Woodhouse K 1998 Cause for concern: women and smoking. In: Doyal L (ed) Women and health services. Open University Press, Buckingham

6

Transition to motherhood: from the woman's perspective

Sally Marchant

INTRODUCTION

This chapter reviews the changing role of women and the effect this has had on the experiences of women as mothers alongside a historical and contemporary perspective of the context of postpartum midwifery care. Postpartum care has been criticised for becoming focused on a series of routine tasks regardless of individual need (Walsh 1997). The low status of postpartum care within midwifery or society in general has also meant there has been little in the way of enquiry into its purpose, achievements or problems (Garcia & Marchant 1996, Garcia et al 1998, Glazener et al 1993). The dilemma for female midwives who support women in their role as mothers while being themselves expected to maintain their integrity as women and mothers within society is explored. The chapter presumes a knowledge of the mainstream feminist and egalitarian principles and based on these, there is enquiry as to their place and potential benefit when considering postpartum services for women and those who provide them.

BACKGROUND TO THE SOCIAL FRAMEWORK OF WOMEN

Sociology theorists have identified models that relate to the roles expected of men and women within the family context. These are described variously but one approach has been to label these as being expressive or instrumental constructs. Expressive is identified primarily by taking the role of a carer and social theorists argue that this work is best undertaken by women as it reflects the qualities associated with femininity. Instrumental includes the work undertaken to gain a wage or money and this function is seen as best undertaken by men, partly because it appears to involve qualities of strength and academic or business achievement (Jorgensen et al 1997). Such concepts underpin the aspects attributed to the roles of the mother and father figure within the framework of the nuclear family by identifying a specific role for each parent within a recognised sociological structure (Parsons 1951).

These social concepts rely on the main attributes identified by gender where the sex of an individual largely depicts or is seen as predictable with regard to their appearance and behaviour. Society only recognises either male or female genetic sex, having no biologically acceptable intermediate state. However, identification by gender relates in practice to a person's outward appearance, their physical attributes and behaviour being mainly aligned to the recognised descriptions for masculine or feminine characteristics. Therefore where gender, as opposed to genetic sex identity, is concerned, individuals can have ambiguous feminine and/or masculine characteristics. Historically it is men, with their masculine characteristics of physical strength, that have dominated the social environment, accruing social advantage through education, wealth and status. This situation continues in various degrees for the majority of cultures today. The female characteristics associated with women are reduced physical strength but greater ability in those qualities related to social and emotional support, advocacy and communication skills. The attributes associated with women continue to be seen as having an inferior status to those of men where women are socially forced to take a lesser or even subservient role. The notion of egalitarian views based on equality with regard to social and personal rights has been a fairly recent development even in the most affluent and developed countries.

In the UK, the public image of women began to change as a result of the involvement of women in the social framework of the country during the First World War and added fuel to the emerging voice of the women's movement. Women demonstrated that they could not only undertake roles of national importance formerly maintained by men, but that they could have greater independence, choice and control in their lives (Gowdridge et al 1997, Llewellyn-Davies 1991). Women were involved in work that was previously considered to be solely the province of men. In addition, some women from the higher social classes undertook menial work previously considered to be only suitable for women from the lower classes. These upsets to the previous social framework for wives, mothers and daughters all contributed to the increasing political activity aimed at raising the social status of women. There was pressure to develop more opportunities for basic and higher education for women and to be actively involved in measures to improve maternal and child health. Women in higher social classes were more able to obtain an independent income from paid work and this contributed to their political voice and a route via Parliament to press for further change (Gowdridge et al 1997, Llewellyn-Davies 1991).

These influences changed the role of women within society with the rising acknowledgement that some women could lead fulfilling lives without the framework of marriage or children. Alongside this, the availability of safer and publicly recognised methods of contraception meant that women could have greater control over their fertility which would in turn have a major influence on their life choices. Instead of it being a foregone conclusion that women would marry and have children, it became more acceptable not to do so. However, this in turn led to a growing friction between women themselves about their role, particularly the place of mothers in society.

MOTHERHOOD: A CONFLICT OF IDENTITY?

The purpose of motherhood has been expressed as one of ultimate fulfilment for a woman with the mother–child relationship being seen as the essence of womanliness and femininity, so that a woman should take pride in this unique role as being her ultimate achievement (Abbott & Wallace 1996, Phoenix et al 1991).

A contrasting view of motherhood is that this is the ultimate example of oppression within a society, the antithesis of liberation where any control over the direction of one's life has to take into consideration the responsibility of children. Some women identify feelings of being shackled or tied down by such a relationship and of being burdened by what they perceive as onerous responsibilities as opposed to opportunities for creative and life-enhancing experiences without the ties of motherhood (Lovenduski Randall 1993). This view is modified by those who consider that where the responsibility for a child is shared, there is then the opportunity for personal growth and freedom alongside the fulfilment of parenting – seen as a different concept from motherhood.

Another aspect of mothering is that of 'owning' or having control over another person's life and opportunities as well as being concerned for their welfare. Although the philosophical framework for this would be one of altruism, where the actions of one person aim to improve the outcome for another, there are examples of mothers who relive their own lives and desires through their children, exerting unwelcome pressures upon them to achieve goals or targets of more importance to the mother than the child (Messenger-Davies & Mosdell 2001).

The mother figure has been illustrated as a powerful influence within the family context, setting moral standards for what is right and wrong. Within some cultures women who have achieved motherhood assume a matriarchal position that has weight and authority with regard to family issues and this authority is often enhanced with advancing age (Symonds & Hunt 1996). There can also be apparent conflict between the role of a woman as a mother and a wife. These two concepts do not always lie easily together within a male-dominated or patriarchal society. The familiar 'mother-in-law' jokes hint at this discord where the son-in-law is faced with a female figure of authority who is not his own mother but where there is an expectation by society that he will in fact bow to her authority as accorded by her 'status' within the family structure.

There has been much greater emphasis on the role of parents and responsibilities for childcare in more recent years. It is arguable that whilst social pressures might be raised for men to have more involvement with childcare and within the family overall, these have not been supported by governmental policies (Giddons 1993). In general, women continue to be disadvantaged by a range of social policies that reduce any potential for them to have less involvement in the areas of childcare and family support by having a reduced capacity as a wage earner. Women are liable to lose promotion opportunities as a result of maternity career breaks, to continue to suffer discrimination with regard to job opportunities and the lack of financially possible and acceptable arrangements for childcare (Lovenduski Randall 1993, Oakley 1980). Women therefore continue to undertake the primary role in child and family care even when they are also undertaking other work in the form of paid employment. Efforts to quantify housework and childcare as equivalent to paid work have not met with success. In addition, there is conflict between women themselves about their role: mothers who want to stay at home and solely undertake the role of mother and family carer in its entirety, those who choose not to do this and those who have no choice about this for financial reasons (Holdsworth 1988, Oakley 1980).

For same-sex couples the gender issues with regard to employment are also evident. Where male same-sex couples have joint childcare it is more likely that the family could live within the income generated from one wage. This is less likely where two women are sharing childcare because of the disparity in earning capacity between single men and women. However, it might be potentially more difficult for men than for women to get time off from their employment for childcare reasons. Where the father undertakes any significant proportion of child or family care, this is still viewed as more of a novelty rather than a viable option (Barclay & Lupton 1999, Jacobs 1997). In some Scandinavian countries the role of the father is identified and underpinned by social policies with regard to paid employment leave and general monetary support for the family unit (Gjerdingen et al 2000).

Women without a resident partner have to juggle their resources to meet the needs of the developing child as well as trying to maintain their own identity as women within their social framework. Society, whilst being more accepting of lone parent families in general, has not sought in any great depth for a social structure that would assist these families with regard to social networks or improved resources (Abbott & Wallace 1996). The overall opinion would still seem to be one of blame where women are seen to have contributed wilfully to their circumstances and therefore are in some way 'lucky' to have any help, let alone that this should be increased. That these women are mothers can also evoke social opinion as to the quality of their mothering, as though society has the right to comment on this because the state is contributing to the family resources. This can be identified by both negative and positive media attention where children's actions are associated with the behaviour or actions of their mothers (Times 2002).

BECOMING A MOTHER

Information about the practical aspects (positive and negative) of having a baby and becoming a mother can be obtained from a range of popular magazines, books and, more recently, Internet websites. The main images portrayed by such literature derive from society's benevolent view of the nurturing mother and the newborn child, often within a stereotypical family environment. Against this rather partial and 'rosy' picture, women themselves have attempted to explain the conflict between the image of motherhood popularised by our society and a woman's need for a personal identity and social freedom (Crowley & Hemmelweit 1992). Literature about women who have used assisted conception or who adopt children has on occasions used language that marginalises these women's experiences as though they are not 'proper' mothers. They may even have less support from benefits and other social mechanisms because of the way in which they became the carer of a child. Such attitudes and conflicts can be viewed as particularly ironic within the midwifery profession where the majority of midwives are women who may be experiencing the very same conflicts as those they are advising and supporting in their professional capacity.

From the confident, pioneering and flamboyant days of the initial women's liberation movement women were encouraged to identify the need for their independence from dependency (of men and children and others). They were exhorted to challenge the status 'given' to women in society as generally being secondary to men, especially in the important areas of education and employment status (Symonds & Hunt 1996). However, recent feminist thinking has identified and debated the real dilemma for some women in balancing the uniqueness of motherhood alongside its inherent dependency whilst trying to retain autonomy as an individual (Crowley & Hemmelweit 1992). The 'state' of motherhood is viewed by society as having a special value that sets women who are mothers apart from those who are not and 'mothering' is seen as inherently 'woman's work', thus reinforcing the differences between the sexes (Phoenix et al 1991). The conflict for women is the distinction between and perhaps protection of this 'special' role and the expectation by society. This is that the woman will take the main responsibility for all the requirements of infant and childcare whilst not necessarily having these same rights when there is dispute over the care or custody of the child (Lovenduski Randall 1993).

It would appear that there are distinct differences between the concepts of mothering and motherhood. Let us look first at motherhood.

Motherhood implies the act of having given birth. This is challenged by those who maybe have subsequent care of children but who have not given birth, by those who have nurtured a pregnancy but from genetic material that was not their own and by women who have become pregnant but never achieved a viable birth as a result of miscarriage. This raises the complexity of trying to explore the concept of being a mother with the societal view leading more towards what the action of being a mother entails and how well (or otherwise) individual women 'achieve' this (see Table 6.1). Society suggests that being a mother requires altruism at its highest level as the child's needs will always come first and will be catered for, sometimes taking priority over the mother's own needs until a degree of independence is reached. Even when the child reaches adulthood

Table 6.1 Concepts around society's values related to 'feminine' qualities (adapted from Oakley 1980)

Women		Mothers	
'Normal'	**'Deviant'**	**'Normal'**	**'Deviant'**
Naturally maternal and home-centred	Reject or find the caring and maternal role difficult	Slaves to their bodies, cannot control their bodies	See childbirth as a physically stressful, life-changing event
Caring for/about families and men	Career orientated	Emotionally unstable, become essentially 'childish' and present-oriented	See childbirth as an emotional and exhausting experience, requiring new skills and hard labour, often with little support
More controlled by their bodies than men	Do not accept 'natural' limits (imposed by body)	Nest-builders, caring urge	Reject social pressure to give up past life with motherhood being the primary role
Inferior to men	Do not accept an inferior position, demand equality		Demand for partner to share responsibility
Deferential/submissive	Aggressive, overassertive		

mothers are seen to have been responsible for the long-term outcomes of their children, positive or negative (Murray 1999). In this respect mothering broadens to include the role of parents. The values held by most developed countries are that the father also has a role in the eventual development of his children and that 'fatherless' children are in some way deprived. Such views lead to the concern that single mothers or couples of the same sex who have children and create a 'family' environment cannot do it as well as the standard heterosexual couple within the nuclear family or, increasingly, the re-formed family. These views have been challenged by social and political organisations and some changes to parenting laws and laws for adoption have taken place and are still evolving. The rights of women to maintain custody and control of their children where a relationship has failed are also subject to great social arbitration, all based upon the highly dubious concepts of what makes 'the good mother' (Price 1988).

Mothering is taken as having a different perspective to that of motherhood. The concept of mothering usually raises images related to care and caring that are benevolent within a relationship totally centred on undemanding, selfless love (Price 1988). Such qualities in the mother–child relationship can, however, also be the subject of ridicule in later years when society considers that the child is no longer entitled to that degree of mothering. At what state or age this might be is not clearly defined as society also recognises that

the selfless aspects of a mother's love have beneficial effects when individuals are distressed or in need of extra support (Alibhai-Brown 1999).

Questions for Reflection ?????

For some people, reflections on their relationship with their mother may be uncomfortable and bring sadness or emotional distress. If you already have insight into your relationship with your mother and have concerns about this, you may prefer not to undertake this activity.

Personal
If you think about your mother (even if she is no longer alive), how would you describe the main characteristics that come to mind? Write these down as you think of them. What comes out from your list? Have you described more about your mother's behaviour than her emotional responses to you or vice versa? Now try and describe the emotions doing this has generated in you. If you had the opportunity, is there anything you would like to say or write to your mother as a result of this?

Professional
Think back to your contact with pregnant or postpartum women. Have you made an assessment of these women's ability to be

mothers? If so, what information might you have used to do this? On reflection, if you feel you do not assess women in this way, why might that be and if you do, what effect might such an assessment (positive or negative) have on the woman's future care? What effect do you think your own experiences of being mothered might have had on your relationship with women in your care?

THE BALANCE OF POWER: WOMEN, MIDWIVES, MOTHERS, MOTHERS-IN-LAW

Within the concept of mothering and of being a mother, when the daughter becomes a mother the balance changes and the mother has anxiety about her child (now to be a mother herself) and wants to advise and protect her in her new experience. At the same time greater pressures are placed upon the new grandmother who has an additional family member to accommodate with regard to care needs. For women with strong mother–son relationships, there is the potential element of competition when the son takes a woman as his companion and she is then seen as being responsible for meeting his needs and raising children of their own, to the same standard or better than his mother.

The role of female midwives and motherhood has received little attention with the majority of studies concentrating on professional issues rather than social ones (Hunt & Symonds 1995, McLoughlin 1997). There is the potential for much confusion about the relationship of the midwife/mother and her ability to give support and advice to women who are about to become mothers. What role does the personal experience of the midwife have in this area? This has perhaps been explored more with regard to advice on breastfeeding, where midwives have been either positively or negatively influenced by their own experiences. The intention of the professional education framework is to encourage research-based evidence to supplant these more anecdotal influences but it would appear that there is much more enquiry required in this area.

MOTHERING AND POSTNATAL CARE

Women have traditionally provided care and support to the newly delivered mother by offering help with domestic chores, personal care and care of other family members. This was to ensure a period of rest and recuperation after the birth (Donnison 1988). Within the multi-layers of society wealth has had an influence on the provision of care where women with greater wealth could pay others for this service while in the poorer communities women had to rely on the unpaid assistance of other women within their social framework. Motherhood was also only valued when it occurred within marriage and women who were not married were not assisted by society or other women to the same extent. Women, often very young women, would be fired from any employment, cast out of their own family network to face a life of destitution in institutions such as the workhouses or on the streets.

Women in general contributed to this view although there were some notable exceptions who advocated reform and a greater degree of humanity. The onus of disgrace was largely placed on the woman, suggesting that as she was the weaker sex she lacked the moral fibre to resist temptation, thereby contributing to her downfall. It is interesting to reflect that although society is less vehement nowadays about women who have children outside an apparent partnership, the pregnancy might still arise for similar reasons today as 200 or more years ago. Unplanned pregnancies still occur through ignorance about safe sex practices, immature infatuation, promises of greater riches to come and the need for affection and belonging where this is seen to be lacking.

The high maternal mortality rate in the latter part of the 19th century that occurred after women had given birth was gradually identified as being in some way associated with the care women received at that time (Donnison 1988). It became apparent that there was no standard knowledge or behaviour that could be attributed to the majority of lay midwives, although some had begun to gain training and greater skills to become certificated midwives (Cowell & Wainwright 1991). Dickens' portrayal of the midwife Sarey Gamp as an unkempt drunkard likely to do more harm than good did much to enlighten his readers about the risk of childbirth (Dickens 1843). Florence Nightingale, amongst others, also contributed to the debate by identifying poor hygiene, malnutrition and high parity as reasons for the high number of postpartum maternal deaths (Loudon 1987).

There was increasing interest in social issues by middle- and upper-class women in the latter part of the 19th century and growing awareness of the inequality of women within society. The persistence and determination of such women was central to the implementation of registration for midwives with the 1902 Midwives Act and the recognition of the need for improved health services for women and children. A number of these women were childless and it is of interest that they chose this course at a time when social pressures on women were more towards taking a place in society and achieving a 'good' marriage. Some of these pioneering women rejected the future planned for them as socialites and encouraged other prominent members of society to pay attention to the needs of lower class women and the influence of poverty upon these women's lives. This was within the context of growing awareness of social injustices and a political background for social change. However, although it was women who were the main protagonists for change and the need for a standardised education and training for midwives, the examination and regulation of this were dominated by medical men and other contemporary male figures of authority (Donnison 1988).

The registration of midwives involved a programme of training for existing lay midwives and the movement towards professional recognition. The activities of the monthly nurse who attended the woman after childbirth were clearly defined as giving support and care to the newly delivered woman and her family. The duties of the midwife at this time included domestic chores as well as administering to the health and well-being of the new mother and her infant (Central Midwives Board 1919).

Such care and attention may have reduced some of the morbidity but the majority of the conditions that led to postpartum mortality were improved with the introduction of blood transfusions and the use of antibiotics in the late 1930s (Loudon 1986, 1987). Midwives were generally paid as independent practitioners, only calling doctors to attend when needed, sometimes being required to pay for their services themselves. Improved nutrition in the population also meant that women approached childbirth in a better state of health than formerly and all this contributed to a reduction in maternal deaths by the time the NHS was introduced in 1948. However, by then the pattern of postpartum care was well established and women were attended by a qualified midwife for the birth and for a defined period after this (Central Midwives Board 1951). Midwifery was an all-female profession at that time and midwives were seen as valued members of the community and wore a distinctive regulated uniform, usually but not always different from the district nursing sisters. District midwives were responsible for the majority of births that occurred in the woman's home and care of the woman and her new baby afterwards. With the introduction of the NHS, women no longer had to pay for the services of the doctor or the midwife and the domiciliary services were made available through the local council. This often included accommodation in the community for the midwife.

The format of postpartum care over this period was designed to identify impending morbidity and pathological conditions as it was these outcomes that had the most impact for society. Developments in maternity care and new treatments for pathological conditions resulted in fewer women encountering such severe pathological disease after childbirth. However, women continued to experience a range of morbidity related to the events of the birth, for example anaemia, pain from perineal sutures, urinary dysfunction and backache, but such outcomes were viewed as minor and to be expected (Glazener et al 1995, McArthur et al 1991). With the emerging freedom of speech and a greater political voice, women themselves began to question the extent of such morbidity and the role of postpartum care in relation to it. What was the midwife doing and what help was there for the new mother in postpartum recovery, infant feeding and childcare?

MIDWIVES AND POSTPARTUM CARE

Midwives were slow to engage with this debate, although the majority of midwives are women and likely to have experienced motherhood themselves. It is of interest that one of the initial articles in the midwifery press discussing the contemporary pattern of postnatal care was written by a male midwife (Lewis 1987).

Alongside the role of women in society in general, the demographic background relating to the midwifery profession has also changed over the past 100 years. In the past, prior to the registration period, the majority of midwives would have been uneducated women from the local community who took a small wage to act as midwife. The new mother was cared for mainly by family members and other women in the community. Legislation requiring midwives to be formally registered raised the status of midwifery as a professional occupation for women who had an appropriate level of education and had undergone a structured training course. This meant that the existing midwives were increasingly supplanted by women who were more often from a middle- or upper-class background. These women were much less likely to be mothers themselves, choosing midwifery instead as a 'career' until they were married. It was not expected that they would continue working as a midwife once they were married.

The celibate midwife who was employed to work within a community setting may have had much to offer women from the point of view of access and continuity of care. It was expected that the midwife would be freely available and 'on call' for the women in the community in return for a wage and often accommodation. With the emancipation of women from the confines of being a wife only within a marriage and, within the profession, the acceptance of married women as employees, the nature of the relationship between mother and midwife needed to change. The movement of birth into hospital also changed the working practices of the majority of midwives to an institutionalised form of employment where work was shared amongst a shift system, reducing the capacity for continuity between the women and the midwives caring for them. Such changes have meant that midwifery practice moved away from being the supporter and carer of the mother to one of mainly monitoring for signs of maternal or infant ill health within an illness model. It is therefore arguable that at this point we lost the sense of caring motherliness towards the new mother, alongside a sharing of the reality of motherhood in relation to selflessness and responsibility.

HEALTH ISSUES

The initiation of the Parliamentary Health Committee investigation into women's health during pregnancy and childbirth was in itself a major step in revision of care for women (Department of Health 1993). The key political figures who were active at this time must be acknowledged as part of this programme of reform. Without such advocates as Baroness Cumberlege and vocal and constructive women Members of Parliament, the process of change might have been very different. It is of interest to note that at this time, the UK's Prime Minister was a woman who had achieved an outstanding professional position as well as being a mother, not to just one child but to twins.

Key advocates within the midwifery profession have done much to support the emerging voice of women, heard initially through the *Changing Childbirth* document (Department of Health 1993) but then increasingly via lay organisations such as the National Childbirth Trust. Where midwives have collaborated with such organisations, the voice of women cannot fail to be powerful, socially and politically. However, at the point of delivery of care, midwifery has not necessarily taken the same route and women continue to be disappointed and critical of their care once the baby has been born. Extracts from the Audit Commission survey *First Class Delivery* should make midwifery bow its head in shame at the lack of care and support shown by some midwives to vulnerable women. Midwives, in their defence, suggest that, particularly with regard to postnatal care, the lack of resources, in the form of more midwives, is to blame for the fragmented and hurried postnatal care women experience particularly within a hospital environment. However, on closer scrutiny, it is perhaps more the very pattern of care that appears to ignore the individual needs of women. Observers and contributors to current postnatal care would describe midwives as still being more concerned to be 'doing to' rather than 'doing for' women within the relationship of giving and receiving care (McLoughlin 1997, Raftos et al 1997).

Salmon (1999) gives a vivid account of women's experiences of perineal pain and trauma in a study that was analysed from a feminist perspective. Salmon's work explored the views of six women whose ages ranged from 25 to 40 years and whose experiences of perineal trauma varied from within 12 to up to 60 months prior to the interview. Where the suturing was undertaken by male doctors, the dominant doctor–patient relationship left women vulnerable and less able to verbalise their feelings about pain or distress. This also occurred where midwives were considered by the women to have greater knowledge than they had, that the midwife knew best, suggesting that where the midwives expressed a view that nothing was wrong, this must be true despite a woman's experiences of pain or discomfort (Bluff & Holloway 1994). The findings suggest that the women had difficulty expressing their views or, if they did, getting them heard and that there was an overall lack of information and advice available for the women about issues of perineal trauma and repair.

Salmon identifies that women's accounts are not valued as reliable by healthcare professionals as a source of legitimate knowledge. It is argued that the women's knowledge is inferior to that gained from textbooks and other conventional sources used within health professional education. Of concern here is the implied suggestion that women cannot therefore be relied upon to know how their own bodies normally function and feel. More important, perhaps, is the view that some discomfort or even pain is to be 'expected' after childbirth but that no values or description are identified for this. That midwives are also collaborating with the general devaluation and marginalisation of women's health by society by failing to initiate more enquiry into these areas suggests that midwifery has lost focus with regards to being 'with women' and has become largely dominated by a male and medical view. It

is ironic if the outcome of continuing educational opportunities for midwives, over time, is the devaluing of qualities more aligned to intuition and empathy, a point also noted by Walsh (2000).

It is only comparatively recently that a woman has had any access to the information recorded about her and her baby during her contact with the maternity services. The context within which such a framework of care existed was not only not challenged by midwives but was to some extent actively resisted as midwives did not consider women were competent to own and be involved in their own care (McGeown & Gardosi 2002). Kirkham (1999) explores the place of the midwife within a professional hierarchy, noting that midwives' loyalty can be greater towards their profession than to the women in their care. In a study about the culture of midwifery in the NHS in England, Kirkham identified that midwives appear to be oppressed as a profession, as a result of domination from the still mainly male medical profession over one that is predominantly female. Kirkham reviews the current context within which midwives work and identifies similar characteristics to other examples of oppression, where disempowering attitudes and values overwhelm those of support and encouragement. Such factors are considered to limit the potential for midwives to improve their working conditions or to substantially change this culture as they are resigned to failure or cannot see change as progression. She notes that midwives demonstrate resigned acceptance of their lot as women and that feelings of helplessness, low expectations and self-blame are common. Attitudes were noted that centred on the midwives' use of self. These ranged from self-blame, where there was an inclination to blame themselves for errors or outcomes regardless of the conditions within which they were working at the time, to identifying other colleagues as selfish for wanting better or different conditions of work and self-sacrifice, making their own (or their families') needs take a lesser role than the needs of the midwifery service. Such factors are not unique to midwives and have been identified as characteristics of women in society in general, suggesting that women are themselves party to their own oppression (Coward 1992).

Such aspects all contribute to the overall status of women in society regardless of whether they are in receipt of or providing assistance or care. Raftos et al (1997) reviewed 21 articles indexed in the CINAHL database from 1993 to 1995 to explore the concept of 'women's health' from a feminist perspective. The majority of the articles were American and four were specifically related to child bearing or motherhood. Women's health was found to be rarely identified holistically but rather as fragmented areas related to a woman's body functions; for example, in relation to reproductive, maternal, family and neonatal health. This was seen as a narrow perspective which incorporated stereotypical views and was biased in favour of a biomedical focus, being disease or problem led. Women were depicted as passive and silent bystanders rather than being the focus of many of the papers. The reviewers note that: 'In many cases, the woman may well not have been there. Indeed, in many papers she was rendered totally invisible (or at best peripheral) to the issue of concern'.

The relevance of health professionals' attitudes to the management of the midwifery services and provision of care for postpartum women must centre around the social position of women within our culture. With regard to clinical care, the whole emphasis of postpartum observations is on the midwife asking questions and undertaking observations on the postpartum woman and her baby. This may have evolved from an initial wish to nurture women back to health after the experiences and dangers of childbirth but appears to have dissolved into a routinised assessment of key factors without any real understanding or knowledge of the normal range for many of these. This again reflects the lack of women's involvement in enquiry and understanding of their own bodies so that they may seek help from others or choose to alter their own lifestyle where this might be necessary.

BREASTFEEDING

Within the constraints of this chapter, it is not possible to explore in any depth specific implications related to feminist theories and women's

choices for feeding their baby (see Chapter 7 for a fuller discussion). It is intended to give a short review of the main factors that appear to face women and midwives in the current context of care.

Breasts are inextricably linked with sex as sexual characteristics. Therefore the significance of this function within any relationship is likely to be affected during pregnancy and postpartum. Society continues to give women conflicting messages about the importance of breastfeeding to infant nutrition and the baby's overall health and yet there is a reluctance to make improvements to enable women who choose to breastfeed to do this with greater societal acceptance. The increased involvement of men in childcare might also have a part to play in some women's confusion over their choice of how to feed their baby. A desire by the partner to share in childcare cannot be total when the baby is breastfed and the total dependence of the breastfed baby on the new mother can be onerous, whereas feeds for a bottle-fed baby can be shared about. Another aspect of breastfeeding that needs reflection is the value given to words such as successful and failure for women who are breastfeeding. Women themselves are liable to attribute these values to the experience and it would be prudent to review the context in which breastfeeding is supported by other female family members.

WHAT CAN MIDWIVES DO?

Increasingly over the past few years, research into women's satisfaction with postpartum services has demonstrated a yawning gap between the intention and the provision of care. Midwives' perception of care has tended to continue along the lines of tasks that identify mainly physical morbidity regardless of a woman's emotional or social needs. This can be seen in the range of research projects that have explored important questions to assist midwives to compile a framework of evidence for practice. This could still be said to fall short of extensively involving both women and clinical midwives to set such an agenda more proactively. Women have increasingly voiced a need for more information and support in order to make the best choices in their new role as a mother, for themselves, their new infant and the family as a whole (Proctor 1999).

Where the women's movement engaged in issues of women's health, motherhood and childbirth were high on the list. Women wanted to have a better experience and to be mothers on their own terms, not in terms of what society considered was good enough for them. For example, consider that only in the past few years, with the introduction of the Child Support Act, has society placed an obligation on the father to make provision for his child and that this approach has not been entirely successful.

The midwifery profession has increasingly seen the need to work more closely with other professional and statutory bodies and lay, self-help groups. The majority of women now receive postpartum care in their own home in their community. Interagency relationships are essential if women's needs are to be identified and met within the social structure and some midwifery services are undertaking important work in this area. Within this ongoing work it is argued that there is an even stronger need for the midwifery profession to address the balance between carer and client. Where the midwife continues to give professional status and knowledge higher status this will reinforce as inferior the place of the postpartum mother. Where the midwife works alongside the mother as advocate and professional friend, much more might be achieved, to the benefit of the service and the individuals. Examples of such an approach can be seen in projects where midwives have identified the need to support women in situations of domestic violence or psychological distress following unexpected events at or around the birth. The extent to which midwives as women will feel able to take part in this aspect of care is still subject to question but the acknowledgement that it is within the remit of midwifery care is of great importance to the place of women in society (Steen & Bharj 2003).

What has been demonstrated in the past as significant discord between the provision of midwifery services and women's postpartum needs will only begin to resolve where midwives treat women as individuals and they are seen as the pivot around which all care needs are organised. Midwives should be involved and active in such change as many are themselves working women who have undertaken educational courses as mature students to become midwives and should be sympathetic and articulate advocates for women in this. Such changes could contribute to women and midwives working together to raise the political status of care after birth and fundamentally alter the context within which postpartum care is undertaken.

Key points

- The changing role of women in society has affected the identity of women and the status of motherhood.

- Contemporary postpartum midwifery care is struggling to keep up with the changing needs of women after birth and to provide women with appropriate support.

- This is further hampered by the continued low status in which postpartum care is viewed by the allocation of resources into maternity services and by society in general.

- There is an increasing dilemma for female midwives who support women in their role as mothers but where they are simultaneously expected to maintain standards of excellence themselves as both a woman and a mother as measured by 'social conscience'.

Questions for Reflection

These are questions that challenge whether midwives should be undertaking postnatal care in its current form at all or whether other healthcare workers could do this just as well. Finding a reason for your existence is a good way to raise your self-esteem and, hopefully, that of postnatal care. Therefore, the more annoyed you are about the above proposal, the more benefit you are likely to gain from this exercise.

Just take a few minutes for private reflection on the following questions. They should act as prompts for further thought or you might want to use some of them for group discussion if you are thinking of reviewing your postpartum services.

Do you enjoy caring for postpartum women in both hospital and community settings? If there are differences between your response for either setting or this aspect of midwifery is not enjoyable, why might that be?

What do you see as the essential aspects of postpartum care? Can you still achieve these all the time or do you have to make choices that are detrimental to the care you feel women should be receiving?

What about your colleagues? If you were asked about the standard of care given to postpartum women by other midwives in your trust, do you feel you give 'better' care than some other midwives? If so, can you explore what makes it better?

If the postpartum care part of your job was undertaken by a non-midwife/healthcare worker, how would you feel about this?

REFERENCES

Abbott P, Wallace C 1996 An introduction to sociology: a feminist perspective. Routledge, London

Alibhai-Brown Y 1999 Alien. In: Cole C, Windrath H (eds) The female odyssey. Women's Press, London, p 40–45

Barclay I, Lupton D 1999 The experience of new fatherhood: a socio-cultural analysis. Journal of Advanced Nursing 29(4): 1013–1020

Bluff R, Holloway I 1994 They know best. Women's perceptions of midwifery care during labour and childbirth. Midwifery 10(3): 157–164

Central Midwives Board 1919 Handbook incorporating the rules of the Central Midwives Board, 5th edn. Central Midwives Board, London

Central Midwives Board 1951 Handbook incorporating the rules of the Central Midwives Board, 20th edn. Central Midwives Board, London

Coward R 1992 Women lash back in anger. The Guardian, March 24, p21

Cowell B, Wainwright D 1991 Behind the blue door – a history of the Royal College of Midwives 1881–1991. Baillière Tindall, London

Crowley H, Hemmelweit S 1992 Knowing women: feminism and knowledge. Polity Press, Cambridge p 11–46, 153–169

Department of Health 1993 Changing childbirth – report of the expert maternity group. HMSO, London

Donnison J 1988 Midwives and medical men. Historical Publications, Hertfordshire

Garcia J, Marchant S 1996 The potential of postnatal care. In: Kroll D (ed) Issues in midwifery care for the future. Baillière Tindall, London, p 58–74

Garcia J, Redshaw M, Fitzsimmons B, Keene J 1998 Audit Commission/National Perinatal Epidemiology Unit. First class delivery. A national survey of women's views of maternity care. Audit Commission Publications, Abingdon, p 30, 51

Giddons A 1993 Sociology, 2nd edn. Blackwell, Oxford

Gjerdingen D, McGovern P, Bakker M et al 2000 Employment and women's work. Women and Health 31(4): 1–20

Glazener C, Abdalla M, Stroud P, Naji S, Templeton A, Russell I 1995 Postnatal maternal morbidity: extent, causes, prevention and treatment. British Journal of Obstetrics and Gynaecology 102(4): 282–287

Glazener CMA, MacArthur C, Garcia J 1993 Postnatal care: time for a change. Contemporary Review of Obstetrics and Gynaecology 5: 130–136

Gowdridge C, Williams AS Wynn M (eds) 1997 Mother courage: letters from mothers in poverty at the end of the century. Penguin, London

Holdsworth A 1988 Out of the doll's house – the story of women in the twentieth century. BBC Enterprises, London

Hunt S, Symonds A 1995 The social meaning of midwifery. Macmillan, London

Jacobs SC 1997 Employment changes over childbirth. A retrospective review. Sociology 31: 577–590

Jorgensen N, Bird J, Heyhoe A et al 1997 Sociology – an interactive approach. HarperCollins, London

Kirkham M 1999 The culture of midwifery in the National Health Service in England. Journal of Advanced Nursing 30 (3): 732–739

Lewis P 1987 The discharge of mothers by midwives. Midwives Chronicle and Nursing Notes January: 16–18

Llewelyn-Davies M (ed) 1991 Life as we have known it. Virago Press, London, p 46–55

Loudon I 1986 Obstetric care, social class, and maternal mortality. British Medical Journal 293: 606–608

Loudon I 1987 Puerperal fever, the streptococcus, and the sulphonamides, 1911–1945. British Medical Journal 295: 485–490

Lovenduski Randall V 1993 Contemporary feminist politics: women and power in Britain. Oxford University Press, Oxford

MacArthur C, Lewis M, Knox G 1991 Health after childbirth: an investigation of long term health problems beginning after childbirth in 11 701 women. HMSO, London

McGeown P, Gardosi J 2002 New pregnancy notes: let us have your views. British Journal of Midwifery 10(5): 260–261

McLoughlin A 1997 The 'F' factor: feminism forsaken? Nurse Education Today 17: 111–114

Messenger-Davies M, Mosdell N 2001 Unconsenting children – the use of children in television reality programmes. School of Journalism, Media and Cultural Studies, Cardiff University, Cardiff

Murray J 1999 Men's Lib for the millennium In: Cole C, Windrath H (eds) The female odyssey. Women's Press, London

Oakley A 1980 Women confined. Martin Robertson, London

Parsons T 1951 The social system. Free Press, New York, p 229

Phoenix A, Woollett A, Lloyd A (eds) 1991 Motherhood: meanings, practices and ideologies. Sage, London

Price J 1988 Motherhood: what it does to your mind. Pandora Press, London, ch 8, 10

Proctor S 1999 Women's reactions to their experience of maternity care. British Journal of Midwifery 7(8): 492–498

Raftos M, Mannix J, Jackson D 1997 More than motherhood? A feminist exploration of 'women's health' in papers indexed by CINAHL 1993–1995. Journal of Advanced Nursing 26: 1142–1149

Salmon D 1999 A feminist analysis of women's experiences of perineal trauma in the immediate post-delivery period. Midwifery 15: 247–256

Steen M, Bharj K 2003 Midwives' reflections exploring attitudes, feelings and experiences when caring for women who have been abused. MIDIRS Midwifery Digest 13(1): 115–118

Symonds A, Hunt S 1996 The midwife and society. Macmillan, London, p 101–123

Times 2002 Jailing of truants' mother sends the right message. May 14th, p7

Walsh D 1997 Hospital postnatal care: the end is nigh. British Journal of Midwifery 5(9): 516–518

Walsh D 2000 Perineal care should be a feminist issue. British Journal of Midwifery 8(12): 731–737

7

Feminism and breastfeeding

Gabrielle Palmer

Feminism encourages women to leave their husbands, kill their children, practice witchcraft, destroy capitalism and become lesbians. (Pat Robertson, US politician 1992)

INTRODUCTION

I ask my confident young neighbour, Alison, a mother of two, what she thinks about feminism and breastfeeding and she replies: 'I don't really know what feminism is'. Alison has been able to plan her life, her births and her career in such a way that she can enjoy motherhood, breastfeeding and the return to paid work. As we talk, another young woman, Amina Lawal, has her sentence of death by stoning upheld. She has been convicted of the crime of giving birth to a baby by an allegedly adulterous relationship. Islamic Sharia law functions in Funtua, Katsina State, in Nigeria where Amina lives and adultery is punishable by death. Amina's baby is proof that she is guilty but there is no such concrete evidence to prove the father's guilt so he goes free. You do not need to know the term feminism to know that this is unjust. Amina was not killed immediately. Whatever her crime, Islamic teaching states that a mother must not be separated from her baby until after she has stopped breastfeeding (McGreal 2002). Can we rejoice in the fact that breastfeeding is so valued and takes priority over punishment?

Much of the control that Alison has over her life has come through years of struggle by generations of women and those rare men who supported them. Maybe it is a sign of progress that many young British women are oblivious of the struggles for women's rights and that the word feminism is meaningless to them. The majority of women are not so free, including women in our supposedly equal society. If Alison had to survive financially on casual employment as a night office cleaner, she might have found breastfeeding difficult to maintain and might have been discouraged from starting. If Amina had resided in another state in Nigeria she might have avoided her ordeal, but baby milk company promotion might have influenced her to stop breastfeeding and her baby might have died. A slogan of feminist thinking of the 1970s was that 'the personal is political'. Both Alison's and Amina's personal lives are shaped by the politics and cultures of the societies in which they live.

The development of human rights legislation and political moves to combat discrimination against women are shunting slowly forward. Many politicians at least pay lip service to women's rights. However, until and unless women have real confidence in themselves and their own bodies, they will feel impeded, not empowered, by their reproductive abilities. The fear of childbirth that leads women to submit to overzealous medical interventions is founded on the fact that a minority of women and their babies might be at risk if they have no access to skilled help. Breastfeeding carries no such risk, indeed it is beneficial for women's health, yet vast numbers of women do not believe that their bodies can function well enough to sustain their babies' lives. The practices and attitudes which maintain this lack of confidence still flourish.

In this chapter I want to show you why I believe breastfeeding is a key feminist issue. Feminism means different things to different people, as the words of Pat Robertson, quoted above, show rather vividly. Key feminist writers have analysed the different approaches to women's bodies and present their own differing approaches (Tong 1998). Astonishingly, breastfeeding is mostly ignored by feminist scholars. It may be linked in a general way to motherhood, to be celebrated or derided, but the subject is absent from most books of feminist discussion. The word 'breast' is far more often indexed or mentioned in relation to breast cancer or surgery than to breastfeeding. How strange that

so many women thinkers view the breast mostly in terms of its vulnerability and not of its power.

You will learn much about feminism from the other chapters in this book and I will give you my perspective. My focus is simple: women suffer injustice and discrimination because they are the sex which creates new life, gives birth and produces milk. Even women who avoid or do not have these experiences suffer the spin-off discrimination simply because they are female.

In the 21st century, women are more or less accepted into male-dominated society but if they give birth, everything shifts and it is usually viewed as an impediment to that god of our times, the economy. Even more than birth, breastfeeding is seen as disruptive to 'normal' life. Theoretically it is viewed as a good thing but its practice is still unaccepted as an essential, necessary, everyday event such as coffee drinking, eating or driving a car. In the British Parliament in the late 1990s, the Speaker (a woman) of the House of Commons forbade politicians to breastfeed their babies in the committee rooms. What does this action say about attitudes to the urgent needs of babies and the status of women, if this denial of rights can be imposed on our representatives?

In the UK only a quarter of babies are breastfeeding at 3 months, in contrast to over 80% in Norway. Finland and Sweden have similar figures (WHO/UNICEF 2000a). Women in these countries have greater equality than in the UK and the rise in breastfeeding matches their rise in power. In 1999 Sweden became the first government to have a majority of female ministers (Seager 2003). Norway is introducing regulations for companies to have at least 40% of women in their boardrooms (Osborn 2002). Scandinavian culture celebrates pride in breastfeeding alongside commitment to further progress in increasing women's economic and political power and sees no contradiction between a complete experience of motherhood and a career which fulfils each woman's potential. Indeed, those countries view both women's equality and the optimum nutrition of babies as essential for sustaining prosperity. They therefore plan working conditions to accommodate all aspects of parenthood.

The feminist economist Marilyn Waring (1989), in her brilliant book *If Women Counted*, describes how economic accounting systems ignore women's major contribution to the global economy. If a woman grows and processes food to feed her family (as millions do) that does not count in national economic data; if processed in a factory, it does. Few people in our country view breastfeeding a baby as a contribution to society's prosperity. Many, even women themselves, do not view breastfeeding as time spent working. In every country, at every level, women are poorer than the men, even though they work longer hours (Egan & Robidoux 2001). As the sex with the impressive power to reproduce and sustain human life, why are they the most disadvantaged? A creature from another planet visiting the Earth might ask, 'If women are the ones that keep the human race going, why do they get the rough deal?' Women produce a miracle fluid which provides complete nutrition for the first 6 months of human life and about half to one-third of nutrients for a child for 2 or 3 years. This fluid contains more effective disease-fighting components than any super drug produced by a pharmaceutical company. Unlike a sportswoman who needs years of training, an ideal diet and extra talent to win medals, almost all women can produce enough milk for more than one baby even in the most adverse conditions.* Women can re-establish lactation years after stopping lactation (WHO 1998a). Women who have never given birth have fed their adopted babies (Elia 1991). Lactation can continue successfully long after the menopause** without any hormonal manipulation. This is 'girl power' indeed, yet many women never feel this power or rejoice in it.

During the past century, male experts have downplayed the miracle of breastfeeding and led thousands to believe that their bodies could not function. Both doctors and manufacturers of artificial baby milk grew wealthy through the exploitation of created inadequacy. Sadly many women involved in the support of new mothers colluded with this denial and destruction of female power. Midwives are in a position to rekindle that sense

of power and to take pride in this subtle skill. They can also undermine women through their own doubts and mixed feelings. No-one has the right to coerce women to breastfeed and any pressure at a personal level is counterproductive. International human rights documents implicitly acknowledge the right of women to choose to breastfeed and the right of parents to have information about breastfeeding (ILO 2000, UN 1979, 1989). This right is violated everywhere through harmful practices in health systems and the community and through widespread subtle commercial tactics (WHO/UNICEF 1990).

No woman has a true choice if artificial feeding is presented as easy and breastfeeding made difficult. Women have the right to choose not to breastfeed but this must be an informed choice. Parents and health professionals need to know that the artificially fed baby requires more medical surveillance because of the greater risk of infection and disease that accompanies this feeding method. There is a tightly spun web of misunderstanding that binds health provision with the vested interests of the baby food companies (Palmer 1993). Why are women not rich through their production of a unique and life-saving substance that outdoes any pharmaceutical or nutritional manufactured product? Why do breastmilk banks struggle to stay funded when the product they provide is far superior to anything produced by an artificial baby milk manufacturer? Why do we have to invest effort in promoting a normal physiological activity? Do we have study days on 'How to promote and protect walking'?

DOES BREASTFEEDING MATTER?

Breastfeeding is a matter of life and death for most babies, because most babies are born into poverty (WHO 2000b). It is a matter of sickness and health for all babies, including the minority who are born into wealth (Howie et al 1990)*. All over the world, poor women deliver a product to their babies which is superior to anything a billionaire could

---

*In a Japanese internment camp in Malaya during the Second World War, undernourished internees gave birth to and breastfed 20 babies, all of whom survived to healthy adulthood. See Palmer 1993, p209.
**In many traditional societies (where menopause occurs earlier), grandmothers breastfeed orphaned grandchildren.

---

*Most human beings (around 80%) are born into poverty. About one-fifth of the human race (1.2 billion people) live on less than a dollar a day. In these conditions not to be breastfeed means, at the very least, severe illness and malnutrition, and usually death.

buy for her child. The causes of infant disease and death are multifactorial so, of course, a breastfed baby may die but her risk of death is far lower than that of an artificially fed baby.

The World Health Organisation (WHO) analysed data from around the world to assess the effect of breastfeeding on survival. They found that in the first 2 months of life, a baby was six times more likely to die if she were not breastfed. Most deaths were due to acute respiratory infection and diarrhoea, but other infections and non-infectious disease contributed to the toll. The risk of death lessens as babies get older but still in the second year of life, a baby who is not breastfed doubles his risk of death. Pakistan had the highest risk (WHO 2000b). Most Pakistani women cannot read the instructions on a tin and live in conditions where it is unsafe to attempt artificial feeding, yet the big transnational companies make Pakistan a focus of the aggressive marketing of artificial baby milks, foods, feeding bottles and teats. These products are pushed at mothers, mainly through health professionals (The Network 1998). The very act of being given, or advised to use, a replacement for her own breastmilk will shatter the floundering confidence of any woman. If she has a breastfeeding problem, such as poor attachment or low milk supply, the use of the product will hasten the end of lactation and result in her baby's illness and often death. Pakistan has one of the world's highest infant, young child and maternal mortality rates and it has recently (2002) passed a law to implement the International Code of Marketing of Breastmilk Substitutes to control the flood of promotion but the law contains weaknesses which undermine its purpose. The baby food companies lobbied the government energetically during the law's drafting process.

It is well known that breastfeeding significantly protects against the commonest causes of infant illness and death such as gastroenteritis and acute respiratory infection. It is less well known that infant feeding affects long-term health. The risk of developing childhood diabetes is far higher if a baby is not breastfed (American Academy of Pediatrics 1994, McKinney et al 1999); so too with certain childhood cancers (Davis 1998). Breastfeeding protects against later obesity (Von Kries et al

1999), hypertension in adulthood (Roberts 2001), malocclusion and the need for expensive dentistry (Palmer 1998). A breastfed baby may be different immunologically for her entire lifetime (Hanson 1999). Out of hundreds of special qualities about breastfeeding, the fact that amazes me most is that a kidney transplant will be more successful if the recipient was breastfed and even more so if the donor was a breastfed sibling (Kois 1984). I could go on about benefits for the whole chapter, but have just picked a few at random.

How many women know that breastfeeding protects their own health? The more a woman has breastfed, the lower her risk of breast cancer (Collaborative Group 2002). Breast cancer is the commonest cancer among women, with a global increase of 26% since 1980 and over half the cases are among the fifth of the world's women who live in Europe and North America (Seager 2003). Breastfeeding may protect against osteoporosis and hip fractures in later life and the development of heart disease and diabetes. There is evidence of reduced risk of ovarian and endometrial cancers (Heinig & Dewey 1997).

Worldwide, more conceptions are prevented through breastfeeding than by all use of modern contraceptive methods. The lactational amenorrhoea method (LAM) is as effective as conventional contraception during the first 6 months after birth, as long as a woman does not menstruate and fully breastfeeds (Labbock 1994). Though the risk of conception increases over time, protection can last into the second year. LAM can be a life saver for women in poor regions who have inadequate access to family planning services. Closely spaced births increase the risk of death for a mother, her new baby and her toddler. When misguided charities send artificial baby milks to a disaster area (such as earthquake, war or famine), besides risking infant death they jeopardise a woman's life through increasing her chance of untimely pregnancy.

It is now widely known that breastfeeding by an HIV-positive mother may transmit the virus to the baby. In the creation of policies concerning the transmission of HIV through breastfeeding, policy makers have had to weigh up several risks. They know that an artificially fed baby is more likely to die of infections and that refraining from breastfeeding increases a woman's risk of pregnancy that would stress her already vulnerable body (UNICEF 1998). Despite the risk of HIV transmission, approximately 85% of HIV-positive women who have breastfed have not transmitted the virus, probably because breastmilk contains factors which combat HIV (Miller et al 2002). Researchers are trying to discover why some women transmit and others do not. Women who breastfeed exclusively are less likely to pass on the virus to their babies. HIV-positive women have the right to make their own infant-feeding decisions according to circumstances and they need support and information to do this. In regions where HIV is commonest, such as Sub-Saharan Africa, more infants are likely to die from artificial feeding than from being breastfed by their HIV-positive mothers (Coutsoudis et al 2002).

ATTITUDES TO RISK

Information about breastfeeding can make people feel angry, guilty or upset and consequently evidence is ignored, denied or even censored. Health professionals routinely communicate the painful facts about the risks of smoking to a pregnant woman. Why do many avoid giving facts about the risks of artificial feeding, even if they know them? Communication skills do not come easily and many health professionals may not have adequate training to deliver health messages tactfully and effectively. Most health decisions are, in the end, taken by the individual and it is well known that receiving information does not always lead to behaviour change so why do so many health professionals censor the facts about artificial feeding (Fleming 2002).

The perils of smoking are clear, yet despite the statistical evidence, people will think of their granny who smoked until 90 with impunity and hope they too will be a lucky exception. Risk assessment is hard to grasp. Why do we fear flying and yet travel blithely in cars, which are far more likely to kill us? Nothing is certain and most of us have a streak of fatalism. Artificial feeding is a less clearcut risk because we believe that any milk is better than no milk at all. Artificial milk can save lives. There will always be some need for

replacement feeding. Other products mimic body fluids and can save lives but they are treated with caution. Artificial insulin is a replacement body fluid which saves the lives of diabetics. Nevertheless, we would not dream of promoting its use as a 'lifestyle choice'. Insulin has negative effects and avoiding or minimising its use is a priority in the management of all types of diabetes. If health protection is our priority we should view the replacement of breastmilk with equal caution.

Most, but not all, babies born into societies like Britain can withstand the risks of artificial feeding. Safe water, sanitation, better housing, education and health services are keys to survival. Our National Health Service (NHS) mops up the results of faulty early feeding. We know thousands of people (including perhaps ourselves) who were artificially fed and are alive and kicking. We rarely consider that their high blood pressure or obesity might have been triggered in infancy. If we suspect this we are too polite to say so. It is only recent research, with improved methodology and clearer definitions of the different patterns of infant feeding, that has led to the discovery of the real impact of breastfeeding on health. There are big differences between the baby who gets a few weeks of breastfeeding together with artificial feeds, water or juices and the baby who is breastfed with no other fluid or food until 6 months and continues breastfeeding after solid foods are introduced. There are many reasons for illness and death and even the breastfed are mortal. What we must question is why the same burden of proof has not been demanded of breastmilk substitutes as has been of breastmilk and women's bodies. We must also ask why an inferior product is promoted and used as the substitute for breastfeeding when maybe donated breastmilk, made safe through pasteurisation, should be the product of choice for babies who do not get their mothers' breastmilk.

Manufacturers who proclaim how close their product is to human milk based it on a rival product which they may have stolen. Most women donate their breastmilk and are delighted to know this saves infant lives, but they may be unaware of trends to exploit their gift for profit. Now products originally derived from human milk, such as lactoferrin or docasahexanoic acid (DHA), are patented and used by the pharmaceutical industry. Are the women who donated their breastmilk earning royalties? A company in California set up to commercialise the provision of donated breastmilk states in its application to the US Patent Office:

Furthermore, milk donors who have weaned their babies or have initiated lactation without pregnancy could feasibly become human labs, becoming exposed through any method to milk strains of disease and producing the appropriate antibody in their milk. Since the breast is reactive to new exposures of pathogens, an array of new immunities can be produced to combat such diseases. Whether these types of donors could produce enough milk to become a primary source remains to be seen, but at least these donors could provide a human lab for biosynthesizing disease specific antibodies that could be replicated later using other methods. (Agennix 2001)

While you ponder the ethics of using women as factory processing plants, we must ask whether the women donating the milk or the company directors are going to be millionaires.

BRITISH CULTURE

Despite the maxim that 'breast is best' few British people are aware that artificial feeding is a risk. It was mostly British 'experts' who introduced the damaging ideas which contributed to breastfeeding decline around the world (Palmer 1993). It was British health bodies who accepted artificial baby milk companies' money early in the 20th century. British doctors, nurses and midwives implemented practices, unknown in breastfeeding societies, which became the norm in most hospitals by the 1930s: '… sometimes you had quite a bit of difficulty getting the baby feeding … Then, we took the milk off with a pump, put it in a bottle and the baby would get breastmilk that way' (Reid 2000). As hospital deliveries increased, so did artificial feeding. Few connected the nipple washing, separation of mother and baby, strict routines and restricted time at the breast with the breastfeeding difficulties, pain and failure that became accepted as inevitable. We carry the social legacy of an experience which has hurt and dismayed thousands of women.

Our culture now presents breastfeeding as an issue of anxiety, ambivalence and even disgust. A study of attitudes to infant feeding as portrayed in the British media found that artificial feeding was represented as 'normal' whereas breastfeeding was discussed negatively in terms of problems or embarrassment or simply seen as comic (Henderson et al 2000). Dr Mavis Gunther's (1971) ground-breaking book, *Infant Feeding*, presented the physiological principles, showing how restricted feeding and poor attachment were key impediments to breastfeeding. We would laugh if we were still advised to wear boned corsets and lisle stockings like our great grandmothers yet, in the 21st century, hospitals still carry out the 1930s practices described above.

The most confident woman might find breastfeeding difficult when she has to run the gauntlet of misinformation and negative attitudes. Her workplace, her family and too often the health system are ill equipped to support her. Information is absent in school education. This particularly influences male attitudes, which often are influential on women's decisions. Mixed messages drive people crazy and it is no help if a blast of pro-breastfeeding propaganda is spread through a maternity unit or health clinic if most staff are unable to provide consistent information and support. If parents' magazines, commercial literature and the general media present artificial feeding as normal and easy and rarely refer to the risks then breastfeeding promotion is discredited. The fact that breastfeeding is seen to be something health professionals must facilitate shows how lost we are. We live in a culture of expertise and dare not suckle our babies without lessons and instructions. When the lessons themselves are inconsistent and the instructors poorly trained, no wonder women collapse.

Imagine a young man embarking upon his first attempt at sexual penetration. Ask him to set about this project in a special sex centre where there are 'experts' he has never met before, ready to supervise and tell him how it ought to be done. Presume that his partner is as inexperienced as himself and that he is asked if he is going to 'try and achieve an erection'. When he starts, a busy 'expert', who may never have personally experienced sexual relations, starts telling him how to do it and inspects his body with a critical expression, prodding him and his partner in an insensitive manner. By the bed is an artificial penis, put there, as the young man is told, 'just in case you can't manage it; many young men can't make it; it's not their fault, nature often fails!' (Palmer 1993)

The negative culture persists, for the most part, not because of lack of good intent from health and social support systems, but because the substitutes for breastmilk are so profitable. Part of these profits are fed back into British health professional bodies, thus keeping them docile and tactful. Even excluding the profits from sales of feeding bottles and related paraphernalia,* the 2001 global value of baby food sales reached US$16 453 million with a predicted 17% rise by 2005 to US$19 823 million. Infant formula accounts for 64% of global sales. In a society which puts the creation of financial wealth as its priority, as long as money can be made through women not breastfeeding, there will be an incentive to undermine their power to do so.

Physiologically more than 99% of women can breastfeed but the majority of babies in Britain are not breastfed for as long as their mothers wanted to. It is remarkable that when an infant death is reported in the media, few dare ask whether the baby was breastfed. We still think it might 'upset the mother', yet it is society as a whole that facilitates breastfeeding far more than an individual woman.

BIOLOGY

When an infant is ejected from the safe womb into the dangerous world outside, milk carries on the work of the placenta. Each mammal's milk is uniquely adapted to the needs of its young, its habitat and its behaviour. For example, a sea mammal, such as a seal, will produce high-fat milk (40–60% fat) for her baby who can gain 23 kg within days and start digesting fish within weeks. Sea mammals need vast amounts of fat

to create the 'blubber' which keeps them warm, stores energy and enables them to swim so skilfully. A seal must get back to sea to feed herself and her rich, fatty milk can sustain her baby for many hours between feeds.

In contrast, the higher primates, such as chimpanzees, produce low-fat, dilute milk designed for frequent feeding. Survival in forests depends on being lean and agile. Chimpanzees breastfeed for around 6–7 years as did our ancestors for the greater part of human life on earth (Dettwyler 1995a). Human milk is also designed for frequent feeding and is uniquely rich in constituents which optimise brain development (Crawford 2002). Jiggling about with the milk of other species in a laboratory cannot match millions of years of evolution.

European culture has been overinfluenced by that most unnatural of mammals, the cow. A modern dairy cow has been intensively bred to produce excessive milk. She needs constant supervision to prevent and cure lactation problems. Her calf could get ill or die if it drank all the milk available. Yet comparisons with cows' behaviour and nutrition still influence ideas about breastfeeding, with damaging consequences.

The 20th century could be characterised by a transition in attitudes to life on Earth. Early on, a dominant belief was that the conquest of nature through scientific discovery and technology would be society's salvation. This exultation in human power gradually transformed into a grudging respect for some of nature's gifts. By the end of the century, awareness of the crucial links between the balance of nature, the health of the planet and human beings had spread. There is argument about the scale of importance, but even the most cynical acknowledge that the natural world is relevant to human welfare and survival. Technology is not intrinsically bad but it can throw nature off balance and do harm.

In the late 1960s, the feminist writer Shulamith Firestone saw women's reproductive traits as the root of oppression and had a vision of a world where women would not need to bear or suckle children (Firestone 1970). Her ideas echoed Aldous Huxley's 1932 novel *Brave New World*, which envisaged with horror a society where

---

*BBC 1 Look East news had an item on the Avent factory. A director boasted that they distributed 20 million bottles a year, 80% of which went to 70 countries. This means that the bottles went to some countries where such feeding is impossible to do safely. When artificial feeding is necessary then cup feeding is recommended by UNICEF and other infant feeding experts. This TV item violated the International Code of Marketing of Breastmilk Substitutes.

babies were hatched in incubators and reared in communal nurseries. Huxley later feared his fantasy was nearing reality. 'Eco-feminists' do not see nature as the enemy, but believe that the only way not to destroy ourselves 'is to strengthen our relationships to each other and the non-human world' (Tong 1998). Both strands of thought co-exist in our society and therefore within the health system. Many women feel more secure with technical tools that 'manage' their reproductive experiences than feel trust in their own bodies. This tension between the implications of our primal animal natures and our sense of what it is to be human influences feelings about breastfeeding.

Television programmes on animal behaviour fascinate millions, especially when they show courtship, reproduction and parenting. The practitioner and writer on childbirth and breastfeeding, Michel Odent, claims that the fact that humans are mammals is accepted in the English-speaking countries as common sense: 'But if you express the same idea in France, even in the most cautious terms, you immediately get a dismayed response in a distinctly Voltairian* tone: "But we are not animals" ' (Odent 1992). Actually I suspect that we might not be as relaxed about our natures as he thinks, but British readers can enjoy the compliment. Michel Odent believes that birth is an involuntary process involving old, primitive, mammalian structures of the brain. He writes that: 'One cannot actively help a woman to give birth. The goal is to avoid disturbing her unnecessarily' (Odent 1992). This statement is also relevant to breastfeeding. Currently I observe that good intentions might lead to too much supervision of breastfeeding and a disregard for the environment before and around birth which interferes with the primal impulses of both a woman and her newborn.

Gorillas reared in captivity who have never witnessed mothering behaviour do not attempt to suckle their young, handle them ineptly and even abandon them. This suggests that breastfeeding is more learned behaviour than instinct for a mother.

Babies certainly have an instinct to suckle and if left to their own devices (Nissen et al 1997) and placed skin to skin, will find their mother's breast and suckle of their own accord (WHO 1998b). Women in so-called 'primitive' human societies are astonished at the idea of lactation failure (Palmer 1993). 'How could a woman be unable to breastfeed?' they ask, amazed, as we would be by someone unable to switch on a television. If you have always seen babies breastfeeding, why would you think that someone could not do this? There is a parallel when singing and dancing are part of everyday life and you just enjoy these activities, spontaneously. You may perfect a few techniques as you grow up, but the basic skills are planted without self-consciousness. I do not want to be overromantic about all traditional environments. In many agricultural societies women do the bulk of the work. The urgent seasonal pressures of sowing or harvesting can force women to restrict or substitute breastfeeding too early, leading to a cycle of infection and malnutrition. But most breastfeeding problems as we know them are associated with hospital delivery, the sustained promotion of artificial feeding and lack of skilled support.

The broad social/medical loss of confidence in breastfeeding has become entrenched in our culture, but a transformation of practices could help give women back the power that is their right. If women have complete confidence that they can breastfeed then they can choose freely to breastfeed or not. A current idea is that breastfeeding can only happen with a health professional's assistance and this concept may itself destroy women's confidence. We need to create an environment that allows breastfeeding to thrive and to end the old medical folklore, maintained in part by the interests of artificial baby milk manufacturers.

The Baby Friendly Hospital Initiative (BFHI; Box 7.1) is one initiative designed to dismantle the practices which damage women's confidence and stop their bodies working. Best practice firstly means 'do no harm'. The first hospital in the UK to request assessment of its practices in relation to 'The 10 steps for successful breastfeeding' (see Box 7.2) was in a deprived area where breastfeeding was alien to the culture of most women because no-one in their families and peer

---

*Voltaire (1694–1778) was a renowned French intellectual and writer who criticised his contemporary Rousseau for his 'attempt to turn us into beasts'.

Box 7.1 Baby Friendly Hospital Initiative

The Baby Friendly Hospital Initiative (BFHI) is a global campaign launched in 1991 by the United Nations Children's Fund (UNICEF) and the World Health Organisation (WHO). BFHI recognises that best practice in health services is crucial to the success of breastfeeding. Best practice is represented by the 10 steps to successful breastfeeding (see Box 7.2).

Box 7.2 The 10 steps for successful breastfeeding (WHO 1998b)

1. Have a written breastfeeding policy that is routinely communicated to all healthcare staff.
2. Train all healthcare staff in skills necessary to implement the policy.
3. Inform all pregnant women about the benefits and management of breastfeeding.
4. Help mothers initiate breastfeeding soon after birth.
5. Show mothers how to breastfeed and how to maintain lactation, even if they should be separated from their infants.
6. Give newborn infants no food or drink other than breastmilk, unless medically indicated.
7. Practise rooming in – allow mother and infants to remain together 24 hours a day.
8. Encourage breastfeeding on demand.
9. Give no artificial teats or dummies to breastfeeding infants.
10. Foster the establishment of breastfeeding support groups and refer mothers to them on discharge from the hospital or clinic.

groups breastfed. You have to be an exceptionally confident woman to behave differently from your friends and family. The Swedish midwife who was training the BFHI assessment team asked a woman in labour if she would be willing to have her baby put skin to skin and to follow his instinct to crawl up to her breast after delivery. The woman was willing but explained: 'I'm not planning to breastfeed'. The midwife replied: 'OK, but please may we just observe your baby's behaviour?'. The baby, left to his own devices, crawled up his mother's abdomen, found her breast and latched on, all in his own time. The team and the mother learned a lot from this baby. This woman, who had not breastfed her previous children and came from a bottlefeeding culture, was still joyfully breastfeeding her healthy son 8 months later. Biology can override culture.

HISTORY
The men who told us how our bodies worked

It is with great pleasure I see at last the preservation of children become the care of men of sense. In my opinion this business has been too long fatally left to the management of women, who cannot be supposed to have a proper knowledge to fit them for the task. (Dr William Cadogan: *Essay on the Nursing and Management of Children*, 1748)

Over recent centuries, we learned much about how our bodies work. Those who complain of the arrogance of medical culture need only live with someone on dialysis who undergoes a successful kidney transplant to modify their attitudes. Modern healthcare, despite its flaws, is on the whole a good thing. It works best as an adjunct to a sound public health infrastructure. Those of us who live in industrialised societies take for granted the sewerage system, water on tap and a consistent supply of energy. Housing, nutrition and healthcare improved dramatically during the 20th century. The low infant and child mortality rates and extended lifespans are a result of these improvements.

The acceleration of discovery and knowledge was led by men. Until the 20th century the majority of women had little access to education or participation in public life. The few who did participate were seldom taken seriously and often later excluded from the history books (Spender 1988). The care and support for mothers and babies carried out by ordinary women, midwives and healers was mostly ignored and often despised. Skilled midwives who saved lives and whose excellent records survived, such as the 18th century Frisian midwife Catharina Schrader (1987), never became famous and influential as male doctors did. A set of values and approaches became established that were essentially masculine. When women eventually, after great struggle, were accepted for medical training, they absorbed the values of the male doctors. Elizabeth Blackwell (1821–1910) was the world's first trained, registered woman doctor. She refused to speak at a women's rights convention because:

I believe that the chief source of the false position of women is the inefficiency of women themselves – the deplorable fact that they are so often careless mothers, weak wives, poor housekeepers, ignorant nurses and frivolous human beings. If they would perform with strength and wisdom the duties which lie immediately around them every sphere of life would soon be open to them. (Forster 1984)

Elizabeth Blackwell's intolerance and lack of empathy echo the attitudes of many male doctors of her time. Her stance is understandable when you read the account of what she had to endure to become a doctor. Elizabeth's achievements can be linked with 'liberal feminism' which tends to the view that if only individual women can enter the ranks of the male elite, then things will get better for all women. This is not true if the culture of that field is already so established that only particular types of women dare enter. In contrast, 'radical feminists' believe that the male-dominated systems that shape our world must be dismantled in order to achieve and fulfil women's rights (Tong 1998).

Many of today's breastfeeding problems come from the misunderstanding of women's bodies by male doctors in the 18th and 19th centuries. This might merely be of historical interest if it were not for the fact that their ideas persist to this day. They have had a profound effect on how women perceive their own bodies. These doctors did some good, but sadly their mistakes have been as influential as their wiser judgements. When someone is clever, there is a great tendency for people to believe that they get everything right and eventually they might believe it themselves. Let me first give an example of one male doctor's idea that deeply affected the lives of women. This is not to do with infant feeding but it illustrates the power of ideas to actually influence our bodies' functions.

The legacy of Dr Sigmund Freud's brilliant ideas

Dr Sigmund Freud (1856–1939) is renowned for creating psychoanalysis, a method of treating emotional, neurotic and mental disorders. His controversial theories had a great impact on ideas about human nature and society. Many of Freud's

concepts, such as the Oedipus complex*, the death wish, penis envy and phallic symbolism, have become familiar. The 20th century development of the professions of psychoanalysis, psychiatry and psychology and the acceptance that mental or neurotic illnesses are not the fault of the sufferers can be traced back to Freud. So hurray for Freud. But, like all great thinkers, his theories sometimes went down one track and forgot to come back.

Freudian theories are interesting, not least because they infuriate many women, and for years they were accepted as dogma in many schools of thought. One Freudian idea was that little boys and girls went through phases of sexually desiring their mothers. In simplistic terms, a little boy renounces his desire through fear that his father will cut off his penis and thereafter he identifies with his father. The little girl realises she does not have a penis so she turns away from her mother and develops a desire for her father. Because of our universal taboos on incest these desires must be suppressed. As I solemnly write about these theories, I want to shout out some joke about men being obsessed with their willies. There is now less reverence for Freud's theories and women thinkers especially have challenged them.

Freud's theory of penis envy glorified the penis as the mighty fulfiller of women's desires and also negated the clitoris as an important organ. The clitoris is homologous** to the penis; in other words, they developed from the same source. The human embryo has the equipment to develop either male or female characteristics. The genitalia look the same until the eighth week of gestation when different hormones (androgens) convert the basic embryonic structures into the glans penis, penis shaft and scrotum. Without these androgens they would become the clitoris, labia minora and labia majora. It is therefore unsurprising that the

---

*The term 'Oedipus complex' is based on the ancient Greek myth of Oedipus who, having been farmed out at birth, did not recognise his parents when he met them nor they him. He fell in love with his mother, killed his father, then married his mother. When he learned the truth about the kinship he put his own eyes out. Freud suggested that little children are in love with their parents.
**Homologous organs are those which have the same evolutionary origin, e.g. the flipper of a sea mammal might have the same origin as the limb of a land mammal.

clitoris is a source of sexual pleasure and its stimulation a key route for most women to achieve orgasm. It may surprise younger readers to know that this was a topic of dispute until research confirmed what, as the biologist Stephen Jay Gould (1995) wrote, 'Women have known since the dawn of time'. Kinsey in 1953, Masters and Johnson in 1969 and Shere Hite in 1981 all did extensive research and confirmed that most women found that clitoral stimulation was the route to joy.

Freud, however, had pondered the intricacies of the different sexes and decided that the clitoral orgasm was infantile and that feminine maturity was only achieved when the woman stopped having 'clitoral' orgasms and had 'vaginal' orgasms only. Why did this notion possess him? I do not know, but scholars of Freud may enlighten us. I always want to ask: 'Did Mrs Freud fake it?'. Stephen Jay Gould (1995) expresses the situation nicely:

Part of the reason must reside in simple male vanity. We (and I mean those of my sex, not the vague editorial pronoun) simply cannot abide the idea that a woman's sexual pleasure might not arise most reliably as a direct result of our own coital efforts.

Well, that was just a theory, so where is the harm? The fact is that Freud's theory of the immature, and therefore incorrect, orgasm was accepted into psychological orthodoxy and the idea infiltrated into relationships. Until the late 1960s, there was almost no good information about sexual techniques. Most women were ignorant about their bodies and men even more so; many did not even know about the existence of the clitoris. If couples suffered unfulfilling sex lives and consulted their doctors, women who could not achieve orgasm during sexual intercourse were labelled 'frigid'. Women who were aware of the Freudian theory feared they were 'immature' if they felt their orgasms were clitorally sourced. Freud's ideas were seen as enlightened reason but they were received into a society full of prejudice and superstition. Taboos against masturbation and bigotry against homosexuality were mingled with Freudian theories and created more confusion and fear. Of course, there must have been women who, through blissful ignorance or good fortune, discovered alone

or together with their partners the means of pleasure. Many older women can tell sad tales about the effects of ignorance on their sex lives. The few confident women who dared to think for themselves and explore their own bodies could ignore social norms and culture. Who cares how and where you get your orgasm?

But women's sexuality was, and is still in much of the world, socially constructed and controlled by a male-dominated society. We still try to feel what we are told we should feel. Freudian thinking implied that if your body did not work in a certain way, you were emotionally immature. The lucky women whose clitorises were positioned so that they received stimulus during coitus could believe that their orgasm originated in their vaginas and judge themselves mature. I can recall from my teen years in the 1960s reading the Agony Aunt's pages in women's magazines. A recurring theme was from 'Worried of Ruislip': a young woman in love and desire with her fiancé would admit guiltily to 'heavy petting', the euphemism for mutual masturbation. The warning response was that if this went on she would never be able to 'fully enjoy married love' and this became a self-fulfilling prophecy. The message was that if you followed your body's impulses now, you would never be a proper woman.

So one doctor published his theory about women's bodies and minds. It caught on and spread into medical, psychological and popular teaching and ruined many women's lives. It was not the worst thing that happened to women; female genital mutilation, lack of reproductive rights or access to safer childbirth are examples of issues which killed and are still killing women. Freud's theory only made them feel inadequate. Nevertheless I have given this account because I want to show how one man's theory could actually make thousands of women believe that their bodies misfunctioned, ignore the scientific evidence of their own experience and prevent them rejoicing in a simple pleasure that nature had provided.

Freud's theory is as an example of how one man's untested theory could influence female feelings, but luckily commercial interests were not involved. The parallel with current breastfeeding culture is clear. Too many women believe that their bodies will not function because erroneous medical and popular culture tells them so. This is endorsed by subtle commercial pressure and money is made from the maintenance of ignorance. The techniques of initiating breastfeeding echo much of the trial and error of initiating sexual activity. Each couple is different, atmosphere is crucial and both individuals have to find the right way for them so as not to get sore or feel pain when new to each other. If every couple who were deeply attracted to each other abandoned sex if it did not go brilliantly the first time, we would have widespread celibacy. Modern sex education has been revolutionised and there are few couples in the UK who could not get some access to information and help for sexual difficulties. No counsellor would dream of telling a woman she experienced orgasm in an incorrect corner of her body. Advice in popular magazines and TV programmes is widespread and vivid. This does not mean everyone is enjoying total sexual fulfillment all the time, but at least information is available.

Breastfeeding, which could transform the health of the nation,* is still not achieved by the majority of British baby/mother couples. If the majority of British women positively do not want to breastfeed whatever the health outcomes, then we might judge this a triumph for women's liberation and choice. The tragedy is that most British parents want to do the best for their child. Women might also be highly motivated to do something that has such significant protection for their own health. Moreover, breastfeeding can be a great pleasure. One of the breastfeeding hormones, oxytocin, is associated with pleasant feelings similar to orgasm. People (men have it too) with higher oxytocin levels have fewer relationship problems. It may be that the good relationship engenders more oxytocin. Experiments which blocked oxytocin flow in rats made them lose interest in their young (Hammand 2001). But if you try to do

---

*In 1995 it was calculated that if all British babies were breastfed for more than 13 weeks, this could save £35 million in reduced costs of treating gastroenteritis. If all women were to breastfeed for 3 months or longer, 400 deaths a year from early breast cancer might be prevented. (National Breastfeeding Working Group 1995).

something and it goes wrong and the common perception is that this is difficult, unpleasant and draining, then it is emotionally sustaining to persuade yourself that it was not really worthwhile. Just as many of our great grandmothers disliked sex because they lived in a climate of ignorance, fear and prejudice, when it comes to breastfeeding, we suffer too.

More learned men and breastfeeding

So what went wrong? The 18th-century doctor William Cadogan, whose words head this section, was also a well-intentioned man who did some good. He saw that babies died when they were not breastfed and did better on their own mother's milk. He stopped pre-lacteal feeds and advised exclusive breastfeeding and both infant and maternal mortality rates fell as a result (Fildes 1986). Called the 'Father of Paediatrics', William Cadogan strove to prevent infant deaths. Unfortunately he also spread his unproven theories through his influence and popularity. William introduced the idea of restricting breastfeeds and frowned upon night feeding. In the 18th and 19th centuries doctors were obsessed by 'overfeeding'. Before Louis Pasteur (1822–1895) discovered the role of bacteria in disease, many believed that too much food caused diarrhoea. When Cadogan told women and wet nurses to breastfeed less often, he seemed unaware of the supply and demand mechanism of lactation. Women would have known it, because a wet nurse feeding two babies (and some fed up to five) would have felt her breasts producing more milk as she suckled more. But Cadogan was not the kind of man to discuss his theories with a mere woman. Cows produced a lot of milk according to their breed and this assumption, that it is the woman who produces milk rather than the baby through his behaviour, still dominates popular perception.

Thereafter it was downhill all the way as male doctors across Europe and North America became experts on infant nutrition. Weighing was introduced to combat overfeeding. It is ironic to learn that weight monitoring was used to admonish a 19th century mother if her baby grew too fast and the 20th-century mother if her baby grew too slowly. Breastfeeding was still valued and women blamed if they did not do it. It was obvious that artificially fed babies got ill and died more often, but women's ability to feed their babies was doubted. 'Lactation is far more likely to go wrong in a woman than in the teetotal, vegetarian, nerveless cow' wrote the renowned Dr Eric Pritchard (1907). Sir Frederick Truby King, another infant feeding guru, was very influential. His methods held sway right into the 1950s. He too was influenced by cows, having observed the high death rate of bucket-fed calves in New Zealand. He was obsessed with routine and it was he who made the clock a god in the nursery. Despite understanding the role of germs in disease, he still held onto the 'overfeeding' theory.

A clean-swept stomach effectively scotches microbes which might otherwise cause fermentation, indigestion, diarrhoea, etc. Babies fed only five times a day will sleep more soundly, run less risk of overfeeding, and have fewer dirty nappies – in itself an important item.

The problem was that mothers 'became absurdly distressed by the sound of a mere hour or so's crying' (Hardyment 1984). We now got to the real problem of breastfeeding: the wrong sex were doing it.

Were the secretion of milk and the feeding of the baby the functions of men and not women, no man, inside or outside the medical profession, would nurse his baby more often than five times in the 24 hours, if he knew that the baby would do well or better with only five feedings. Why should it be otherwise with women? Mothers have too much to do in any case: why should they throw away time and leisure by frequent useless nursings? (King 1924)

The destructive effect of this medical misinformation is poignantly illustrated in an account from the end of the Second World War. Julia Kraut, a homeless German woman, gives birth to her fourth child in a cellar: 'Every day I went to the command post and begged milk for my baby who was barely alive. No success … I made tea for the baby by boiling nettle leaves'. Julia believed that she could not breastfeed. Her culture may have taught her that she must wait for the milk to 'come in'. She was unaware that putting her newborn to the breast would have stimulated her breastmilk supply.

Instead she risked her baby's life and suffered terrible anguish (Townsend & Townsend 1990).

If it were men who had to breastfeed, believe me, there would be scientific evidence tomorrow that babies should not be breastfed at all. (Gina Ford, Guardian 28.8.2002)

We live with this legacy of ignorance today. However much breastfeeding is valued in nutritional or health terms, the cultural message is that there are better things for women to be doing. I am not talking about High Court judges and surgeons. Poor women must return quickly to low-paid cleaning or catering jobs in deregulated service industries because that is seen as good for the economy. How the economy benefits those mothers and babies is another matter. How many midwives get the amount of paid maternity leave they really need? How many British hospitals provide the childcare facilities, support and flexible work patterns that make breastfeeding easy? Health professionals all over the world are models of health practice for communities. How can midwives fulfil their role as protectors of women's and babies' health if they and their own babies suffer discrimination? How can we expect society to change if midwives cannot achieve mutual support systems which make them leaders in making breastfeeding happen? It may not be easy, but nor was getting women the vote, equal wages and access to education. If we accept the current constraints on women's lives, then we are betraying our great grandmothers who fought so hard for equality.

The average British woman can expect to live for 84 years and may have two babies in her lifetime. European society accepts that people take time out from their jobs or at least adjust their work schedules for a range of activities. Middle-class youth take 'gap years'; academics take sabbaticals and sportsmen and women train for competitions. People are expected to do jury service, military service and a whole range of education and training packages. These ventures cost money to the state, the sponsor or the individual yet are viewed as essential investments in society's welfare. Yet when a woman adjusts her life in order to provide the optimum nutrition, health and psychological nurture for her baby she may be viewed as demanding and self-indulgent. The current approach to infant feeding still reflects the culture of the early 20th century. The approach can be summarised as: 'Breastfeeding is, in theory, a good thing, but most women are not really willing and able to do it and they have better things to do; it is all rather difficult so let us put our energies into artificial feeding'.

Artificial feeding techniques have influenced breastfeeding. How many women hold their babies sideways and try to suckle 'round the corner' because they bottle fed a relative's baby when they were younger or practised with their dolly's feeding bottles? How much 'nipple sucking' has been tolerated in agony because women saw more babies sucking on teats than breastfeeding? Why is a baby who sleeps for hours drugged by the indigestibility of artificial baby milk viewed as 'good' and the normal breastfed baby's feeding patterns viewed with alarm? Are we more inept and less competent mothers than our closest relatives, chimpanzees? If so, why? Billions of pounds of profits are made by artificial baby milk manufacturers through women's supposed impotence. We still value success in male terms. The money we make for ourselves or our employers, the official targets we reach, the qualifications or ranks we achieve give us our self-respect and social status.

Perhaps the most powerful constraint against breastfeeding is the way it is simply ignored. In 1998, a doctor from the USA, Ferid Murad, the winner of that year's Nobel Prize for Medicine, was interviewed by Tim Sebastian on BBC TV World Service. He was asked for his views on solving the world's health problems. Ferid replied: 'Diarrhoea is the biggest killer of babies, but no one will find a cure because there is no market in Africa'. This Nobel Prize-winning doctor was unaware of the significant health effect of exclusive breastfeeding from birth and continuing to breastfeed into the second or third year on preventing deaths from diarrhoea. There is so much documented evidence. If such a life-saving fluid as breastmilk came out of Ferid Murad's own body, would he be as oblivious of its qualities? When the honoured elite is so oblivious, no wonder ordinary citizens are too. Shamefully,

many British health professionals are equally indifferent to the simple facts of breastfeeding's contribution to health.

Sadly many women health professionals collude with this essentially masculine approach and duck the challenge. There is still resistance to the abandonment of unproven rituals (or provenly damaging rituals) such as top-up feeds, timed feedings and routine biochemical investigations (such as blood glucose tests) in full-term healthy babies who show no signs of illness. The risks of using the man-made substitutes is downplayed as it was a century ago. The discovery of dangerous products is not a priority news item. There is documentation of chance findings (Walker & Heiser 2002). In November 2002 the United States Federal Drug Agency (FDA) alerted the public and all relevant healthcare facilities to the danger of infant formula contaminated with *Enterobacter sakazakii*, a foodborne pathogen that can cause sepsis, meningitis and necrotising enterocolitis. Wyeth announced a voluntary recall of 1.5 million cans in the USA. Whether they recalled or tested all their exported stocks I have not yet discovered. The FDA only initiated an investigation because in Belgium in 1998, two babies became ill and another two died as a result of being fed contaminated infant formula. The thriving relationships, glued with social contacts, lunches, gifts and financial support, between artificial baby food companies and health professional organisations endorse the doubts and wobbling confidence of most British women. Artificial feeding is promoted as controllable and easy whereas breastfeeding is presented as problematic and complicated. All mothers, however they feed their babies, need support which could be in the form of acknowledgement and reward for the skill and dedication which most mothers strive for. Poor and single mothers are urged to find waged employment in workplaces unsupportive of breastfeeding soon after their babies' births, thus completely devaluing any commitment to breastfeeding (Leach 1994).

FEELINGS ABOUT BREASTS

Why is it in the papers everyday
That soft-porn on page 3 is still OK?

If you don't stick them out with a wriggle and a pout
You're told in no uncertain terms put them away.
(From the song 'Breastfeeding baby in the park' by
Janet Russell in 'No Bed of Roses', Fellside Records,
1992)

The obsession with the breast as a sexual object
became so widespread in North America and
Europe during the last century that many of us
think this is normal for the whole human race, but
this is not so. Katherine Dettwyler, in her essay
'Beauty and the Breast', gives examples of societies
where the concept of the breast as an erotic part
of the body is viewed with indifference or amazement. I too have met people who laugh at the idea
that grown men suckle and knead breasts like a
small baby. Katherine Dettwyler shows the contrast of perception in the United States and quotes
an article in *Time Magazine* where women's breasts
are referred to as 'human genitalia' (Dettwyler
1995b). This extraordinary statement was echoed
by a male friend who, during a discussion about
public breastfeeding, said: 'But you wouldn't
want men to go about with their penises exposed'.
Most societies, however minimal their clothing,
usually conceal their genitals, whether for mod-
esty or protection. Breasts, however, have been
viewed with such alarm only in recent times. Even
in societies where women are veiled, exposure of
the breast is accepted as necessary for feeding a
baby. Sadly, this is dying out. Readers from cultures where attitudes to breasts are saner than in
Britain may be able to contribute enlightening
ideas to their colleagues and reflect on the social
trends in other societies. One helpful development
is that in the USA and Europe, legislation has been
adopted to give women the right to breastfeed in
public. We can be glad about this but it is amazing
that we have had to pass laws to enable women to
do what is urgent, essential and natural.

'Topless' beaches may be widespread in Europe
but it is mostly women with breasts that conform
to the current standards of youthful beauty who
frequent them. There is nothing wrong with
youth wanting to display its beauty, but when it
becomes such a fixation that society discourages
the original use of an organ then we have a problem. We do not feel shocked by the sight of legs,
the nape of the neck or a bare tummy, yet all these

body parts can be viewed as sexy. They can all
be displayed even if imperfect. My sense is that
breast obsession evolved in societies where
breastfeeding almost died out and that there is
a connection.

We cannot reflect on attitudes to breasts without
considering how we feel about our own bodies.
The development, or not, of breasts at puberty is
for many women a more significant event than
the onset of menarche or the growth of body hair.
Even if a woman wears loose or flattening clothes,
it is hard to hide her fundamental body shape
and breasts or their absence are noticed. In discussions about the pains and pleasures of adolescence, few men seem to recall the exact timing of
physical changes but many women remember
vividly. Many women perceived a sense of inse-
curity and self-consciousness about their breasts
developing too early, too late, too small or too
large. Those who developed breasts which con-
formed to the stereotypical shape displayed in
tabloid newspapers would then find themselves
privileged or burdened with a badge of sexuality.
Many women do not feel proud and confident
of their bodies and particularly their breasts. We
know this because of the increasing numbers of
women who pay for surgery to enlarge or reduce
their breasts (Seager 2003). If a young woman
feels bad about her body because she believes it
must conform to a stereotypical ideal, then she
may well lack confidence when she first breastfeeds. Midwives play a major role in making
women feel good about their bodies, yet we know
that negative and demeaning statements are made
about women's bodies by health professionals.
This is a taboo subject because it is an unprofes-
sional practice. This has to be tackled and I believe
that part of this is for midwives themselves to
explore how they feel about their own bodies.

Many women may enjoy and relish the power
they have to attract attention and arouse sexual feeling with the sight of their breasts. In the
Stephen Frears film 'My Beautiful Launderette'
(Frears 1985), the hero's young cousin exposes
her breasts and exhibits them at a family gather-
ing in such a way that he can see and other family
members cannot. One can admire the young
woman's daring and empathise with the hero's

embarrassment and fascination. In private sexual relationships many women enjoy the erotic power of their breasts not just for their own physical pleasure but because it is a good feeling to be able to trigger reactions in a partner simply by presenting a part of your body. Of course, this is not confined to breasts alone. Dettwyler argues that the fact that breasts arouse erotic sensations both in ourselves and others is culturally constructed. My reaction is that this could be said of a lot of sexual experiences and takes us back to Freud. Culture is dynamic as well as diverse. In some parts of the world kissing is not a part of sexual activity, but this does not mean kissing is a bad thing.

I see no problem with breasts being used for both feeding babies and for erotic pleasure. Pleasure in contact with our babies is natural. There is a crossover of the sensuality of physical contact with our babies and sexual feelings. Because we live in an era of extreme anxiety about child sexual abuse, some women feel disturbed by the sensuality of breastfeeding. It is rarely discussed. Fiona Giles (2001) is researching the culture of lactation. She describes a series of photographs by David La Chapelle for *Playboy*. Naomi Campbell is depicted pouring breastmilk over herself. Later Fiona describes a vision of someone's mum tipping 'a bucket of her own expressed breastmilk in joyful abandon over her naked body'. If these concepts are disturbing, I suspect it may be that we feel breastfeeding has to be controlled … particularly by health professionals.

CONCLUSION

I started this chapter by describing Alison and Amina. Their lives could not be more different, but both breastfed their children. Alison grew up in a bottle-feeding culture but had access to the National Childbirth Trust's information and support system. She also had good self-esteem and a supportive partner. Amina comes from a breastfeeding culture and takes the process for granted but she is subject to an entirely discriminatory system of justice and is oppressed. Alison's privilege does not mean breastfeeding itself is a privilege. Amina's oppression does not mean

breastfeeding itself is oppressive. Breastfeeding has been perceived as a symbol of women's domestication and oppression, but it is an act of power and strength. Yet we still see breastfeeding as something to do with domestication and, however unwillingly, accept that if we venture outside the home, then it has to be curtailed.

Women have been economically productive since the dawn of time and the great majority have breastfed their children. In pre-industrial societies, a range of mutual support systems and flexible patterns of work enabled women to do this. Even today in some of the poorest regions it is still the norm for neighbours and families to rally round and help with other tasks when a new mother is establishing breastfeeding. Women mind each other's machines, pluck each other's tea plants, weed each other's vegetable patches while the other breastfeeds. If babies are artificially fed they get ill and work time is often lost through taking a baby for medical treatment and also sadly for funerals. Even in industrialised countries companies find benefits in supporting breastfeeding. A typical study from the USA found 25% of one-day absenteeism episodes were by breastfeeding mothers and 75% by bottle-feeding mothers (Cohen et al 1995). UK calculations show that if all babies were breastfed for more than 13 weeks, £35 million would be saved on the costs of hospital admissions for gastroenteritis (National Breastfeeding Working Group 1995).

But I do not want to justify breastfeeding by proving its economic value to governments and corporations. Breastfeeding is a woman's right wherever she comes from, whether she is an African farmer or an American factory worker. Breastfeeding is neither a lifestyle choice of the middle classes nor the oppression of peasants; it is the right of every woman whether she is in Parliament or in prison, is a lawyer, a cleaner or a schoolgirl, or a midwife.

We all have the responsibility to protect, respect, facilitate and fulfil the right to breastfeed. We must also accept that women have the right not to breastfeed. We cannot coerce women to use their bodies in the way we think best, however painful it is for us to accept that. This is an issue both of human rights and practicality. If a woman truly does not want to breastfeed, she cannot be forced to do so. However, if we succeed in removing all the constraints that prevent women from breastfeeding, we would realise how few are the women who really do not want to breastfeed and how rare are those who really cannot. We should be determined to succeed because it is important.

In ancient times, the great Islamic scholar and doctor Avicenna (980–1037) complained that curbs on women wasted the potential of half the world. In the late 20th century, a North American historian wrote: 'In general, the best clue to a nation's growth and development potential is the status and role of women' (Landes 1998). Avicenna probably took breastfeeding for granted and saw no conflict with women's full contribution to society and breastfeeding. I would like to be wrong but I suspect David Landes, in common with many male thinkers, is unaware of this important aspect of women's rights and this multifaceted contribution to individual and social well-being.

The world will not change through moaning and complaining. We will only achieve women's right to breastfeed through enlightening the powerful, supporting other women and respecting our own rights. Midwives, through their special role, have the skills to lead women to experience their rights and through this, the world can be a better place. They can do this through working together.

Questions for Reflection ?????

Invite an older relative or friend to talk about her life as a young woman. Reflect on the difference and similarities between her experiences and your own. How much did culture and politics shape those experiences?

Think about your own or another woman's experience of breastfeeding after a return to paid work. Did you (or she) feel supported by the government or the employers? Did you (or she) feel proud of contributing to society's wealth?

Do you or your family have a different attitude to breastfeeding than the usual British one? If you do, why do you think that is?

How do we humans differ from other animals? What do you think the term 'natural' means?

Can men and women help each other or is the 'battle of the sexes' inevitable?

List some famous women athletes, sportswomen, sailors, mountaineers, dancers, skaters and others who are models of physical skills. Then reflect on why so many women still lack confidence in their bodies.

How do you feel about your own breasts? Reflect on what contributed to these feelings.

Do you believe that you can contribute to making life better and fairer for women?

Key points

- Women who wish to breastfeed may suffer injustice and discrimination because of a perception within society that breastfeeding disrupts 'normal' life and does not contribute to the national economy.

- The negative culture around breastfeeding persists, for the most part, not because of lack of good intent from health and social support systems but because the substitutes for breastmilk are so profitable.

- Breastfeeding benefits the short- and long-term health of both mother and baby but, despite being a physiologically normal activity, it is often presented as being complex and requiring medical intervention and surveillance.

- Contemporary social beliefs, such as an expectation that babies should learn to sleep through the night, and medical practices, such as monitoring babies' blood sugar levels, add to the belief that breastfeeding is problematic.

REFERENCES

Agennix Fact Sheet 2001: http://www.agennix.com/pdfs/agennix_fact_sheet_fall2001.pdf

American Academy of Pediatrics 1994 Infant feeding practices and their possible relationship to the etiology of diabetes mellitus. Pediatrics 5: 752–754

Cohen R, Mrtek MB, Mrtek RG 1995 Comparison of maternal absenteeism and infant illness rates among breastfeeding and formula feeding women in two corporations. American Journal of Health Promotion 10: 148–153

Collaborative Group on Hormonal Factors in Breast Cancer 2002 Breast cancer and breastfeeding: collaborative reanalysis of individual data from 47 epidemiological studies in 30 countries, including 50 302 women with breast cancer and 96 973 without the disease. Lancet 360: 1871–1895

Coutsoudis A, Goga AE, Rollins N, Coovadia HM on behalf of The Child Health Group 2002 Free formula milk for infants of HIV-infected women: blessing or curse? Health Policy and Planning 17(2): 154–160

Crawford MA 2002 The role of nutrition in human evolution. The Caroline Walker Lecture

Davis MK 1998 Review of evidence for an association between infant feeding and childhood cancer. International Journal of Cancer (Preventive Oncology) 11: 29–33

Dettwyler KA 1995a A time to wean: the hominid blueprint for the natural age of weaning in modern human populations. In: Stuart-Macadam P, Dettwyler KA (eds) Breastfeeding: biocultural perspectives. Aldine de Gruyter, New York

Dettwyler KA 1995b Beauty and the breast: the cultural context of breastfeeding in the United States. In: Stuart-Macadam P, Dettwyler KA (eds) Breastfeeding: biocultural perspectives. Aldine de Gruyter, New York

Egan C, Robidoux M 2001 Women. In: Bircham E, Charlton J (eds) Anti-capitalism, a guide to the movement. Bookmark Publications, London

Elia I 1991 Adoptive lactation. East Anglian Film Archives, University of East Anglia, Norwich

Euromonitor International 2001

Fildes VA 1986 Breasts, bottles and babies: a history of infant feeding. Edinburgh University Press, Edinburgh

Firestone S 1970 The dialectic of sex: the case for feminine revolution. William Morrow, New York

Fleming A 2002 A little knowledge is good for your health. The Guardian 17th September

Forster M 1984 Significant sisters. Penguin, Harmondsworth

Frears, Stephen D (director) 1985 Working Title/SAF/Channel 4.

Giles F 2001 The nipple effect. smh.com.au-Spectrum.htm.13

Gould SJ 1995 Male nipples and clitoral ripples. In: Adam's navel. Penguin, London

Gunther M 1971 Infant feeding. Methuen, London

Hammond C 2001 Brainwaves. BBC Radio 4 17th September

Hanson LA 1999 Human milk and host defence: immediate and long term effects. Acta Paediatrica 88: 42–46

Hardyment C 1984 Dream babies. Oxford University Press, Oxford

Heinig JM, Dewey KG 1997 Health effects of breastfeeding for mothers: a critical review. Nutrition Research Reviews 1: 35–36

Henderson L, Kitzinger J, Green J 2000 Representing infant feeding: content analysis of British media portrayals of bottle feeding and breastfeeding. British Medical Journal 321: 1196–1198

Hite S 1981 The Hite Report: a nationwide study of female sexuality. Macmillan, New York

Howie PW Forsyth J, Ogston S et al 1990 Protective effect of breastfeeding against infection. British Medical Journal 300: 11–16

International Labour Organisation 2000 Maternity Protection Convention No. 183. International Labour Organisation, Geneva

King FT 1924 The expectant mother and baby's first month. Macmillan, London

Kinsey AC 1953 Sexual behaviour in the human female. Institute of Sex Research, Indiana University

Kois WE 1984 Influence of breastfeeding on subsequent activity of a related renal allograft. Journal of Surgical Research 37: 89–93

Labbock M 1994 The lactational amenorrhea method (LAM): a postpartum introductory family planning method with policy and program implications. Advances in Contraception 10: 93–109

Landes DS 1998 The wealth and poverty of nations. Little, Brown, London

Leach P 1994 Children first. Penguin, Harmondsworth

Masters WH, Johnson VE 1969 An analysis of human sexuality. Panther Books, London

McGreal C 2002 Woman faces death by stoning 'after weaning'. The Guardian 20th August

McKinney PA, Parslow R, Gurney KA, Law GR et al 1999 Perinatal and neonatal determinants of childhood type 1 diabetes. A case-control study in Yorkshire, UK. Diabetes Care 22(6): 928–932

Miller M, Iliff P, Stoltzfus RJ, Humphrey J 2002 Breastmilk erythopoietin and mother-to-child HIV transmission through breastmilk. Lancet 360: 1246–1248

National Breastfeeding Working Group 1995 Guidance to the NHS. Department of Health, London

Nissen E, Widstrom AM, Hilja G et al 1997 Effects of routinely giving pethidine during labour on infants' developing breastfeeding behaviour. Acta Paediatrica 86: 201–208

Odent M 1992 The nature of birth and breastfeeding. Bergin and Garvey, Westport

Osborn A 2002 Norway sets 40+ female quota for boardrooms. The Guardian 1st August

Palmer B 1998 The influence of breastfeeding on the development of the oral cavity: a commentary. Journal of Human Lactation 14 (2): 93–98

Palmer G 1993 The politics of breastfeeding. Pandora Press, London

Pritchard EL 1907 Infant education. Marylebone Health Society, London

Reid L 2000 Scottish midwives, 20th century voices. Tuckwell Press, East Linton

Roberts SB 2001 Prevention of hypertension in adulthood by breastfeeding? Commentary. Lancet 357: 406–407

Schrader C 1987 'Mother and child were saved'. The memoirs (1693–1740) of Catharina Schrader (trans Martland H). Rodopi, Amsterdam

Seager J 2003 Women in the world: an international atlas. Myriad Editions, Brighton

Spender D 1988 Women of ideas and what men have done to them. Pandora Press, London

The Network 1998 The feeding fiasco: pushing commercial infant foods in Islamabad, Pakistan. Available from Baby Milk Action, Cambridge, UK

Tong RP 1998 Feminist thought: a more comprehensive introduction. Westview Press, Colorado

Townsend C, Townsend E 1990 War wives: a Second World War anthology. Grafton Books, London

UNICEF, UNAIDS, WHO 1998 HIV and infant feeding: guidelines for decision-makers. UNICEF, New York

United Nations General Assembly 1979 The Convention on the Elimination of all forms of Discrimination against Women (CEDAW). United Nations, New York

United Nations General Assembly 1989 The Convention on the Rights of the Child. United Nations, New York

Von Kries R, Koletzko B, Saurerwals T et al 1999 Breastfeeding and obesity: cross sectional study. British Medical Journal 319: 147–150

Walker M, Heiser B 2002 Selling out mothers and babies. Appendix C. National Alliance for Breastfeeding Advocacy, Weston, MA

Waring M 1989 If women counted: a new feminist economics. Macmillan, London

WHO 1998a Relactation: review of experience and recommendations for practice. Department of Child and Adolescent Health. WHO, Geneva

WHO 1998b Evidence for the ten steps to successful breastfeeding. WHO, Geneva

WHO Collaborative Team 2000b The role of breastfeeding in the prevention of infant mortality. Lancet 355: 451–455

WHO Europe/UNICEF 2000a Feeding and nutrition of infants and young children. WHO Regional Publications Series No. 87. WHO, Copenhagen

WHO/UNICEF, SIDA, USAID 2001 The Innocenti Declaration on the protection, promotion and support of Breastfeeding. WHO, Florence

8

Depression in the postnatal period: a normal response to motherhood

Jane M. Ussher

YINTRODUCTION

Depression following childbirth is not a rare phenomenon. Depressed mood, referred to as 'the blues', in the immediate period following the birth of a child affects up to 80% of women. Postnatal depression that is severe enough to require treatment is said to affect between 7% and 35%. Are these women ill and suffering from a psychiatric disorder, as the traditional biomedical view would have it? Or, as many feminist critics would argue, are they experiencing an understandable response to a major life change, which is one of the greatest stressors found in family life? Is depression during the postnatal period a specific syndrome, needing special diagnosis and treatment? Or is it no different from depression experienced by women at any other point in life, or not even accurately defined as 'depression' at all? This chapter will address these questions and examine the different aetiological explanations for postnatal depression, as well as the implications for prevention and treatment.

POSTNATAL DEPRESSION – AN UNDERSTANDABLE RESPONSE?

Traditionally, medicine and psychiatry have categorised depression experienced by women in the period following the birth of a child as 'post partum'. Uncontroversial, you might think. However, as many feminist critics have argued (e.g. Nicolson 1998), this diagnosis pathologises women who are tired, unhappy or overwrought following the birth of a child (or during the early years of child rearing). It implies that they are suffering from an illness, a condition that is abnormal and deserving of biomedical cure, rather than a completely understandable response to the reality of early motherhood.

How many women can say, with all honesty, that they have not experienced despair in the months following the birth of a child? Absence of sleep, disruption of routine, putting the needs of the baby above all others (including self), hours of breastfeeding (or endless preparation of bottles), crying – wouldn't depressed mood be an understandable natural response? In one study of 50 healthy non-depressed mothers in the immediate period after childbirth, all of the women described their lives as 'hectic' and 86% reported extreme fatigue (Ruchala 1994). If it is a woman's first child, this transition to motherhood brings a whole host of other challenges in addition to tiredness and lack of time. Loss of work or needing to cope with both work and motherhood; loss of identity as a childless woman; severe curtailment of freedom; dramatic changes in the relationship with partner, friends and family; shock at the disparity between the fantasy and reality of motherhood – I could go on but the point is made.

I was in shock. It had been a difficult birth, and I was exhausted. All I wanted to do was sleep for a week, but sleep was the last thing on the agenda. I'd got a baby to look after, to attend to, and when it dawned on me that I'd have this responsibility for the next 20 years, I wondered what on earth I'd let myself in for. It took months for the sense of disbelief to lift. (Alison)*

If we conceptualise depression as a reaction to a stressful life event, more likely to occur if there are a series of stressful life events (Brown & Harris 1989), it is not surprising that women experience depression in the period after childbirth, as it is a life event that requires major adjustment. Research has shown that women who have experienced additional life events, particularly those involving family members, are at higher risk of postnatal depression (Aderbigbe et al 1993, Areias et al 1996).

---

*All the interviews without specific references to other sources were conducted by myself.

Equally, motherhood involves multiple stressors, occurring simultaneously. And they are impossible to escape from, unless a woman has the luxury of handing over the baby and escaping to a health spa for a weekend to recuperate. This is part of the paradox of motherhood – exhaustion, never-ending responsibility, negation of selfishness and independence yet at the same time, the desire to be with the child, to care, protect and nurture. In her eloquent and moving memoir about the first year of her daughter's life, Rachel Cusk captures the contradictions and dilemmas, the difficulties, of new motherhood, as is illustrated by the extract below.

Her eyelids begin to droop. The sight of them reminds me of the possibility that she might go to sleep and stay that way for two or three hours. She has done this before. The prospect is exciting, for it is when the baby sleeps that I liaise, as if I were a lover, with my former life. These liaisons, though always thrilling, are often frantic. I dash about the house unable to decide what to do: to read, to work, to telephone my friends. Sometimes these pleasures elude me and I end up gloomily cleaning the house or standing in front of the mirror striving to recognise myself. Sometimes I miss the baby and lie beside her cot while she sleeps. Sometimes I manage to read, or work, or talk, and am enjoying it when she wakes up unexpectedly and cries. And then the pain of moving from one life to another is acute. Nevertheless, watching her eyelids droop, my excitement at the prospect of freedom buzzes about my veins. I begin manically to list and consider things I might do, discarding some ideas, cherishing others. Her eyelids droop again and close altogether. In repose her face is as delicate, as tranquil, as a shell. As I look, an alarming colour spreads rapidly over it. The skin darkens, promising storms. Her eyes flip open, her body writhes, her small mouth opens like a yawning abyss of grief and pain. She roars. She bellows. She cries out in anger, agony, outrage, terror. I feel as if I have been discovered in some terrible infidelity. My thoughts of freedom cover themselves and scatter and I am filled with fury and shame. (Cusk 2001, p 65–66)

The transition to motherhood brings with it a dramatic change in the way a woman sees herself, her body and her relationship to the world. Activities which were taken for granted previously – reading a book, calling a friend, sitting quietly alone listening to music – become prize jewels that sit elusively just out of reach. As Rachel Cusk describes above, these activities exist only as mere memories of a former life, which can be glimpsed as a possibility when the baby sleeps, to be stolen away when the crying starts. The life that a woman knew before her first child, is turned upside down – everything changes. And it is completely out of the woman's control.

I was used to being in control, not at someone else's beck and call. I worked for twenty years, studied at university twice. I don't like relinquishing control. It's like bananarama land. (Adelle, in LeBlanc 1991, p 140)

Feeling out of control, when there is an expectation of control, is a major factor in lowering a woman's self-esteem, potentially leading to anxiety and depression. This is not something unique to women in the immediate postnatal period. In interviews I have conducted with women who present with moderate to severe premenstrual symptoms (PMS), the major themes that emerged were feeling out of control and unable to cope premenstrually, particularly in relation to family demands (Ussher 2002). What these women have in common with women reporting postnatal depression is extremely high expectations of self.

Questions for Reflection ?????

Are images of perfect smiling mothers media fantasies or an accurate depiction of life?

How would you describe a normal reaction to early motherhood?

Should women be able to cope with a new baby because motherhood is 'natural'?

Is a woman ill if she is tired, stressed and anxious when dealing with a new baby?

THE PERFECT MOTHER

Society tells us that motherhood is natural and blissful. The beatific Madonna adorns church frescos. Smiling sun-kissed supermodels hold their babies in a modern mimicry of this ancient motif. Is it surprising that women see and believe? Representations in high and popular culture – in

art, film, magazines, television – play a significant role in creating scripts of femininity that women follow from an early age. From childhood, fairy tales tell us that romance and love, followed by the 'happy ever after' of marriage and motherhood, are our route to happiness and fulfilment (Ussher 1997a). Research shows that young women still cite motherhood as an aim in life, alongside career and financial independence (Lees 1993). Modern women want it all. And what do they get? An impossible conundrum: if they continue to do paid work after childbirth, they invariably have two full-time jobs – home and work – with no acknowledgment of the difficulties involved, often little support and a deep sense of shame and guilt for 'failing' to live up to the fantasy that looks so simple and sexy from the outside.

So what does the fantasy say? Motherhood is easy and natural – what women are made for, bonding happening at the moment of birth. It is fun – images of toddlers on the beach, laughing children in the park. It is rewarding – the first smile, first word, first step of your child is a moment to cherish forever. That contact, connection and overwhelming love between mother and child, is something that can never be matched. It is magical – reading stories, playing games, a return to our own childhoods, with the wisdom of adulthood to allow us to repeat it.

Motherhood *can* be all of those things but it is also exhausting, frustrating, alienating, difficult and lonely. It is hard, relentless work, and probably the most difficult thing any woman will do. It involves endless sacrifice, patience and self-control and when that is impossible (for no-one can be patient and calm at all times), the ability to forgive oneself, for not being perfect. Winnicott (1971) had it right when he talked about 'good enough mothering'. The problem is, many women try to be perfect or they think they are the only ones who are not coping and end up feeling a failure as a result.

When you are not coping you wind up leading a double life – OK on the exterior, dying inside. (Madelaine, in LeBlanc 1991, p 140)

If everyone spoke up and was honest you would realise that you are not alone, not the worst off. Women do hold a lot in and do not talk because they feel that they are alone in not coping. (Charmaine, in LeBlanc 1991, p 141)

There's a conspiracy of silence surrounding motherhood. I thought that I was a failure, that it was just me who couldn't cope, until I broke down and admitted it all to my best friend, and she said all mums feel like that. (Debbie)

Feminist critics (Nicolson 1998, Ussher 1989) have argued that it is the idealised social representations of motherhood that surround us that keep women silent, blaming themselves, rather than speaking out and saying that sometimes they feel as if they cannot cope. Looking at other mothers and seeing only the surface appearance – the mask of perfection and coping – that hides the exhaustion and ambivalence within.

I'm a bad mother because I sometimes hate my child. I just want to shut the bathroom door and have five minutes peace. (Clare)

I try my best, but can't always keep a smile on my face. When things get too much, I lose my temper, then hate myself as a result. That makes me feel bad, and I'm more likely to snap, so it's a vicious cycle. (Susan)

These women have internalised the idealised representations of motherhood and as a result, experience themselves as failing. In reality, they are only human and experiencing completely normal reactions. Most parents dislike – even hate – their children at times. It is not surprising; parent–child relationships are one of the most intense engagements that we can experience. With heightened love and affection comes heightened anger and disappointment. Mostly, the anger passes. A 'good enough' parent will contain her dislike or anger and not take it out on the child, most of the time. If she loses her temper – and all parents do at some time or other – it does not mean that all is lost, that she is a failure. She is only human, with human reactions and pressures.

The harder we try to be perfect, the more likely we are to fail – so paradoxically, it is better to be easy on ourselves, to not expect too much, to try and be 'good enough', not the Madonna personified. This way, women are more likely to be able to anticipate irritation or anger, knowing that it occurs when they, and the child, are tired. Or when there are multiple demands – trying to cook supper, stop a child crying, talk to a partner who wants to discuss a problem, all at the same time; even Superwoman could not do all of this with a smile. Yet so many women try and feel as if they are at fault when irritation flares or they cannot juggle everything. It is not surprising that self-blame, guilt and depression can be the result.

Questions for Reflection ?????

How would you feel if you had to cope with a new baby as well as a husband who felt usurped?

Should men help with young children or is motherhood woman's work?

How would you feel if you suddenly had to cope with 24-hour care of another person, with no support, little sleep and no time for yourself?

TIMING OF POSTNATAL DEPRESSION

Feminists may be critical of the pathologisation of women who are deeply unhappy after the birth of a child but this does not mean that we dismiss their despair. Postnatal depression is a real phenomenon.

Depression can occur at any point following the birth of a child (see Box 8.1). The *Diagnostic and Statistical Manual* of the American Psychiatric Association (DSMIV) (APA 2000) categorises depression as 'post partum' if it occurs in the first 4 weeks after birth. Others argue that depression that occurs in the first 12 months following birth can be diagnosed as 'postnatal depression' (Nicolson 1998).

There is general agreement that the 'blues', a conglomeration of symptoms which include tearfulness, mood swings and irritability, occurring in the first few days after the birth, is related to medical procedures during childbirth and the hormonal changes of the early postnatal period (Harris 1994) and should be distinguished from postnatal depression as it generally passes within 10 days after the birth. Found in similar rates across cultures (Kumar 1994), it appears to be a

Box 8.1 Timing of depression following childbirth
• The blues: weeping and anxiety occurring between 2 and 10 days following birth. Transitory. • Depression and anxiety on arriving home with a new baby. Lasts a week or two. • Depressed moods with good and bad days. Up to 3 months after birth. • Clinical depression. Enduring symptoms such as anxiety, sleep and appetite disturbance.

Box 8.2 Signs of clinical postnatal depression
• Prolonged sense of hopelessness • Feeling that life isn't worth living • Thoughts of harming self or child • Appetite and sleep disturbance • Uncontrolled expressions of emotion, such as weeping • Overwhelming tiredness • Decreased energy • Feelings of worthlessness and guilt

normal reaction to the birth of a child (Lee 1998) and occurs at a rate that is similar to that found after any gynaecological surgery (Iles et al 1989), suggesting that it may be related to the physical trauma of birth.

For some women, the shock of adjustment to motherhood turns into a depression that can last for months, if not years, particularly if there is a continued disparity between their expectations and reality. For example, for many women, 'bonding' is not an automatic process, happening at birth. It may happen after the first few weeks, first few months or even after a few years. For some women, it does not happen at all. This can be a major cause of depression.

It was a really strange feeling, and I expected to feel something for her and I didn't. I kept thinking, 'Oh God – a total stranger!' I didn't feel anything. (Samantha, in Nicolson 1998, p 62)

Alex is 5 now, and I've only just started to appreciate him, to really love him. Up until recently, there wasn't a day went by when I didn't regret having him. It was like having a weight attached to my back the whole time, and I just resented him. (Sarah)

It has been suggested that the difference between postnatal depression (PND) and the blues is one of degree (Barnett 1988), with PND being diagnosed when the symptoms fail to resolve over time. It has also been suggested that women with more intense symptoms of the blues may be more at risk of prolonged depression (Sutter et al 1997). Women who have been depressed during pregnancy are also at high risk of developing depression postnatally (Da Costa et al 2000) (Box 8.2).

However, there may be a gap of some time before depression develops postnatally. For some women, depression may occur at the point of returning to work, when the competing demands of motherhood and work are experienced as impossible (Taylor 1996). There can be role strain, due to the contradictory nature of work and home identities – needing to keep emotions at bay at work due to 'professionalism' adding extra strain and pressure, leading women to collapse, or to snap, when they get home. The sheer physical toll of getting up early caring for a young child, getting older children ready for school, organising childcare and the school run before the working day has even started, and having to keep silent about it, so as not to be seen to be different from colleagues without children, cannot be over estimated (Ussher et al 2000).

'It's as if parenthood is invisible in the workplace' Annie told me. She felt as if she would be dismissed as not being serious about her work if she left early to pick up her children from school or if she took a day off when they were sick. So Annie used after-school care and sent her young son off to his lessons when he had a bad cold, that eventually turned into pneumonia. This was a turning point – the overwhelming guilt she experienced as a result of this incident led her to revert to part-time work and to give her home life priority. Annie might not get promoted as quickly as some of her colleagues but her mental health has taken a positive turn for the better.

However, depression is not something unique to the immediate postnatal year. The rate of depression in mothers of toddlers has been reported to be the same as that found in mothers with new babies (Cox et al 1993). And fathers are not immune either. One study reported that 9% of fathers were depressed 6 weeks after the birth of a child, with

5.4% depressed at 6 months (Ballard & Suedfeld 1988). Men whose partners were depressed were at higher risk. This highlights the important role of relationships in depression following the birth of a child, both as risk and as an ameliorative factor.

Questions for Reflection ?????

How would you feel if you had an important meeting at work and your child was sick at home?

What if you gave birth and found that you didn't like your child – you just wanted to sleep and be left alone?

RELATIONSHIP ISSUES AND SOCIAL SUPPORT

Case study 8.1 Alice

Alice gave birth to Toby 6 months ago. He was a much longed-for child, Alice hoping that his arrival would heal some of the difficulties in her relationship with Tom, her husband of 3 years. Nothing could have been further from the truth. Whilst there had been tensions and friction between the couple before Toby's birth, now there was a complete void. Tom resented the time that Alice spent with Toby. He felt usurped. He didn't like the smell of nappies, found his son's crying irritating, and thought that Alice had let herself go. She used to look attractive and slim. Now she was overweight – her stomach still round after the pregnancy – and her hair often unwashed. Tom knew Alice didn't like the amount of time he spent at the pub. But what else could he do? Home was no longer a refuge – it was a noisy nursery.

Alice found motherhood difficult and stressful. Toby seemed to do nothing other than feed and cry. The moments when he was asleep were filled with rushing around trying to keep the house clean, preparing the supper and, if she had a moment, attending to her own appearance. She wouldn't have been that bothered herself, but knew that Tom minded. Trying to keep him happy and look after Toby as well seemed an impossible task, but Alice did her best. Then she got mastitis. Breastfeeding became agony, but she was determined to persevere. Bottles weren't good for a baby, she knew, and she wanted to have the physical connection with Toby when he was feeding. The pain was so severe that she often cried throughout his feed. This seemed to distress Toby and he would cry too. Alice would try to put him down to settle him, but this just made him more

distressed. If Tom came in at this point, he'd get furious with Alice, telling her she was pathetic–couldn't she manage such a natural thing as feeding her own child? And where was his dinner? After a month of this, Alice collapsed with a severe viral infection. Her doctor told her she had postnatal depression and gave her antidepressants.

Family tensions, particularly with a partner, are a major factor in depression during the postnatal period. If, like Alice above, you are a new mother, coping with the challenges of a baby and your partner is angry and judgemental, the likelihood of depression will be increased. The isolation and powerlessness experienced by women in a traditional heterosexual marriage, where the woman is at home, serving her family and her man, is a major cause of depression throughout the lifespan, as feminist critics have argued (e.g. Stoppard 2000). In the postnatal period, this powerlessness can have much more far-reaching effects.

Feeling torn between partner and child is a common experience for new mothers; the postnatal period is one of the more perilous in relationships, as the focus of the mother is on the infant and her partner can feel rejected, ignored and usurped, as Tom did, above. If the partner has awareness and tolerance, this can be worked through. It may bring up unresolved issues for the partner – being rejected in the past, childhood feelings of a new baby taking mother's attention, the fear of never being noticed – and a considerable degree of psychological sophistication is needed to contain these and not project them onto the current situation. Some couples manage it; others struggle and eventually split up. Dealing with a relationship crisis will add to the risk of depression for the new mother – another stressful life event added to the existing pile.

In her study of Australian women following the birth of a child, Wendy LeBlanc (1999) identified the main relationship issues facing women as being financial dependency that they had not expected and did not like; physical, mental and emotional dependency; feeling that the man was selfish and did not empathise; communication difficulties; sexual problems; lack of intimacy; reverting to traditional male/female roles; lack of power. Paula Nicolson (1998) identified similar themes in her study of British women. Violence towards women also increases during the pre- and postnatal periods. One study of 1014 women who had experienced domestic violence reported that 18% experienced their first physical abuse from their partner during pregnancy, with 24% saying that previous abuse escalated at this time (Webster et al 1994). After the birth of a child, the added stress and strain, and the inability of the woman to give the same amount of attention she previously did to her partner, can precipitate violence (Connelly et al 2000). Mental and emotional abuse is also not uncommon; constant put-downs and criticism, insults, humiliation, lack of co-operation and support, and belittling of motherhood (LeBlanc 1999), as illustrated in the case study above. It is not surprising to find that the years following the birth of a child are a time when separation and divorce statistics peak – many couples do not survive the transition unscathed or united.

I guess having children magnified all the flaws in our relationship. I certainly did not expect the jealousy and over-demanding behaviour that came with the stress of a first baby with whom my husband had to compete. (Emma, in LeBlanc 1999, p 206)

Conversely, social support ameliorates depression; the more social support a woman has in life generally, the more likely she is to cope with stress and to avoid the pit of despair that characterises depression (Bebbington 1996). Women who receive good social support in the period prior to and following childbirth, and in the early years of a child's life, are less likely to experience depression (Collins 1993, Seguin et al 1999). This support can come from partner, family or friends. It can come from health professionals, from organised support groups or childcare centres. If women rely on one person for support – invariably their partner – the situation is more perilous. It is a great responsibility for one person to bear, particularly when they have their own emotional reactions to and investments in the mother and child. This is why, paradoxically, research has shown that single mothers with good support networks experience less depression than married or co-habiting women whose husbands do not play a major role in childcare (Brown et al

1986). The latter are more likely to rely on one person and to feel let down or resentful when that person does not or cannot deliver. However, other research has found that single mothers are at risk of depression if they carry the whole burden of childcare alone.

The type of support a woman receives can be a key factor in preventing depression. Researchers have found that practical help is perceived by many women as being more important than emotional support (Jordan 1989). Having help with shopping, babysitting for an hour or two or help with cooking and cleaning may be more important than a shoulder to cry on, particularly for women who do not have a partner to share the burden with.

RAGING HORMONES

Knowing the multifarious causes of depression in the postnatal period is vital for women and for health professionals. Unfortunately, despite the compelling evidence that social factors are a major cause, the historical legacy of 'raging hormones' theories is still with us, with biology being given the blame.

This is an explanation with a long lineage. Plato and Hippocrates both attributed women's moodiness and illness to the wandering womb, recommending pregnancy as a cure (Ussher 1989) – an irony in a discussion of postnatal depression. In the 19th century, the womb was seen to be the seat of a woman's power, with reproduction robbing her brain of its capability to think, making women unfit to be doctors or lawyers, according to medical 'experts'. The modern version of the wandering womb is the adoption of a narrow biomedical model to explain depression in the postnatal period, with the attribution of symptoms to hormones (Dalton 1989, Garnett et al 1990) or genetics (Bebbington 1998).

It is not disputed that women experience hormonal changes in the period immediately following childbirth. These have been directly connected to 'the blues', changes in oestrogen (Harris 1994) leading to a postbirth high that is followed by a crash, that lasts for about a week. However, feminist and social science researchers have contested the role of hormones in the aetiology of depression after this period (Nicolson 1998, Taylor 1996, Ussher 1992). Psychiatrists now agree; the DSMIV (APA 2000) does not have a specific diagnostic category for 'postnatal depression', as no hormonal or obstetric variable has been found to be associated with non-psychotic postnatal depression (Albright 1993). The risk factors for depression in the postnatal period are thus the same as at any other time in life, with the added strains of early motherhood acting as a stressor, as is argued above. Postnatal depression is thus seen to be an understandable response to the realities of motherhood. Indeed, some would see it as a rational response (Nicolson 1998), with women who do not experience it being abnormal, statistically speaking at least. Postnatal psychosis, a condition that affects less than 0.01% of women giving birth, is a very different disorder, associated strongly with previous experience of psychosis and a biological predisposition to future psychotic episodes, with birth acting as a trigger (Harris 1994).

PSYCHOLOGICAL FACTORS ASSOCIATED WITH DEPRESSION DURING PREGNANCY AND THE POSTNATAL PERIOD

Whilst there is a danger in pathologising women who experience more serious or prolonged depression in the postnatal period, individualising what may simply be a normal response to motherhood, there is some evidence that specific psychological factors may put women at greater risk of depression postnatally. One of the biggest risk factors is a previous history of depression (Gotlib et al 1989) and women who have previously been depressed are slower to recover, and more likely to relapse, than those who have not (Bell et al 1994). It has also been suggested that women with low self-esteem, insecure emotional attachments and who are obsessive, overcontrolled and perfectionist are more likely to experience depression postnatally (Albright 1993). However, as archetypal representations of motherhood position women as perfectly in control at all times, and motherhood as blissful, as was argued above, we may deem 'overcontrolled' a normal aspect of femininity and should

---

Box 8.3 Risk factors for postnatal depression
• Lack of social support
• Conflict with a partner
• Presence of other life stresses
• Unrealistically rosy expectations of motherhood
• Family history of PND
• High expectations applied to self
• Anxiety and depression during pregnancy
• Negative attitudes or ambivalence towards pregnancy
• Previous history of depression

be wary of positioning women as abnormal or dysfunctional if they are attempting to control their lives, often against all odds.

If it is the case that clinical depression in the postnatal period is no different from depression at any other time in life, the psychological factors which make women vulnerable at any time will also apply here (Whiffen 1992). Social or environmental factors which have been associated with higher reporting of depression include marital status, with married women reporting higher rates of problems than single women or married men; caring roles, with women looking after small children or elderly relatives being at higher risk; employment status, with work generally providing a protective factor, particularly for working-class women; absence of social support and economic or social power; gendered role socialisation, which leads to depressogenic attributional styles and an emphasis on affiliation rather than achievement, leading to vulnerability when relationships are under threat; multiple role strain and conflict, as well as the devaluation of traditional feminine roles; and sexual violence or abuse, in adulthood or childhood (Bebbington 1996, Stoppard 2000). Any assessment of a woman who presents with depression postnatally should include an evaluation of these factors to evaluate risk of prolonged or clinical depression.

DECONSTRUCTING POSTNATAL DEPRESSION

How do we make sense of these different explanations for postnatal depression? Before proposing a feminist-inspired model that allows us to do so, I would like to take a critical look at expert accounts of PND, starting with the definition of the disorder itself.

Within medicine and psychology, the desire for valid and reliable comparison across epidemiological and treatment studies and the need to facilitate research into aetiological mechanisms have precipitated the establishment of consensus definitions of mental health problems and PND is no exception. The diagnostic categories reified in DSMIV are the archetypal case. The desire for uniform definitions of mental health problems may appear on the surface to be a necessary first step for both research and clinical intervention. However, the very notion of categorisation of experience into psychiatric syndromes has been criticised from many different avenues.

The focus on diagnostic categories reifies the notion of PND as a clinical entity that occurs in a consistent and homogeneous way, that has an identifiable aetiology and is perceived to have *caused* the symptoms women report. This acts to deny the social and discursive context of women's lives, as well as the gendered nature of science, which defines how women's bodies and lives are studied. In contrast, as many critics have argued, PND can be conceptualised as a social category created by a process of expert definition (Nicolson 1998), similar to other mental health problems (Ussher 1991). In this view, PND is a socially constructed label, based on value-laden definitions of normality. Parallel arguments have been made about many other 'disorders', both physical and psychological (Foucault 1967), leading to a deconstruction of expert diagnosis and a questioning of the existence of many 'syndromes'.

Within mainstream psychology and medicine, if a phenomenon cannot be objectively observed and measured using reliable, standardised techniques, then it cannot be 'known'. This has resulted in a methodology-driven, rather than a theory-driven, analysis of PND and its possible aetiology. For example, the role of unconscious factors cannot be easily assessed within a hypothetico-deductive frame and so they are not included in the majority of mainstream analyses (for example, see Bebbington 1996). Equally, as historical, political and wider societal factors are

not easily operationalised and assessed, they are only addressed within social constructionist or feminist critiques (Chesler 1998, Stoppard 2000, Ussher 1991). According to a positivist paradigm, PND is construed as an individual problem – a disorder affecting an individual woman, on whom biomedical or psychosocial factors impact and produce symptomatology.

The woman who presents with problems is implicitly positioned as passive and devoid of social context in traditional analyses of PND, since agency is not easy (if at all possible) to observe. So it is inevitable that it is her body, or her symptoms, that are the entire focus of attention. Yet women are not passive objects in relation to either interpretation of physical or psychological symptoms or in relation to the discursive construction of PND. Self-referral for treatment is a process of active negotiation of symptomatology, current life events and lifestyle, and cultural, medical or psychological discourse about PND. Many women make sense of their experiences through positioning themselves as suffering from depression, anxiety or problems such as PND; others may experience symptoms but not make ascriptions of any of these problems. In one study of new mothers (Small et al 1994), one-third of those who met the criteria for PND did not want it labelled as such. They said that they were not experiencing an illness but dealing as well as they could with overwhelming tiredness, isolation, lack of support and physical strain (Lee 1998). To position these women as 'false negatives', as they are in the case of PMS research (Hamilton 1990), is to misinterpret the active negotiation and resistance of dominant discourse associated with madness in which many women engage. It is to reinforce the notion of women as passive dupes, rather than active agents who continuously make sense of and interpret the social sphere and their own psychological or bodily experiences (Ussher 1997a).

As psychological symptoms are not visibly apparent, they have to be observed through the interface of subjective accounts. As these may easily fall outside the required standards of objectivity and replicability, in empirical research they are collected through the use of standardised instruments. This is why there has been an inordinate amount of attention given to developing reliable and valid standardised questionnaire measures for assessing the incidence of specific mental health problems, such as depression, anxiety or PND. In mainstream research in this area there is almost total reliance on quantitative methods of data collection and statistical analysis of results. Thus, the complexity and contradictions evident within women's subjective accounts are negated and a potentially rich source of data is left uncollected and unexamined.

Equally, within mainstream psychology and medicine, women are made to fit the researcher's model of PND, in contrast to grounded methods of data collection and analysis where the constraints of a priori assumptions are not imposed upon participants' accounts, which are collected in a more open, qualitative manner. This is why I have quoted women extensively in this chapter. The use of questionnaires also assumes that 'symptoms' can be categorised and classified in a dichotomous manner as existing or not, with the only added complexity being the notion of a *degree* of symptomatology. That a woman might reply that she sometimes has a symptom and sometimes does not, that it depends on what is happening in her life, whether she has recently eaten, what she is thinking or how recently she has had sex, amongst other factors, is not acknowledged at all; neither is her own assessment of the meaning of her symptoms.

A MATERIAL-DISCURSIVE-INTRAPSYCHIC ANALYSIS OF POSTNATAL DEPRESSION

Yet a feminist deconstruction of PND, where we position it as normal and understandable, is not enough, many women do experience extreme distress in the postnatal period. Is this a specific illness or simply a depression that occurs postnatally? If psychological, social and physical factors have been found to be associated with symptoms, which one is the most important? What I would suggest is a move towards a material-discursive-intrapsychic analysis, where material, discursive and intrapsychic aspects of experience can be examined without promoting one level of analysis above the other. 'Material-discursive' approaches have recently been developed in a number of areas of psychology, such as sexuality, PMS and mental or physical health (Ussher 1997b, Yardley 1997). This is a result of both frustration with traditional medicine and psychology, which have tended to adopt a solely materialist standpoint, thus negating discursive aspects of experience, and dissatisfaction with the negation of the material aspects of life in many discursive accounts. This integrationist material-discursive approach is to be welcomed, yet arguably does not always go far enough, as the intrapsychic is often still left out because it is seen as individualistic or reductionist or not easily accessible to empirical investigation. Equally, when intrapsychic factors are considered (for example, in psychoanalytic or cognitive theorising) they are invariably conceptualised separately from either material or discursive factors.

It is time that all three levels together are incorporated into academic theory and practice, in order to provide a multidimensional analysis of women's lives, of postnatal depression as a discursive category and of the mental health symptoms many women experience. So what is meant by a material-discursive-intrapsychic approach?

The level of materiality

To talk of materiality is to talk of factors which exist at a corporeal, a societal or an institutional level, factors which are traditionally at the centre of biomedical or sociological accounts. This would include biological factors associated with psychological symptomatology; the physiological changes that take place during pregnancy, childbirth and in the postnatal period; the physical presence of a baby; difficulties the child may experience; lack of sleep and other physical consequences of pregnancy and motherhood; material factors which institutionalise the diagnosis and treatment of PND; gender inequalities and inequalities in heterosexual relationships, legitimating masculine power and control. The latter would encapsulate economic factors which make women dependent on men; presence or absence of accommodation which allows women in destructive relationships to leave; support for women of a legal, emotional and structural kind, which allows protection from further harassment or abuse. It would include issues of social class which lead to expectations of 'normal' behaviour for women and men and which are implicated in educational or employment opportunities available to both, as well as in the way individuals are treated by external institutions such as social services or the mental health professions. How many children are present (or are, in custody battles, withheld) and the material consequences of being married (or not) are also part of this level of analysis. Equally, previous history of abuse or of bereavement is partly a material event, as is family history – the number of siblings, parental relationships and factors such as parental divorce or separation from parents in childhood. There are also many material consequences of experiencing or being treated for PND, in terms of physical or psychological vulnerability, as well as powerlessness at an economic or societal level.

The social isolation which can be a consequence of mental health problems or which can act to exacerbate its effects is also partly a material issue. Sex, ethnicity and sexuality are also associated with materiality – with the reproductive body, gendered or sexual behaviour and physical appearance. Within a feminist perspective it is recognised that material factors often militate against women: women are often economically, physically and socially disadvantaged in relation to men.

The level of the discursive

To focus on the 'discursive' is to look at social and linguistic domains – talk, visual representation, ideology, culture and power. What is arguably of most relevance in analyses of PND is the discursive construction of depression, of medical or psychological expertise (Foucault 1967), as well as the analysis of the relationship between representations of 'motherhood', 'fatherhood', 'woman' and 'man' and the social roles adopted by individual women and men.

As the discursive construction of 'PND' as illness, as individual problem and as justification

for expert intervention has already been explored above, I will focus only on the discursive construction of gender here. Within a discursive account, rather than femininity being seen as innate, here it is seen as something which is performed or acquired. In the process of becoming 'woman', it is argued that women follow the various scripts of femininity which are taught to them through the family, school and the myriad representations of 'normal' gender roles in popular and high culture, as well as in science and the law (see Ussher 1997a). They have to choose between the contradictory representations of femininity which are available at any point in time, in order to find a fit between what they wish to be and what is currently allowed (Ussher 1997a). The fact that many women take up the archetypal position of 'woman' – always positioned as secondary to 'man' – is attributed to the dominance of patriarchy and the fact that gender is constructed within a 'heterosexual matrix' (Butler 1990).

Within a heterosexual matrix, the traditional script of femininity tells us that women live their lives through a man. To have a man, and keep him, is the goal of every girl's life. The good girl is invariably self-sacrificing but she always gets her man. In the 21st century, 'getting' still means monogamy and usually marriage or motherhood; this is the script for the 'respectable' woman. *Not* getting means being positioned as sad or bad; the spinster on the shelf or the shameful whore. And the sexual woman, the whore, is always deemed to deserve all the condemnation that she gets (see Ussher 1997a).

In the traditional discursive construction of heterosexuality 'man' is positioned as powerful and 'woman' as passive and beholden to man. The institutionalised couple they together form is positioned as immune from scrutiny or intervention from outside. At the same time, 'man' is idealised as the answer to a woman's dreams: the fairy-tale prince who will sweep her off her feet; 'Mr Right' who will bring happiness, contentment and fulfilment of her heart's desires – the 'happy ever after' ending we are promised at the end of romantic fiction and fairy tales. Yet it is also acknowledged that this relationship can result in violence, oppression and neglect. The traditional discursive representation of heterosexuality provides an explanation for this which ensures that many women stay in it: the myth of 'Beauty and the Beast'. We are taught that a good woman can always tame or transform the monstrous brute or beast; through her ministrations or example, the frog will turn into the prince, the violent man into the charming thoughtful lover. The woman who cannot enact this transformation is positioned as being to blame; she must try harder, be more self-sacrificing or attempt with greater vigour to be the 'perfect woman'. Yet even if she fails at this and the beast is never transformed, we are reminded by the fairy stories and by romantic fiction that underneath it all the brute is a vulnerable and needy man and that he is the most sexy or desirable partner a woman could find (Mr Darcy, Rhett Butler ...). And if all else fails, women still have the hope that motherhood will provide true fulfilment, as will the security of knowing that they are safe within the boundaries of a 'normal' heterosexual life (see Ussher 1997a).

This is not merely an analysis of fairy stories or of an outmoded script of heterosexual femininity that many women have rejected in their quest for a more autonomous or agentic life. It is one of the explanations put forward for why women stay in unhappy, neglectful or violent relationships with men and arguably one of the explanations for why women internalise marital or family difficulties as depression (Ussher 2000). Women are taught to gain happiness through relationships, invariably with men. They are also taught that it is their fault if it fails.

The level of the intrapsychic

Intrapsychic factors are those which operate at the level of the individual and the psychological, factors which are traditionally the central focus of psychological analyses of PND (see above). This would include analyses of the way in which women blame themselves for problems in relationships and psychological explanations for why this is so, incorporating factors such as low self-esteem, depression, the impact of previous neglect or abuse, guilt, shame, fear of loss or separation and the idealisation of both heterosexuality and

of men. It would include an analysis of psychological defences, such as repression, denial, projection or splitting, as mechanisms for dealing with difficulty or psychological pain. For example, we see evidence of splitting in the way women see themselves, or their man, as all good or all bad, with no acknowledgement that everyone can exhibit both positive and negative characteristics at the same time; or in the way women blame themselves, or their bodies, for problems which they experience. It would also include women's internalisation of the idealised fantasy of motherhood and of the expectations of being 'woman' in a heterosexual social sphere.

Thus depression during the postnatal period cannot be simply attributed to one factor. A complex interaction of material, discursive and intrapsychic factors determines whether a particular woman will experience depression or not (see Figure 8.1). It is the combination of these factors that leads to depression – no one single factor is the 'cause' and thus no one single factor can be the 'cure'.

Why is this a feminist approach? It acknowledges, and takes seriously, women's pain and despair; it takes the myriad causes of this despair

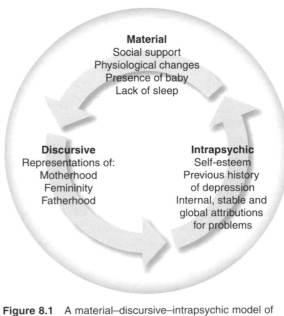

Material
Social support
Physiological changes
Presence of baby
Lack of sleep

Discursive
Representations of:
Motherhood
Femininity
Fatherhood

Intrapsychic
Self-esteem
Previous history
of depression
Internal, stable and
global attributions
for problems

Figure 8.1 A material–discursive–intrapsychic model of postnatal depression.

on board; it does not blame the woman or her body; it does not position her as 'mad' or 'abnormal'; and it is strongly critical of a society in which women are expected to be perfect, to be super-mothers, meaning that women feel a failure when the reality does not match the fantasy.

HOW TO SUPPORT WOMEN LIVING THROUGH DEPRESSION POSTNATALLY

In addition to challenging the myths of motherhood, as many feminist critics have done, there are many things that can be done to prevent and ameliorate depression during pregnancy and in the postnatal period. These include practical support, medical support of an orthodox or alternative nature, and psychological support. These can be offered without positioning women as 'ill'. Indeed, as we have seen from the discussion above, experiencing symptoms that would be deemed 'depression' in the postnatal period is so normal that it would be inappropriate to categorise women as 'ill' unless we see motherhood itself as an illness.

Medical support

Whilst there is no evidence of a hormonal or obstetric cause of depression in the postnatal period, we cannot so easily dismiss the role of neurotransmitters in depression, whether it occurs during the postnatal period or at any other time in life. There is a substantial amount of research suggesting that moderate to severe depression is linked to changes in dopamine or serotonin levels (Bebbington 1996). This is not to say that these changes *cause* depression – both depressive symptoms and neurochemical changes could be caused by a third factor, such as stress or negative cognitions. For some women, antidepressants can be an effective treatment for PND. They can help to lift the woman's mood, to help her sleep and increase her appetite, which in turn gives greater strength and stamina for coping with the day-to-day tasks of motherhood. However, if antidepressants are the only solution offered to a woman, and the factors that have lead to her depression are not fully examined, this could be seen as a 'sticking plaster' approach which will not be effective in the long term.

Natural remedies which focus on the body can also be effective in alleviating depressive symptoms, including herbs, acupuncture and homeopathy (McIntyre 1994). Other 'self-help' remedies, such as rest and relaxation, diet and exercise, are also important. However, if there are underlying psychological issues associated with depression, or if there are major stresses in a woman's family environment, interventions of a psychological nature may be more effective.

Psychological interventions for depression

There are now myriad psychological therapies available to treat depression. Psychoanalytic psychotherapy, cognitive behaviour therapy, family therapy and group therapy have all been found to be effective. The decision on which therapy is appropriate for a particular woman may be based on availability of services, on what a woman can afford, on a match between woman and therapist or whether she wishes her partner to be part of the intervention. Self-help groups where women can meet other mothers can be very beneficial, demonstrating to women that they are not alone in feeling depressed. Practical support is also invaluable (see Box 8.4). Women can also benefit from basic advice about self-care and taking time out, as well as not expecting too much of themselves (see Box 8.5).

Box 8.4   Practical support for women

Childcare
Babysitting
Help with shopping and cleaning
Meeting other women with young children
Financial assistance
Couples counselling
Transport for hospital appointments
Self-help books on depression

> **Box 8.5**   Advice to women (adapted from the Royal College of Psychiatrist's website, with permission, http://www.ropsych.ac.uk/info/help/pndep/)
>
> **DON'T** try to be a superwoman.
> **DO** make friends with other couples who are expecting or have just had a baby.
> **DO** identify someone in whom you can confide.
> **DO** take every opportunity to get your head down. Try to learn the knack of cat-napping.
> **DO** get enough nourishment.
> **DO** find time to have fun with your partner.
> **DO** let yourself and your partner be intimate, even if you don't yet feel like sex: at least kiss and cuddle, stroke and fondle.
> **DON'T** blame yourself or him: life is tough at this time.
> **DON'T** be afraid to ask for help when you need it.

CONCLUSION

This chapter has argued that depression following childbirth is not a pathological condition. Rather, it is an understandable response to the difficulties of motherhood. It results from a complex interaction of material, discursive and intrapsychic factors, which differ between women and thus need to be assessed on an individual basis. Many women who experience depression in the early years of their child's life can be helped by social support, having realistic expectations of themselves and of the difficulties of the mothering role, and practical help with childcare. For other women, where the depression may be more severe or long lasting, medical treatment (of a traditional or complementary nature) or psychological therapy can be beneficial. There are also a number of agencies that specialise in offering advice and support for women (see Box 8.6). For clinicians, the most important thing is to validate the woman's feelings, to be empathic and understanding, to reassure her that she is not unusual or abnormal and to avoid any notion of blame. This means being sensitive to the strong influence of idealised expectations of motherhood, which position women who are unhappy postnatally as failures. Whilst avoiding a pathological framework where a woman is positioned as 'ill', it is also important to offer support and help of a psychological, medical and practical nature, as is appropriate for a woman's individual circumstances and desires.

> **Box 8.6**   Organisations that can help (UK)
>
> **Association for Post Natal Illness:** 145 Dawes Road, Fulham, London SW6 7EB. Helpline 020 7386 0868.
>
> **BM CRY-SIS:** London WC1N 3XX.
> For help and support with a crying baby.
>
> **Meet-A-Mum-Association (MAMA):** Waterside Centre, 26 Avenue Road, South Norwood, London SE25 4DX. Tel: office 020 8771 5595; postnatal depression helpline (Monday to Friday 7pm to 10pm) 020 8768 0123. Fax: 020 8239 1153.
> Email address: meet-a-mum.assoc@blueyonder.co.uk
> Self-help groups for mothers with small children and specific help and support to women suffering from postnatal depression.
>
> **National Childbirth Trust:** Alexandra House, Oldham Terrace, Acton, London W3 6NH. Tel: 020 8992 2616; enquiry line 0870 444 8707; breastfeeding line 0870 444 8708.
> Fax: 020 8992 5929. Advice, support and counselling on all aspects of childbirth and early parenthood.
>
> **The Samaritans:** 10 The Grove, Slough SL1 1QP. Tel: 08457 909090 in the UK or 1850 609090 in Eire (the number of your local branch can be found in the telephone directory).

Key points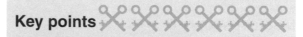

- Depression after childbirth is a normal and common experience.

- Cultural representations position motherhood as easy and blissful – in reality it is a major source of stress.

- Women who try to be the perfect mother set themselves up to fail. It's impossible.

- Women with social support are less likely to be depressed.

- Clinical depression in the postnatal period is no different from depression at any other time in life.

- Depression is caused by a combination of psychological, biological and social factors.

REFERENCES

Aderbigbe YA, Gureje O, Omigbodun O 1993 Postnatal emotional disorders in Nigerian women: a study of antecedents and associations. British Journal of Psychiatry 163: 645–650

Albright A 1993 Postpartum depression: an overview. Journal of Counseling and Development 71(3): 316–320

APA 2000 Diagnostic and statistical manual of mental disorders, edition IV. American Psychiatric Association, Washington DC

Areias MEG, Kumar R, Barros H, Figueiredo E 1996 Correlates of postnatal depression in mothers and fathers. British Journal of Psychiatry 169(1): 36–41

Ballard EJ, Suedfeld P 1988 Performance ratings of Canadian Prime Ministers: individual and situational factors. Political Psychology 9(2): 291–302

Barnett PAG 1988 Psychosocial functioning and depression: distinguishing amoung antecedents, concommitants, and consequences. Psychological Bulletin. 104: 97–126

Bebbington P 1996 The origins of sex differences in depressive disorder: bridging the gap. International Review of Psychiatry 8(4): 295–332

Bebbington P 1998 Sex and depression. Psychological Medicine 28(1): 1–8

Bell AJ, Land NM, Milne S, Hassanyeh F 1994 Long-term outcome of post-partum psychiatric illness requiring admission. Journal of Affective Disorders 31(1): 67–70

Brown GW, Harris TO (eds) 1989 Life events and illness. Guilford Press, New York

Brown GW, Andrews B, Harris TO, Adler Z 1986 Social support, self-esteem and depression. Psychological Medicine 16(4): 813–831

Butler JP 1990 Gender trouble: feminism and the subversion of identity. Routledge, New York

Chesler P 1998 Women and madness, 2nd edn. Doubleday, New York

Collins NL 1993 Social support in pregnancy: psychosocial correlates of birth outcomes and postpartum depression. Journal of Personality and Social Psychology 65(6): 1243–1258

Connelly CD, Newton RR, Landsverk J, Aarons GA 2000 Assessment of intimate partner violence among high-risk postpartum mothers: concordance of clinical measures. Women and Health 31(1): 21–37

Cox JL, Murray D, Chapman G 1993 A controlled study of the onset, duration and prevalence of postnatal depression. British Journal of Psychiatry 163: 27–31

Cusk R 2001 A life's work: on becoming a mother. Fourth Estate, London

Da Costa D, Larouche J, Dritsa M, Brender W 2000 Psychosocial correlates of prepartum and postpartum depressed mood. Journal of Affective Disorders 59(1): 31–40

Dalton K 1989 Depression after childbirth: how to recognize and treat postnatal illness, 2nd edn. Oxford University Press, London

Foucault M 1967 Madness and civilisation: a history of insanity in the age of reason. Tavistock, London

Garnett T, Studd JW, Henderson A, Watson N, Savvas M, Leather A 1990. Hormone implants and tachyphylaxis. British Journal of Obstetrics and Gynaecology 97(10): 917–921

Gotlib IH, Whiffen VE, Mount JH, Milne K 1989 Prevalence rates and demographic characteristics associated with depression in pregnancy and the postpartum. Journal of Consulting and Clinical Psychology 57(2): 269–274

Hamilton JAG 1990 Problematic aspects of diagnosing premenstrual phase dysphoria: recommendations for psychological research and practice. Professional Psychology: Research and Practice 21(1): 60–68

Harris B 1994 Biological and hormonal aspects of postpartum depressed mood: working towards strategies for prophylaxis and treatment. British Journal of Psychiatry 164: 288–292

Iles S, Gath D, Kennerley H 1989 Maternity blues: II. A comparison between post-operative women and post-natal women. British Journal of Psychiatry 155: 363–366

Jordan PL 1989 Support behaviors identified as helpful and desired by second-time parents over the perinatal period. Maternal Child Nursing Journal 18(2): 133–145

Kumar R 1994 Postnatal mental illness, a transcultural perspective. Social Psychiatry and Psychiatric Epidemiology 29: 250–264

LeBlanc W 1991 Naked motherhood: shattering illusions and sharing truths. Random House, Sydney

LeBlanc W 1999 Naked Motherhood: shattering illusions and sharing truths. Random House, Sydney

Lee C 1998 Women's health: psychological and social persepctives. Sage, London

Lees S 1993 Sugar and spice: sexuality and adolescent girls. Penguin, London

McIntyre A 1994 The complete women's herbal. Gaia, London

Nicolson, P 1998 Postnatal depression: psychology, science and the transition to motherhood. Routledge, London

Ruchala PLH 1994 The post-partum experience of low risk women: a time of adjustment and change. Maternal-Child Nursing Journal 22: 83–89

Seguin L, Potvin L, St Denis M, Loiselle J 1999 Socio-environmental factors and postnatal depressive symptomatology: a longitudinal study. Women and Health 29(1): 57–72

Small R, Brown S, Lumley J, Astbury J 1994 Missing voices: what women say and do about depression after childbirth. Journal of Reproductive and Infant Psychology 12(2): 89–103

Stoppard J 2000 Understanding depression: feminist social constructionist approaches. Routledge, London

Sutter AL, Leroy V, Dallay D, Verdoux H 1997 Post-partum blues and mild depressive symptomatology at days three and five after delivery: a French cross-sectional study. Journal of Affective Disorders 44(1): 1–4

Taylor V 1996 Rock-a-by-baby: feminism, self-help and postpartum depression. Routledge, New York

Ussher JM 1989 The psychology of the female body. Taylor and Francis/Routledge, Florence, KY

Ussher JM 1991 Women's madness: misogyny or mental illness? University of Massachusetts Press, Amherst, MA

Ussher JM 1992 Reproductive rhetoric and the blaming of the body. In: Nicolson P (ed) The psychology of women's health and health care. Macmillan, London, p 31–61

Ussher JM 1997a Fantasies of femininity: reframing the boundaries of sex. Penguin, London

Ussher JM 1997b. Body talk: the material and discursive regulation of sexuality, madness and reproduction. Routledge, London

Ussher JM 2000 Women's madness: a material-discursive-intrapsychic approach. In: Fee D (ed) Psychology and the postmodern: mental illness as discourse and experience. Sage, London, p 207–230

Ussher JM 2002 Processes of appraisal and coping in the development and maintenance of premenstrual dysphoric disorder. Journal of Community and Applied Social Psychology 12: 1–14

Ussher JM, Hunter M, Browne SJ 2000 Good, bad or dangerous to know: representations of femininity in narrative accounts of PMS. In: Squire C (ed) Culture and psychology. Rontledge Falmer, New York, p 87–99

Webster J, Sweet S, Stolz TA 1994 Domestic violence in pregnancy: a prevalence study. Medical Journal of Australia 161: 461–472

Whiffen VE 1992 Is postpartum depression a distinct diagnosis? Clinical Psychology Review 12(5): 485–508

Winnicott DW 1971 Playing and reality. Tavistock, London

Yardley L (ed) 1997 Material discourses of health and illness. Taylor and Francis/Routledge, Florence, KY

9

Midwifery practice:
ways of working

Carol Bates

INTRODUCTION

Ann Oakley argues that the way in which child-birth is managed affects the position of women in society (Oakley 1993). This chapter will demonstrate that it also affects the position of midwives in society and the ways in which they work. A feminist analysis of midwifery practice has been slow in coming which may be because midwives as a group, despite having been recognised as exhibiting behaviours attributed to oppressed groups (Kirkham 1999), have yet to embrace feminism.

Over the years there has been a political backlash against feminism. Oakley & Mitchell (1997) think this backlash, whilst grounded in a fear of feminism, is also recognition of the power that feminism has exercised in changing women's lives. Faludi (1992) argues that because of the huge changes that have occurred in society over the last century (and feminism cannot take responsibility for them all), the basis of the backlash is a desire to systematically undermine women and their progress in society. According to Oakley & Mitchell (1997), at the heart of the backlash against feminism are beliefs, held by both men and women, that:

- women are no longer discriminated against
- feminists exaggerate(d) the extent of such discrimination
- feminism has never represented the interests of women as a group
- feminism is principally, and unhelpfully, a language of 'victimisation'

- feminism ignores the social and personal importance of the family, including to women
- feminists inaccurately portray discrimination against women as a male conspiracy (Oakley & Mitchell 1997, p 33–34).

Question for Reflection ?????

What are your views of feminism and its contribution (or otherwise) to society? Think about your own life experience and decide which of these arguments you agree or disagree with and why.

Coward (1999), for example, author and columnist for *The Guardian*, dismisses centuries of discrimination against women by men and suggests that the feminist movement has denied men equality. She considers that feminism has demonised men and has damaged relations between men and women. For Coward, the feminist movement is now an irrelevance.

Feminist thinkers and writers such as Oakley (1987), Oakley & Mitchell (1997) and Faludi (1992) vigorously oppose such arguments and remain of the view that women are still discriminated against. Women may have entered the public sphere but not on equal terms (Figes 1995, Oakley & Mitchell 1997). They are present in the workplace and in many institutions but they are subordinated within them. Midwives are a good example of this. The domestic division of labour continues as before and women are subject to domestic violence (Bewley et al 1997, Walby 1990).

Capitalism is the driving force of the Western world. A Marxist feminist analysis of capitalism shows it to be a system of power relations as well as economic relations (Barrett 1980). Marx was not particularly interested in the problems of women in society because women were primarily concerned with reproduction rather than economic production and early radical feminists such as Firestone (1979) began to consider this to be the root cause of women's oppression (Tong 1989).

The driving force of capitalism is patriarchy and Oakley later highlighted that it was not women's ability to give birth that was the problem but the need of patriarchy to control it (Oakley 1980). As scientific knowledge advanced and the use of technology became the norm, radical feminists argued that the management of childbirth inevitably became inextricably linked to capitalism as men produced expensive technology to monitor women's reproduction. Postfeminists are unlikely to agree with this analysis.

Postfeminists argue that the early feminist movement is no longer relevant to women's lives. Coward (1999) is a good example of postfeminist thinking. Critics of postfeminism argue that it is purely antifeminist propaganda, part of the backlash against feminism. The prime movers are often disillusioned women who have reaped the benefits of feminism but are now finding, to coin a media phrase, that they 'cannot have it all'. Women are encouraged to believe that feminism is the enemy (Oakley & Mitchell 1997) because it has gone too far and is the underlying cause of their unhappiness (Faludi 1992). The problem for women is not feminism but patriarchy which, rather than helping women to achieve equality, has consistently and systematically moved the goalposts to hamper women's progress in society (Faludi 1992, Oakley & Mitchell 1997).

The backlash against feminism is also characterised by patriarchal practices being justified rather than criticised. Kenda Crozier (2001) gives a good example of this when discussing postfeminist thinking and child-bearing practices. She is a midwifery lecturer and argues that to say women were dominated by the patriarchal medicalisation of childbirth is a disservice to women because it implies women were passive and submissive in allowing themselves to be controlled. She also considers that the time has come to re-examine the argument about technology being used to control women in the light of a growing demand from consumers for technology because it allows them to take control of the birthing process.

Prior to the late 1990s women did not have a choice about the use of technology; it was, as demonstrated in the Short Report (HMSO 1980), thrust upon them (Oakley 1980). The use of technology can never give women overall control of the birthing process because someone else is always in control of the technology. Crozier has also omitted to mention the impact of technology on childbirth; for example, rising caesarean section rates (Parliamentary Office of Science & Technology 2002), rising maternal morbidity rates (Bick & MacArthur 1995, MacArthur et al 1991), the impact of iatrogenic distress on mothers and babies (Robinson 1995) and the culture of midwifery produced by the medicalisation of child bearing (Kirkham 1999).

This chapter, using a radical feminist perspective, will explore the connections between changes in the management of childbirth and the ways in which midwives work. It will show how patriarchy has systematically and persistently undermined midwives, which has restricted our progress in society and created problems for child-bearing women. As you read this chapter, decide for yourself if feminism is relevant to you both personally and professionally.

MIDWIFERY: IN THE BEGINNING

Midwifery practice has evolved over many centuries. Historically the care of women in childbirth and infants was an integral part of the female healing role. All women, regardless of class, were dependent upon the midwife to see them through childbirth. In their role as healers, these women had considerable knowledge of anatomy and pharmacology. They used analgesics, digestive aids, anti-inflammatory agents, ergot, belladonna and digitalis. Their work was highly valued (Oakley 1976).

Midwives came under attack primarily from the Church in its drive to support and control an emerging medical profession. Female healers also challenged the male hegemony of the medieval Church because disease was considered to be a God-given affliction and therefore it had to be seen to be under strict religious control. Consequently many midwives were persecuted and accused of practising witchcraft.

Medical practice required a university education. This effectively excluded women because they were barred from universities. During the 13th century, male medical groups such as the barber surgeons and apothecaries began to consolidate their position by forming guilds and professional associations, which enabled them to demand exclusive rights to practise. State regulation of medical practice began in the 16th century overseen by the Church, which was responsible for surveying the competence of medical practitioners (Oakley 1976). The Church also licensed midwives during the 16th and 17th centuries but it was never rigorously enforced (Witz 1992).

Midwifery skills were acquired through experience and an informal apprenticeship. Often skills were passed on from mother to daughter. Although there were many midwives who did not have any formal training, apprenticeships were available, some lasting as long as 7 years. The instructing midwife would receive payment (Oakley 1976).

Denunciation by the male medical profession of the female midwife as ignorant and untrained began in the 17th century, which also saw the emergence of the male midwife. Initially they were only called upon when intervention was required but eventually, as they became more fashionable, especially among upper-class women, they began to compete directly with the female midwives for care of women in normal labour. The majority of midwives were unlicensed but during the 17th century, because of the threat of male midwives to their sphere of practice, they made various attempts to organise themselves, including seeking a Royal Charter in the hope of protecting their practice (Donnison 1988).

During the 18th century male midwifery practice thrived and by the 19th century, once midwifery was included in general medical training, doctors began establishing obstetrics as a specialism within the medical profession (Donnison 1988). In 1858 the Medical (Registration) Act was passed giving professional status to the numerous male medical practitioners, i.e. physicians, surgeons and apothecaries. The female group of healers and midwives was not included.

The Female Medical Society and Obstetrical Association of Midwives attempted unsuccessfully to resist the limited sphere of practice for midwives and the professional subordination of midwifery to the medical profession (Witz 1992). Women were excluded from medical training until 1876 and the majority of female midwives still did not have access to any recognised training. Consequently as scientific knowledge developed the female midwife was excluded and her role was further eroded. This marginalisation of female midwifery practice continued and culminated in the passing of the Midwives Act 1902.

STATUTORY CONTROL OF MIDWIFERY PRACTICE: THE BEGINNING OF THE END?

Statutory control of midwifery practice began with the first Midwives Act in 1902. The Act provided for state registration and mandatory training of midwives. It established the setting up of the Central Midwives Board (CMB) and the regulations for the training and supervision of midwifery practice. It legitimised control of female midwifery practice by male medical practitioners.

Prior to 1902, because of centuries of marginalisation by the medical profession, of the female healers who practised midwifery, working-class, lay midwives dominated midwifery practice. There was a minority of midwives who had undergone a formal course of midwifery training but there was little standardisation of such courses until 1872 when the London Obstetrical Society (LOS) established a midwifery examination and diploma but this diploma would not have reflected the intuitive, female knowledge of childbirth developed over many centuries.

The women involved in the formation of the Midwives Institute in 1881 (later to become the Royal College of Midwives), which was proactive in campaigning for legislation to regulate midwifery practice, had the LOS qualification in midwifery but, unlike the lay midwives, few of them had ever practised midwifery. They came from the upper and middle classes and had been drawn into midwifery reform through their links with a network of social and professional activists committed to welfare work and social reform (Heagarty 1990).

The Midwives Institute, in their eagerness for legislation, accepted the limited sphere of competence and subordinate professional status envisaged for midwives by the medical profession. Witz (1992) believes they did this in good faith, believing that by clearly confining the sphere of practice to normal labour they would be preserving a degree of autonomy for midwives. They also believed Parliamentary recognition of midwives would raise the status of midwifery practice and it would then become 'an occupation for educated, refined gentlewomen' (Witz 1992, p 122).

Legislation, which made registration and formal training a prerequisite for midwifery practice, eventually was to force the lay midwife out of practice, but the Act included a period of grace during which lay midwives could register as legitimate practitioners. This measure was also needed as a stopgap until sufficient numbers of midwives had been trained.

Eventually midwives fell into one of three categories: the trained midwife, the lay midwife and the uncertificated midwife. To be registered the lay midwife had to provide evidence that she had been practising for at least one year prior to implementation of the Act and, reminiscent of the medieval Church's control of medical practice, provide a certificate of 'good character' from a church minister. Lay midwives were known as 'bona fide' midwives. The uncertificated midwives were only allowed to practise until 1905. Bona fide midwives constituted the majority of the Midwives Roll, which was published for the first time in 1905 (Towler & Bramall 1986).

The medical profession was divided over the issue of midwifery regulation. A minority group was entirely opposed to legislation, wanting to abolish the role of the female midwife. Those doctors supporting midwifery legislation, however, wanted it on their own terms, with a 'rigidly demarcated and de-skilled sphere of competence' (Witz 1992, p 109). Witz likens the campaign by doctors for midwifery legislation to the spider legislating for the fly. Legislation was not going to give the midwives professional autonomy or status but ensnare them in a web of legislation that controlled and supervised a sphere of practice defined by the medical profession.

The focus of midwifery practice was to be attendance on normal labour, thus preserving female midwifery practice 'as a distinct occupation role within the medical division of labour' (Witz 1992, p 112). Witz describes this as a deskilling strategy and it could be argued that this strategy has continued throughout the 20th century. Versluysen (cited in Hearn 1982) considers the Act to have confirmed the subordinate status of midwives because the Central Midwives Board 'put a majority of medical men on the council responsible for the training and registration of midwives, thereby making clear that neither skilled women nor mothers could regard birth as their own concern any more' (p 43).

Witz considers that the decision to retain the role of the midwife, albeit through a deskilling strategy, was made for pragmatic reasons; midwives already attended a high proportion of births, especially poor women who could not afford the doctor's fees. Witz also suggests that doctors were reluctant to place themselves in a position where they could be called upon to meet the demand for midwifery services. Labour was unpredictable and time consuming or, to quote the medical profession of the time, 'tiresome and unremunerative work' (Witz 1992, p 22).

THE INTRODUCTION OF ANTENATAL CARE AND ITS IMPACT ON MIDWIFERY PRACTICE

At the turn of the century infant and maternal mortality rates were high. The annual infant death rate was 120 000. The chief causes of death in the first 3 months of life were prematurity and immaturity. Infant diarrhoea accounted for 28% of infant deaths. Various reports published at the time considered that many infant deaths were avoidable and could be prevented by antenatal and intrapartum care. Maternal ignorance was also considered to be part of the problem (Oakley 1986).

Maternal mortality was 1 in 264 births. Approximately 3000 women died annually. A senior medical officer responsible for maternity and child health within the newly created Ministry of Health, Janet Campbell, published a report in 1924 that described maternal mortality as a major public health problem. Campbell considered many

maternal deaths to be avoidable; to prove her point she instigated the very first national 'confidential enquiries' into maternal death. Medical officers of health in different parts of the country were asked to investigate all cases of puerperal fever (both fatal and non-fatal) and all other maternal deaths occurring in their areas between October 1921 and December 1922.

This investigation showed that of 380 deaths, 256 were due to puerperal fever. Campbell considered one of the most likely causes of maternal mortality was the quality of professional attendance in pregnancy, at delivery and during the postnatal period. She thought the solution to the problem was the provision of antenatal care and she proposed improvements in medical education and midwifery training that included antenatal care. She effectively brought maternal mortality and morbidity to public attention (Oakley 1986).

Once maternal death began to be reported as being 'avoidable', many women's groups, such as the Women's Co-operative Guild, Women's Labour League, the National Council of Women and the National Union of Women's Suffrage Societies, began to campaign for better maternity care. The ensuing expansion of antenatal care put increasing demands on the midwife and the ultimate aim of preventing infection led to the call for midwives to also be trained as nurses (Kirkham 1996). Heagarty (1990) considers this supported the use of nurse training to legitimise the expanded role of the midwife and also reinforced the medical profession's dominance in maternity care.

During the 1930s subsidised midwifery services began and by 1936 around half of practising midwives were salaried or subsidised. Inevitably independent midwives experienced financial hardship. The 1936 Midwives Act required local authorities to provide a salaried whole-time midwifery service. It also enabled the incorporation of antenatal care into midwifery practice and the provision of analgesia. The Act also provided for midwives to be engaged as maternity nurses in cases where the doctor was in charge of the delivery. This effectively brought to an end the role of the unqualified handywoman. Following this Act the CMB extended midwifery training and refresher courses began.

THE IMPACT OF THE NATIONAL HEALTH SERVICE ON MIDWIFERY PRACTICE

The introduction of the National Health Service (NHS) in 1948 heralded the beginning of changes in midwives' working patterns that were to continue throughout the 20th century. The NHS gave GPs a strong incentive to develop antenatal care by giving them a separate fee for midwifery services. Women would also have direct access to GP care independent of the midwife and the obstetrician. This meant that the first point of contact for pregnant women became the GP rather than the midwife and, according to Oakley (1986), this 'permanently altered the midwives' control over maternity care' (Oakley 1986, p 143). GPs began to see women in early pregnancy, giving them, rather than the midwives, the opportunity to define normality.

Women now had the opportunity for a hospital confinement and ultimately this resulted in fragmentation of care and fundamentally affected the role of the domiciliary midwife. The home-birth rate dropped significantly during the 1950s and while the midwives attending these births expressed greater job satisfaction than the hospital midwives, in some areas domiciliary midwives were expressing dissatisfaction at just providing postnatal care. These midwives had effectively been reduced to the role of maternity nurse.

THE IMPACT OF GOVERNMENT REPORTS ON MIDWIFERY PRACTICE

This situation was exacerbated with the publication of the Cranbrook Committee Report (HMSO 1959), which recommended a 70% hospital confinement rate but stressed that the domiciliary midwifery service should be maintained (Towler & Bramall 1986). This of course was necessary to accommodate care of the increasing number of women who were being discharged ever earlier after hospital delivery because of a shortage of beds. The role of the midwife was becoming increasingly ill defined.

In 1970 the Peel Report (DHSS 1970) was published. The Peel Committee had been set up at the recommendation of the Department of Health to look at the domiciliary midwifery service and the hospital maternity bed situation, in the light of the falling birth rate and the increasing popularity of hospital confinement. The Peel Report recommended 100% hospital confinement in the interests of safety.

The Peel Report further fragmented midwifery care and enabled the medicalisation of childbirth to begin in earnest and was to fundamentally change the nature of midwifery practice (Bates 1993). Following its implementation care became very fragmented and eventually interventions became so commonplace that they came to be regarded as the norm; for example, active management of labour supported by continuous electronic fetal heart rate monitoring. The World Health Organisation published a report called *Having a Baby in Europe* (WHO 1986) that outlined the problems of the high levels of fragmented care which had developed since the publication of the Peel Report.

The publication 2 years later of the Briggs Report (Briggs 1972) heralded sweeping changes to the professional structure of education, the control and government of nurses, health visitors and midwives. Despite fierce opposition from the CMB, who considered the report to be a threat to the identity of midwifery as being separate from nursing, the government accepted the findings of the Briggs Report and the Nurses, Midwives and Health Visitors Act was eventually passed in 1979. The Central Midwives Board handed over its functions to new statutory bodies, the main one being the United Kingdom Central Council for Nursing, Midwifery and Health Visiting (UKCC) in 1983.

The Short Report (HMSO 1980), *Perinatal and Neonatal Mortality*, compounded the problem for midwives because it gave continued support to the notion of a 100% hospital confinement and the maximum use of technology. This report devotes nine pages to discussion concerning midwifery practice. The discussion entitled 'Midwives and their training' begins with the following quote from a letter to *The Times*: 'It does not seem to be sufficiently appreciated by society as a whole that midwives are a dying species' (HMSO 1980, p 71).

The Committee cites the need for 'absolute safety for mothers and more recently babies' and the new 'investigative approach' to maternity care as being the cause of the demise of the midwife. The Committee considered that this new approach to maternity care made it inevitable that obstetricians would be required to undertake practices traditionally assigned to the midwife and that included care of 'normal' women.

They enquired of the RCM representative whether midwives needed to rewrite their job description. The College response was that they did not and midwives ought to be 'allowed' to fulfil their existing job description (p 71). The use of the term 'allowed' is very revealing. It reflects the RCM's awareness of where the power lay, with the medical profession and the Parliamentary committee. Feminists would argue that the College was dealing with powerful patriarchal forces.

The Short Committee was committed to routine use of technology in the belief that it would reduce perinatal mortality rates and expressed the view that women (and midwives) had to embrace the use of technology even though the committee was aware that:

Inevitably the intensive care approach has led to some dissatisfaction – mothers who have not been adequately prepared may feel that the process of delivery is being dehumanised by technology, and midwives may regret that they are displaced by doctors in the supervision of labour. Nevertheless much of the new technology is of accepted benefit to the mother and baby and we regard it as an integral part of modern maternity care. (HMSO 1980)

The RCM comment that midwives ought to be allowed to fulfil their existing job description clearly struck a chord with the Committee because they made efforts to appear supportive of midwifery practice. For example, they recommended that steps were taken to make better use of midwifery skills, that midwives should be given greater responsibility for the care of women with uncomplicated pregnancies, and that efforts should be made to re-establish midwifery as a profession (p 76). But the overall strategy of the Committee was the same as that used by the doctors prior to the passing of the Midwives Act in 1902 – a process of deskilling:

Overall supervision of the care of the pregnant woman is the responsibility of the doctor and we do not consider that midwives should become more active in their role as independent practitioners, but should become effective members of the maternity team. (HMSO 1980)

This ensured that midwifery would remain 'a distinct occupation role within the medical division of labour' (Witz 1992, p 112), thus maintaining medical control of both child bearing and midwifery practice. The Committee expressed their approval of DOMINO deliveries and stressed the need for adequate numbers of community midwives because of the inevitable increase in workload in the postnatal period, indicating that the future primary role of the community midwife was to be postnatal care (HMSO 1980).

In response to the recommendations of the Short Report, the government established a Maternity Services Advisory Committee whose brief was to address issues surrounding perinatal death rates and ways of improving care for women in maternity hospitals. Consumer groups were complaining about the impersonal nature of both maternity hospitals and the care women received. This resulted in the publication of the *Maternity Care in Action Reports, parts I, II and III* (HMSO 1982, 1984, 1985). Their stated intention was to act as a guide to good practice but in reality they exacerbated the problem for women (and midwives), as making a clear distinction between antepartum, postpartum and postnatal care enabled obstetricians to isolate antenatal and intrapartum care for themselves further isolating the postnatal period.

Oakley (1986) considers the Short Report displayed a profound change in attitude towards women (the chair was a woman – the late Renee Short). Previous reports had been sensitive to women's preferences, whereas the Short Report dismissed the preferences of women as irrelevant to policy formulation. Policy developments included antenatal care becoming a screening exercise for place of birth and women's preferences being seen as incompatible with the medical determination of risk. The Short Committee's deliberations confirm Ann Oakley's belief that: 'The achievements of male obstetricians over those of female midwifery are rarely argued empirically, but always *a priori*, from the double premise of male and medical superiority' (Oakley 1980, p 11).

The move from community-based care to hospital-based consultant-led care had an enormous impact on the work of midwives. Midwives accommodated the changes and embraced the routine use of technology, perceiving it as an extension of their skills. Midwives have been criticised for not realising that this would result in erosion of their skills (Donnison 1988) but midwives did not have the status and consequently the power to challenge two powerful male groups – the medical profession and the House of Commons. They had been subject to patriarchal forces working against them since the turn of the century. Eventually the oppressed become their own oppressors (Bartky 1998).

A lone voice in the wilderness was a medical statistician, Marjorie Tew. She analysed all available data, including the Registrar General's statistics, and came to the following conclusion: 'There is no causal relationship between hospital birth and lower perinatal mortality rate' (Tew 1978). She also considered that analysis of the statistics supported the hypothesis 'that reductions in mortality are more likely to result from improvements in the general health of the mothers and their fitness to reproduce than from innovations in scientific obstetrics no matter how sophisticated' (Tew 1981).

Initially Marjorie Tew had difficulty in getting her main work, *Safer childbirth? A Critical History of Maternity Care,* published because she was opposing 'the establishment' (Tew 1990, p. viii). This demonstrates the pervasive nature of patriarchy (Lowe & Hubbard 1983, Rich 1977).

The Midwives Act of 1902 was never going to give midwives opportunities to develop professional status through education, training and practice. The deskilling strategy successfully employed by the medical profession contained the midwife's sphere of practice to the normal and ensured medical control over the occupational infrastructure of midwifery, thus maintaining medical control of midwifery practice (Witz 1992). It was because of this that the Short Committee, having endorsed obstetric control of normal pregnancy and birth, felt able to ask if the midwives needed to rewrite their job description. Male medical superiority over female midwifery

practice was *a priori* and not yet open to challenge but this was to change in the 1990s.

Question for Reflection ?????

If midwives as a group had a feminist consciousness, what impact might this have on the organisation of maternity services?

SEPARATE LEGISLATION FOR MIDWIVES?

The 1979 Nurses, Midwives and Health Visitors Act resulted in the dissolution of the Central Midwives Board and the General Nursing Council, which were replaced by the United Kingdom Central Council for Nursing, Midwifery and Health Visiting (UKCC). Periodically disillusioned midwives call for a return of separate legislation for midwives. The Association of Radical Midwives (ARM), founded in 1976, published a Midwifery Legislation Manifesto in 1991. The document argued that since the 1979 Act the midwifery profession had seen a further erosion of its autonomy and was experiencing difficulty in meeting the needs of child-bearing women.

The root cause of the problems midwives were experiencing was not the 1979 Act per se but the fact that birth in hospital had become the norm and this had reduced midwives from giving total care to women throughout the child-bearing process to being contributors to fragmented systems of care. They had effectively been deskilled (Witz 1992). Hunt (1996) believes the publication of *Changing Childbirth* in England (Department of Health 1993), with its focus on giving women continuity of care, plus choice and control of the child-bearing process, had the potential to reinstate midwives' autonomy but much depended on the midwives' willingness to resume their former responsibilities and accept accountability for their actions. But Hunt considers this could be an unrealistic expectation because 'Most midwives in Britain have still trained first as nurses and are more familiar with the role of helper in care than leader of care' (Hunt 1996, p 204).

Whilst this is true, a feminist analysis reveals that at a fundamental level, midwives were and remain an oppressed group. Bartky (1998, p 48) describes psychological oppression as being 'weighed down in your mind'. She considers it to be institutionalised and systematic and results in the oppressed becoming their own oppressors. Working in hospitals over many decades has institutionalised midwives and laid them open to patriarchal forces.

It is extremely unlikely in the present climate that midwives will get separate legislation. The Nurses, Midwives and Health Visitors Act (1979) began the process of integrating the statutory control of healthcare workers. The passing of the Nurses, Midwives and Health Visitors Act (1997) consolidated this position. This Act dissolved the UKCC and the four national boards and replaced them with a new body, the Nursing and Midwifery Council (NMC). This has effectively centralised the control of healthcare workers although local supervision of midwives continues through local supervising authorities. The stated purpose of the NMC is public protection through 'rigorous regulation'. The President, Jonathan Asbridge, envisages the NMC becoming 'an efficient, modern and effective regulatory machine' (Asbridge 2002, p 3). It is a patriarchal machine.

There is now a plethora of NHS organisations exercising patriarchal control of all aspects of the clinical practice of all healthcare workers, including the medical profession. These include the National Institute for Clinical Excellence (NICE), NHS Litigation Authority (NHSLA), which established the Clinical Negligence Scheme for Trusts (CNST) in 1994, the Audit Commission, National Clinical Assessment Authority, National Patient Safety Agency, Commission for Health Improvement, Patients Advice and Liaison Services (PALS) and the NHS Modernisation Agency which, together with the NHSLA, is leading the Delivering Healthy Babies Project in trusts with a focus on multidisciplinary care. These organisations have been implemented in response to either the NHS Plan (Department of Health 2000a), or the recommendations of the Kennedy Report (Bristol Royal Infirmary 2001, Dimond 2002a).

Eventually there will be a regulatory body to regulate the regulators. The NHS Reform and Health Care Professions Act 2002 will establish the Council for the Registration of Healthcare Professionals (Dimond 2002a). There is to be a Commission for Healthcare Audit and Inspection which will have overall responsibility for auditing, regulating and overseeing all care given in the NHS and this will include midwifery care.

Separate midwifery legislation, certainly for the time being, is at odds with political will that is driving government policy towards a centralised, multidisciplinary approach to regulation. Patriarchal forces are scrutinising and regulating clinical practice as never before.

Question for Reflection ?????

Think about your own practice. What impact have the many government agencies had on your professional practice?

IS MIDWIFERY A PROFESSION?

Feminist interpretations of professional status have shown it to be a patriarchal concept (Heagarty 1990, Oakley 1993, Witz 1992). Professions promote and extend their power by claiming an exclusive body of knowledge and expertise, e.g. medicine, law and the church. They organise and control themselves by establishing standards of ethics, knowledge and skills for licensed practitioners (Oakley 1993). Professionals usually consider their work to be for the public good. This enables them to distance themselves from any accusations of self-interest that may occur as a result of their demand for professional control.

Traditional approaches to professionalism do not acknowledge that it is linked to a dominant social elite. Membership of professions tended to come from the upper and middle classes and at the turn of the century the UK still had an Empire and society was divided into a clearly defined class structure. Melosh (cited in Heagarty 1990) considered professions were more than just special organisations of work but rather particular expressions and vehicles of dominant class and culture.

The original membership of the Midwives Institute demonstrates the truth of this observation. It was composed mainly of middle- and upper-class women who joined forces with male professional groups in their efforts to achieve legislation for midwives. Heagarty is critical of the Institute for this. She thinks that to focus on the struggle between midwife and medical man deflects attention away from alliances made between a female midwifery elite and male doctors and the result of these alliances on the rank and file of mainly working-class female midwives. She also considers that although the women of the Institute joined the suffrage cause in the name of all women, their attitude towards working-class women displayed more kinship with men than women (Heagarty 1990).

At a fundamental level the women of the Midwives Institute were social reformers as opposed to being midwives (although they held midwifery qualifications). They were also pawns in a patriarchal power game. They were being used as scapegoats to enable the medical profession to maintain control of midwifery practice. There was an urgent need to address vital issues such as maternal and infant mortality rates, which were high. The practices of the uneducated bona fide midwives were probably considered to be part of the problem. Consequently the women of the Institute, by instinct social reformers rather than practising midwives, felt allegiance to social reform rather than the plight of the midwives. Feminist scholarship would later reveal the all-pervasive nature of patriarchy and the ways in which it operated. Hubbard (1983), for example, describes patriarchy as being:

Completely intertwined and hidden in the ordinary truths and realities that the people who live in the society accept without question. This tends to obscure the fact that these beliefs are actively generated and furthered by members of the dominant group because they are consistent with that group's interests. (p 1)

Hearn (1982) explores issues surrounding females and professional status. He describes primarily female occupations such as midwifery, nursing, health visiting, radiography, speech therapy, etc. as 'paramedical semi-professions to service the full profession of medicine'. He puts social workers into the same category because they spend their time serving the needs of doctors, lawyers and the courts.

Hearn highlights the development of hospital-based medicine as being of special significance for the medical semi-professions. The form and layout of the buildings and the sexual division of labour within and outside them reinforce each other. Hospital-based maternity care has certainly had a profound impact on midwifery practice. He considers that structural arrangements are developed with the specific intention of enabling a semi-profession to serve a particular profession and this is a major way of defining the space within which the semi-profession is expected to function. A good example of this is the ongoing reorganisation of midwifery care and the maternity services to meet developments in obstetric and neonatal paediatric practice.

Hearn singles out midwives as being of great significance because we work within the private sphere of women's lives, e.g. giving birth, but we do so within a public arena and this creates potential for conflict. He considers professionalisation is not some evolutionary natural process (as men would have women believe) but is merely a term for a variety of processes by which men move into and increase their influence on the semi-professions (Hearn 1982).

Hearn argues that female semi-professional occupations can never have full professional status until the activity they undertake is fully dominated by men in both management and the ranks. It will then become 'masculinised'. Jonathan Asbridge, President of the new Nursing and Midwifery Council, used this term in a news item about the numbers of men in nursing. He considers nursing is becoming 'masculinised' because a record number of male nurses are now working in UK hospitals. More than 10% of nurses are men compared to 1% 50 years ago (*Daily Mail* 30th October 2002, p 18).

Men were excluded from midwifery until the passing of the Sexual Discrimination and Equal

Opportunities Act (1975). The number of male midwives remains small but in the light of Hearn's argument, if the numbers were to rise significantly, theoretically this could enable midwifery to achieve full professional status. Hearn (1982) considers that becoming masculinised is 'the fate that awaits the semi-profession' that aspires to full professional status. If midwifery became masculinised it would become absorbed into obstetrics and women would be subjected to an entirely masculine view of birth.

So what is the solution to this seemingly insoluble problem? Midwifery has not been helped by being continually linked to nursing, especially since the mid-20th century. Nursing and midwifery are two entirely separate occupations with entirely different roots. Whereas nursing has its roots in domestic work (Oakley 1993), midwifery has its roots in the female healing role (Mitchell & Oakley 1976).

Oakley is sympathetic to the plight of nurses. She thinks the underlying cause of their problem is that doctors are associated with curing whereas nursing is associated with caring. Even though caring is fundamental to curing, society places greater value on the ability to cure. Despite nursing becoming highly specialised it has yet to achieve full professional status. Oakley thinks this is because advances in medical science have made nurses invisible (Oakley 1993).

The medical profession has tried unsuccessfully, over many centuries, to make midwifery practice invisible. It has not yet succeeded because against all the odds, midwifery has managed to maintain fundamental skills that embrace the emotional, psychological and physiological aspects of child bearing. Midwives do not need to become embroiled in arguments about what constitutes professional status. It is a spurious argument because the obsession with professional status has its roots in patriarchal power and control which has alienated women from the child-bearing process (Bates 1993). Women need confident, articulate midwives with highly developed skills. The erosion of the role of autonomous midwifery practice over many decades has restricted the options available to women and has promoted child bearing as a pathological medicalised process (Oakley & Houd 1990).

Question for Reflection ?????

What do you think constitutes professional midwifery practice?

PATRIARCHY AND GENDER RELATIONS

Midwifery's struggle for survival over many centuries demonstrates the all-pervasive nature and power of patriarchy and how it has enabled gender inequality to be maintained.

Feminists initially used the concept of patriarchy to:

- analyse the systematic organisation of male supremacy over women
- analyse the exploitative relations which affect and subordinate women
- provide a conceptual framework for the nature of the dominance of men in society.

Adrienne Rich, a radical feminist from the 1970s, gave an all-embracing definition of patriarchy. She described it as:

A familial-social, ideological, political system in which men – by force, direct pressure, or through ritual, tradition, law and language, customs, etiquette, education, and the division of labour – determine what part women shall or shall not play, and in which the female is everywhere subsumed under the male. (Rich 1977, p 57)

Sylvia Walby later defined patriarchy in more simple terms. She described it as 'a system of social structures and practices in which men dominate, oppress and exploit women' (Walby 1990, p 20). She considered patriarchy to be both private and public. Private patriarchy was based on gender inequalities in the home and public patriarchy based on inequality and discrimination in public life.

Postmodern feminists have criticised (perhaps unjustly) Walby's theory as being too generalist (Pilcher 1998, Rogers 1998). They argue that society has become too complex, i.e. age, class, race, ethnicity, and there are different kinds of femininities and masculinities but the theory remains useful for shedding light on gender inequalities if the complexities of society are taken into consideration (Pilcher 1998).

Walby argues that whilst the feminist movement was a key factor in shifting patriarchy from the private to the public arena, it still exists. Her definition of patriarchy specifies systems, structures and practices. Midwives have been subject to ever-changing systems of care and restructuring of the maternity services that have defined the space and consequently the way in which they practise. Their practice has also been controlled to a significant degree by the practices of the medical profession. Walby would argue that obstetric practice is a form of public patriarchy that has effectively controlled child-bearing women and midwifery practice. The patriarchal control of child bearing has been well documented by many feminist writers (Doyal 1995, Ehrenreich & English 1979, Oakley 1976, 1980, 1986, 1993, Pratten 1990, Rich 1977).

Connell (1987) takes Walby's theories of patriarchy and gender relations a step further. Rather than explaining why there are gender inequalities, he is concerned with how they are maintained. Connell does not consider gender relations to be fixed. Rather, he thinks they are an ongoing process and are subject to resistance as well as conformity. Gender relations, he suggests, can be contested or accepted and patriarchy therefore can be subject to challenge.

Midwives have been attempting to challenge patriarchy for many centuries. The real difficulty is knowing how to mount a successful challenge to medical hegemony, which continued during the latter half of the 20th century despite increasing numbers of women entering the medical profession (Elston 1993). The problem for women entering a predominantly male discipline such as obstetrics is that collectively this group will express a masculine view of childbirth. If the women wish to be successful they must subscribe to this view.

It is sometimes difficult to understand this collusion, especially when it is midwives subscribing to it. The feminist philosopher Bartky suggests that collusion arises through what she describes as 'a divided consciousness'. Women, although seeing themselves as victims of an unjust system of power, can nevertheless perceive it as being natural, inevitable and inescapable. Consequently they remain blind to the extent to which they themselves are implicated in the victimisation of other women (Bartky 1990, p 11–12). Midwives have been subject to medical hegemony for many decades.

Medical hegemony

The concept of medical hegemony and how it works is worth a brief exploration. Connell (1987) describes the term 'hegemony' as a social ascendancy, which he considers is achieved in an ongoing play of social forces. Ascendancy is usually achieved within a balance of these forces, which must be kept in a state of play if ascendancy is to be maintained.

The story of midwifery's ongoing struggle for survival provides a good example of medical hegemony in action. For many centuries doctors strove for social ascendancy over the midwives, aided and abetted by the Church. The balance of forces, the midwives versus the doctors and male midwives, remained roughly equal until the male doctors and male midwives gained social ascendancy over the female midwives. Eventually the educated female healers and midwives as a group were driven out of practice (Donnison 1988, Oakley 1993, Towler & Bramall 1986). Poor women could not afford the doctors' and male midwives' fees so local women through necessity took on the role of lay midwife for these women.

When the campaign for midwifery legislation began the state of play came into sharp focus again with the doctors struggling for ascendancy over the midwife, this time aided and abetted by the House of Commons and various other agencies. In the deliberations of the Short Committee 80 years later, technology was the major patriarchal force.

Raymond DeVries predicted the demise of traditional midwifery practice once the application of technology to pregnancy and childbirth became the norm. He believes relentless use of technology can create a uniform culture that will render midwifery skills obsolete (DeVries 1993). Unfortunately the belief persists that modern obstetric practice is responsible for the huge reduction in maternal mortality that occurred during the 20th century (Shorter 1983).

Maternal mortality was reduced by 50% during the 1930s and 1940s. The reduction was a result of better living conditions, water supply, better nutrition, contraception, the discovery of sulphonamide drugs and penicillin, and the use of ergometrine and blood transfusion (Tew 1990). All of this occurred long before modern obstetrics got into its stride. The fact that belief in obstetric practice persisted for so long despite evidence to the contrary demonstrates the power of patriarchy.

The prime source of patriarchal power towards the end of the 20th century was no longer the medical profession. Whilst still powerful, it did not exercise the same degree of control as in the past. There were a variety of reasons for this. The reorganisation of the NHS in the early 1990s gave greater power to other sources of patriarchal power, for example general managers and chief executives of trusts.

A powerful driver for change was the revision of the Legal Aid rules in 1990. From here on, all claims on behalf of infants became state funded (Capstick 1993). Inevitably this boosted the number of claims. The ensuing fear of litigation made it equally inevitable that a more formal approach to risk assessment and management would be adopted. Huge expenditure on clinical negligence claims led to the setting up of the NHS Litigation Authority and the implementation of the Clinical Negligence Scheme for Trusts (CNST) in 1994 (NHSLA 2002). This has led to defensive practice by both midwives and obstetricians and has further eroded the role of the midwife. The legal profession and the state are a powerful source of patriarchal power within the maternity services.

CONSUMER IMPACT ON MIDWIFERY PRACTICE AND WAYS OF WORKING

Following the publication of Janet Campbell's report on maternal deaths in the 1920s, women began to realise that maternal death was avoidable. Campaigning by the many women's groups, based on the findings of Janet Campbell's confidential enquiry into maternal death due to sepsis at the beginning of the century, resulted in the introduction of antenatal care and eventually the

provision of hospital beds. This had a profound effect upon midwifery education and the ways in which midwives were employed. In the second half of the 20th century consumer groups such as the National Childbirth Trust and the Association for Improvements in Maternity Services have campaigned relentlessly on behalf of child-bearing women.

This culminated in the setting up of a House of Commons Select Committee chaired by Nicholas Winterton. The report of this committee (House of Commons 1992) highlighted the importance of the social context of child bearing and the impact of health inequalities. The report expressed the view that the outcome of pregnancy for both mother and baby was largely dependent on the woman's social environment and it questioned the indiscriminate use of technology.

The findings of this report did not subscribe to the patriarchal view of child bearing and therefore they were not implemented. Instead another committee was convened chaired by Baroness Cumberlege. This committee published the *Changing Childbirth* report (Department of Health 1993) which, although recommending that women should have choice and greater control of the child-bearing process, continued to support a medical view of pregnancy and birth.

During the 1990s, the other three countries of the UK reviewed their provision of maternity care. Each country published a report that supported woman-centred care and recommendations that women should have greater choice and control of the care they received (DHSS Northern Ireland 1994, Scottish Office 1993, Welsh Office 1991).

All of these reports brought a wind of change to the maternity services and midwives, in efforts to provide a degree of continuity of care within fragmented services, sought opportunities to rethink models of midwifery care. This took place against a backdrop of reorganisation of the NHS and increasing litigation.

CHANGING PATTERNS OF MIDWIFERY CARE

Following the implementation of the Community Care Act (1990), most district general hospitals converted to trust status. In the majority of these

NHS trusts midwives practise in an obstetric-led environment. Hospital-based midwives provide care for all pregnant women regardless of risk. Obstetric practice and the routine application of technology to all aspects of the child-bearing process evident in many trusts have effectively marginalised midwifery practice within the hospital environment.

Ever more sophisticated methods of antenatal screening resulted in an increase in fetal medicine, high-dependency and neonatal intensive care units throughout the UK. Specialist midwifery posts were created for care of diabetic women, bereavement counselling and risk management. More recently, following the implementation of a nationwide antenatal screening programme, regional antenatal screening co-ordinator midwives have been appointed (Janecek 2002).

Since 1997 the main thrust of NHS care has been towards reducing health inequalities through public health, health promotion and meeting the health needs of the socially disadvantaged (Department of Health 1999, 2001). Social and health inequalities are a major cause of poor pregnancy outcomes for both mother and baby. Midwives now work within programmes such as SureStart, which was set up in response to concern about a lack of parenting skills. Traditionally preparation for parenting was integral to the role of the midwife but it too became a casualty of the medicalisation of child bearing as the focus of antenatal classes became preparation for labour rather than parenting.

The *Patient's Charter* (Department of Health 1994) advocated that each pregnant woman should have a named midwife who would be responsible for providing care throughout pregnancy, labour and delivery and the postnatal period. This strengthened the recommendations of *Changing Childbirth* and gave midwives another opportunity to develop different systems of care to enable greater continuity of care and choice for women by enhancing the role of the midwife as lead professional (Department of Health 1993).

Team midwifery

There were three main models of team midwifery developed throughout the late 1980s and early 1990s: teams in the hospital setting, in the community and teams providing care in both the hospital and community setting. Teams usually consisted of a small core of midwives providing care for both high- and low-risk women. This was based on the assumption that all women, regardless of risk and type of delivery, would benefit from midwifery input into their care. Caroline Flint is a great proponent of this model of care and she led the well-known Know Your Midwife scheme. A group of four midwives aimed to provide exclusive care for 250 low-risk women per annum. The aim was for the women to get to know all four midwives, one of whom would be with her in labour (Flint 1993b, Flint & Poulengeris 1987).

Team midwifery has been problematic for both women and midwives. A contentious issue for hospital-based midwives was the requirement that they should rotate through all shifts and around all areas of clinical practice. Whilst this enables midwives to maintain their skills in all areas, many disliked the lack of stability and felt it prevented them from building specialised expertise in an area of their own choosing (Ball et al 2002). Small teams achieved the intended aim of continuity of care but at great cost to individual midwives, who had to work increasingly longer hours to maintain continuity. Larger teams resulted in the very problem for women that they had been set up to rectify – fragmented care.

A national study of team midwifery confirmed that it is associated with higher levels of staff burnout because the midwives, as well as working longer hours than midwives working in traditional patterns, felt it gave them less control over their decision making and working patterns and they were paid less (Sandall 1996). Working patterns can be problematic for both team and caseload midwifery practice. Providing woman-centred care may not be midwife centred.

Caseload midwifery

This consists of small groups of midwives working with a defined group of women to provide a full range of care. The midwife is responsible for the planning and management of care in partnership with the woman, including liaison with medical colleagues and other professionals in the multidisciplinary team. These midwives may be based in hospital or the community, with a caseload of 30–40 women a year. Caseload midwifery practice is sometimes referred to as midwifery group practice. The midwives are expected to be available for their women when required and are known to work long hours. Job satisfaction for these midwives can be very high but like team midwives, burnout rates are high (Sandall 1995, 1999).

A small study of group midwifery practice in a London hospital highlighted the need for flexibility of working patterns and midwives had to be prepared to work long shifts. Nonetheless, the job satisfaction was high. Interestingly, none of the midwives in this study had dependent children. The midwives without children considered it would be impossible to continue with this way of working once they did have children. The majority of midwives in the study agreed that part-time work was not really an option for group practice working because it might lead to a decrease in continuity of carer for women (Fenwick 1998).

A letter from a practising midwife to the *British Journal of Midwifery* (July 2002, p 424) considers that caseload midwifery is a working style that only a few midwives can comfortably manage. The author considers that it leads to midwives working to exhaustion levels, creating unsafe practice levels, undermines family life and the remuneration is poor. She takes great exception to the notion that non-interventionist, supportive midwifery care can only be provided by caseload midwives and she objects to Lewis's (2000) view that hospital midwives are 'guardians of the medical model'. She suggests rather that they are individuals doing a difficult job and reminds us that they are 'the backbone of maternity services in Britain today'.

One-to-one midwifery practice

This project took the concept of continuity of care a step further by aiming to provide continuity of carer. Twenty midwives were deployed for 800 women, giving each midwife a caseload of 40 women. The midwives worked in partnerships and were given a high degree of autonomy and flexibility in the management of their workload. Arrangements for being available to women were personal and varied but were mainly organised within their partnerships. Midwives were able to reorganise their planned work and ensure rest time following night calls. Flexibility included an absence of fixed duties such as antenatal clinics and they were never used as a reserve workforce for hospital (Stevens & McCourt 2002).

Key to the success of the project for midwives was the inbuilt flexibility of working patterns that were not apparent in standard team midwifery working patterns. Having control over working patterns enables midwives to integrate their home life and be more responsive to women's needs (Sandall 1996).

Flint acknowledges that midwives working in both team and caseload practice often feel as if they are on duty all the time and this is because they probably are. She suggests they may be partly to blame by not turning off their bleeps. She suggest that this demonstrates they have 'a great interest in their subject' and 'they are fulfilling the role of a professional woman who needs to think through and think forward about her profession' (Flint 1993a, p 144).

Flint is well known for her commitment to midwifery and woman-centred care but here she seems to be suggesting that feeling overworked is the price midwives have to pay if they are to fulfil their professional role. But midwives are women too (Kirkham 1999) and they can have problems trying to juggle work and family commitments that, if unresolved, can lead to occupational stress (Birch 2001).

Theoretically, team midwifery should offer greater flexibility of working for midwives, e.g. as in one-to-one midwifery. Any system of care that is detrimental to midwives will ultimately be detrimental to women. It could be argued that this is an exploitation of women but in reality it is probably grounded in the 'caring' stereotype of feminine occupations that persists. Caring is often equated with 'self-sacrifice'. Hearn (1982) considers that this stereotyping of femininity as being caring is central to the maintenance of patriarchal control.

A structured review of several studies of mid-wifery models of care, commissioned by a group seeking evidence-based information about the best way to organise their midwifery services, found no evidence to support a long-held belief that ideally a woman needs to know the midwife who cares for her in labour (Flint & Poulengeris 1987, McCourt & Page 1996). This review suggests that women rate a competent carer as being of greater importance than knowing the midwife. The report concludes that the atten-dance in labour by a known midwife should not be the main determinant of the service (Green et al 1998).

Unfortunately this review gives no insight into the nature of the care women received. Team/caseload and one-to-one midwives usually care for women regardless of risk and therefore are required to provide midwifery care that supports obstetric practice according to degree of risk. Once midwifery care is grounded in the routine use of technology it is likely that women will give priority to competence in the manage-ment of the technology over the personal touch (Bates 1998).

Birth centres

Birth centres are a more recent innovation. These centres, managed and run by midwives, care for low-risk women with little or no medical inter-vention. Birth centres can be located within an NHS trust or be a stand-alone unit. Crowborough Birthing Centre, for example, was once an under-subscribed GP unit threatened with closure in the 1990s. It is now a thriving midwifery-led birth centre. The Alexander Birthing Centre is a small self-contained unit within an acute trust in Watford. Lichfield has a stand-alone birth centre within the community hospital which has a nor-mal birth rate of 92% (Godfrey 2002).

Birth centres are seen as the way forward for promoting midwife-led care and the role of the midwife as lead professional. They improve morale among midwives frustrated by the interventionist model of care to be found in most consultant-led units. Because birth centres enable midwives to practise to their full potential, it increases their job satisfaction and self-esteem (Godfrey 2002). Birth centres have also been shown to reduce intervention rates. For example, Barnet Health Authority (2000) evaluated the outcome of care in the Edgware birth centre and found a dramatic reduction in intervention rates.

This demonstrates the potential of offering women a clearly defined alternative choice to med-ical care. Once the benefits of a non-interventionist, midwifery model of care for women with uncom-plicated pregnancies becomes apparent, govern-ment as well as women are likely to opt for midwifery care. It is inevitable that not all mid-wives (or all women) will subscribe to this model, especially those who have become entrenched (through no fault of their own) in a medical model of birth.

Independent midwives

A very small number of midwives choose to work outside the NHS. These self-employed midwives offer a full range of care to women who pay them directly for their services. Women who choose an independent midwife often do so because they want a home birth but some trusts give independent midwives honorary contracts to enable them to work within the NHS. Some independent midwives work in partnership with each other or in a midwifery group practice (Flint 1993a).

The number of independent midwives remains very small. According to the UKCC, out of 32 291 practising midwives in 2000–2001, only 65 were recorded as being self-employed in private prac-tice. The cost of indemnity insurance is an issue. Insurance premiums can be as high as £8000 per year and consequently some independent mid-wives cannot afford to take out cover. This means that in the event of harm occurring to a woman or her baby, she would not get compensation and the personal property of the independent midwife would be at risk (Dimond 2002b). This effectively keeps the numbers of independent midwives very low (Gillen 1995).

HOME BIRTH: THE REBIRTH OF COMMUNITY MIDWIFERY?

Since the early 20th century the number of babies born at home gradually decreased as more hospital beds became available. Following the publication of the Cranbrook Report (HMSO 1959) and finally the Peel Report (DHSS 1970), which recommended 100% hospital confinement in the interests of safety, the number of women giving birth at home fell to less than 1% (Campbell & MacFarlane 1994). This began the process of relegating the community midwife to maternity nurse. The Short Report (HMSO 1980) almost completed the process. The fortunes of the community midwives began to change following the publication of *Changing Childbirth* (Department of Health 1993) and they have been undergoing a long-awaited revival. One of the recommendations of *Changing Childbirth* was that women should have greater choice and that included choice in place of birth.

An initial hurdle for women was GPs, who are usually the point of entry into the maternity services for most women. GPs' reluctance to support home birth stems from their concern about where the limits of their responsibility lie in relation to intrapartum care (Bates 2002). This was resolved by the publication of a joint statement issued by the RCM and the Royal College of General Practitioners (RCGP), confirming that in an emergency the midwife would refer directly to an obstetrician and that women wishing to arrange a home birth should be able to do so (RCM/RCGP 1995).

A further hurdle for women was the attitude of acute NHS trusts. Hospital confinement was more convenient for them. It kept pregnant women under one roof and enabled the medicalisation of all aspects of child bearing that was central to risk management strategies. There were also implications for workforce planning because home birth required the deployment of midwives into the community.

Some trusts questioned their legal obligation to provide a home birth service. This was a dilemma for midwives as well as women and created considerable conflict among consumer groups such as the Association for Improvements in Maternity Services (AIMS), who pointed out quite rightly that women could not be forced into giving birth in hospital against their will.

In response to the conflict that ensued, the UKCC issued two statements entitled 'Supporting women who intend to give birth at home'. The UKCC confirmed that whilst women may believe they have a right to home birth and midwives believed they were duty bound to attend a woman at home, legally this was not the case (UKCC 2000, 2001). The upshot of the argument was that whilst there was no statutory requirement for the NHS to provide a home birth service, national policies supported maternal choice and therefore trusts had an obligation to support women in their choices. The number of home births continues to rise, albeit sporadically, throughout the UK (Bates 2002).

Unlike alliances forged by the Midwives Institute in the 1880s, the alliance between the RCM and the RCGP in the 1990s appears to be in the interests of midwives and women. Without it, GPs are unlikely to have co-operated. In reality, medical hegemony was on the wane. Funding of the NHS and developing a new affordable, practical workforce was high on the government agenda. Consumer demands had increased. Litigation costs were rising so much that the NHSLA had been established in the early 1990s and implemented CNST standards into most trusts by 1994. The new source of patriarchal power was the NHS Management Executive and the legal profession through the NHSLA.

The election of the New Labour government in 1997 compounded the problems of the medical profession. They continued with the drive for clinical and cost effectiveness and greater consumer involvement in all aspects of healthcare. The medical profession became further destabilised by events in Bristol and Alderhay in Liverpool. Like the lay midwives 100 years previously, doctors were being seen as part of the problem. The medical profession had always had considerable political skills that had enabled them to redirect or neutralise managerial attempts to control them (Hunter 1994) but this was coming to an end.

AUDIT: A PATRIARCHAL AGENT FOR CHANGE

Despite the different models of midwifery care that emerged during the 1990s, obstetric practice in consultant-led units continued to control women and midwifery practice through policies, protocols and guidelines. The routine application of technology had become the norm and caesarean section rates began to rise. Risk management strategies were developed dependent upon intervention, which was applied to all women on a 'just in case' rather than an evidence basis (Pratten 1990). Audit of the outcome of maternity care was to become a powerful patriarchal agent for change.

The Audit Commission was set up in response to a government drive for maternity care that was both clinically and cost effective. The Commission conducted an audit of 2376 women, 500 GPs and 13 NHS trusts. Their 1997 report, *A First Class Delivery Service*, confirmed a high level of intervention rates and increasing caesarean section rates.

This report was the first document to acknowledge that there were two entirely different philosophies of maternity care: childbirth considered normal until it proved itself otherwise and childbirth only being considered normal in retrospect. And each one would result in an entirely different rationale for maternity services. The Audit Commission was of the view that whilst safety should always be of prime concern, maternity care should reflect that we are now a predominantly healthy nation and the nature of the service should be to provide care and support through a normal life event (Audit Commission 1997).

This was followed by an audit of midwifery practice in 124 maternity units carried out by the now defunct English National Board. The findings of this audit confirmed wide variations in intervention rates throughout England, suggesting blanket policies rather than individually tailored care and demonstrating that care was not woman centred. The audit also highlighted that the proportion of normal deliveries undertaken by midwives was falling. In some units the normal delivery rate was only 52%.

The audit also confirmed a rise in intervention rates and in some areas the caesarean section rate was up to 27% (ENB 1999). A further audit carried out in 1999–2000 highlighted that caesarean section rates in 56% of maternity units remained at over 20% and only 36% of services had midwife delivery rates of above 70% (ENB 2001).

The findings of this audit demonstrated that despite the variety of models of midwifery care that had been evolving since the 1980s in efforts to improve the quality of maternity care, overall the many reorganisations of maternity services were not working for the majority of women or midwives. Problematic for midwives was the introduction of NHS trusts, which introduced management practices that created increasingly stressful demands within both the job itself and the working environment (Ball et al 2002).

Trust managers began implementing government directives to extend the use of specialist midwifery skills and this coincided with continued efforts to reduce employment costs. Midwives in many units were working longer shifts, had greater workloads and a serious reduction in the number of experienced colleagues. Morale was very low, sickness and turnover rates high (Bates & McNabb 1996). The findings of the research project *Why do Midwives Leave?* (Ball et al 2002) confirm that these same problems continue.

CAN MATERNITY CARE EVER BE WOMAN CENTRED?

A good relationship based on mutual trust and respect is central to providing woman-centred care. The group of midwives most likely to feel they achieve this is community midwives (Ball et al 2002). The way in which community work is organised enables midwives to establish and develop good relationships with women although since the majority of births have taken place in hospital, few community midwives provide intrapartum care. The rise in the home birth rate is an opportunity for community midwives, if they have the skills required for attending home births, to redress the balance.

The research of Ball et al highlights the many problems for midwives working in the NHS. They feel they have very little, if any, control over the way they practise and this has resulted in many of them deciding to leave the service (Ball et al 2002). The findings of this research confirm that midwives as a group do not have a feminist consciousness because the majority continue to have the unrealistic expectation that on registration they will take responsibility for their own work and function as autonomous practitioners. Autonomous midwifery practice has been systematically phased out since the passing of the Midwives Act 1902.

Feminist research

The use of feminist approaches to research would also enable a more woman centred approach to maternity care. Feminist research endeavours to find out the questions women need to ask if they are to get the information they require to make informed choices. The scientific paradigm relies upon the results of the randomised controlled trial or quantitative research on which to base practice, i.e. it gives a generalized answer. Scientific knowledge prides itself on its objectivity but childbirth is a subjective experience, different for each woman and it can only be evaluated personally. Feminist research takes women's needs and experiences into account and aims at being instrumental in improving women's lives in some way (Webb 1993).

Walsh highlights how women seeking to work out control and choice for themselves are frequently caught up in what he calls the 'middle ground', that inevitable space that occurs when views have become polarised, e.g. normality against abnormality, intervention against non-intervention (Walsh 2002). Different women will want to make different choices (Raphael-Leff 1991). If we want to enable women to make choices we must not replace one dominant discourse with another. The challenge for midwives is to open up options for women rather than close them down (Walsh 2002). This means offering women a variety of care pathways and a choice in place of birth. This will also enable the implementation of flexible and supportive family-friendly working hours for midwives (Department of Health 2000b). For care to be woman centred it must also be midwife centred.

CONCLUSION

Rich argued in the 1970s that motherhood was no longer an experience for women because it had become institutionalised (Rich 1977). Modern obstetrics has consolidated this position by placing birth in an institution and turning the fetus into a patient. A mechanistic view of women's bodies is maintained through reproductive technologies, family planning and care during pregnancy and birth (Corea 1988, Doyal 1995, Martin 1987, Spallone 1989). The institutionalisation of midwives has rendered them apparently oblivious to this and we have unwittingly colluded in the process (Bartky 1990) because as a group we do not have a feminist consciousness (Bates 1993).

The majority of women have the potential to give birth normally. Placing midwifery practice in the community would greatly assist in putting childbirth back into its social context. The biomedical model of child bearing does not lend itself to choice, continuity and control for the majority of women or midwives. The needs of women and midwives would become central to the care we give rather than the needs of the institution. Part of the role of the midwife is to encourage self-confidence and help a woman to develop an internal locus of control, thus raising levels of self-esteem that stand a woman in good stead during the early months of motherhood.

The position of midwives within the NHS mirrors the secondary role of women in society. A feminist consciousness would enable midwives to actively seek liberation from the patriarchal ties that bind us to a masculine view of pregnancy and birth.

Key points

■ Patriarchy has systematically and persistently undermined midwives, creating problems for child-bearing women.

■ Government policy in the mid and late 20th century was instrumental in moving childbirth into hospital, despite a lack of evidence that this reduces the perinatal mortality rate. The move into hospital led to fragmentation of care.

■ In recent years different models of care have emerged that promote normality and holistic care.

■ Placing midwifery practice in the community sets it within its social context.

REFERENCES

Asbridge J 2002 A new organisation with a purpose. Nursing and Midwifery Council News 1: 3

Audit Commission 1997 A first class delivery service: improving maternity services in England and Wales. Audit Commission, London

Ball L, Curtis P, Kirkham M 2002 Why do midwives leave? Royal College of Midwives, London

Barnet Health Authority 2000 Evaluation of Edgware birth centre. Barnet Health Authority, London

Barrett M 1980 Women's oppression today: problems in Marxist feminist analysis. Verso Editions and NLB, London

Bartky SL 1990 Femininity and domination: studies in the phenomenology of oppression. Routledge, London

Bartky SL 1998 On psychological oppression. In: Rogers MF (ed) Contemporary feminist theory. McGraw-Hill, New York

Bates C 1993 Care in normal labour: a feminist perspective. In: Alexander J, Levy V, Roth C (eds) Midwifery practice: core topics 2. Macmillan, London

Bates C 1998 Continuing to care. British Journal of Midwifery 6(9): 597

Bates C (ed) 2002 Home birth handbook: volume 1. Promoting home birth. Royal College of Midwives Trust, London

Bates C, McNabb M 1996 Governing midwifery practice. British Journal of Midwifery 4(3): 119–120

Bewley S, Friend, F, Mezey G (eds) 1997 Violence against women. RCOG Press, London

Bick DE, MacArthur C 1995 The extent, severity and effect of health problems after childbirth. British Journal of Midwifery 3: 27–31

Birch L 2001 Stress in midwifery practice: an empirical study. British Journal of Midwifery 9(12): 730–734

Briggs A 1972 Report of the Committee on Nursing. HMSO, London

Bristol Royal Infirmary 2001 Learning from Bristol. Report of the Public Inquiry into Children's Heart Surgery at the BRI 1984–1995. BRI, Bristol

Campbell R, MacFarlane A 1994 Where to be born: the debate and the evidence, 2nd edn. National Perinatal Epidemiology Unit, Oxford

Capstick B (ed) Litigation: a risk management guide for midwives. Royal College of Midwives in conjunction with Capsticks Solicitors, London

Connell RW 1987 Gender and power. Basil Blackwood Ltd, Oxford

Corea G 1988 The mother machine. Women's Press, London

Coward R 1999 Sacred cows: is feminism relevant to the new millennium? Harper Collins Publishers, London

Crozier K 2001 Technology: is it killing the art of midwifery? RCM Midwives Journal 4(12): 410–411

Department of Health 1993 Changing childbirth: report of the Expert Maternity Group. HMSO, London

Department of Health 1994 The Patient's Charter: maternity services. HMSO, London

Department of Health 1999 Saving lives. Our healthier nation. HMSO, London

Department of Health 2000a The NHS Plan. HMSO, London

Department of Health 2000b Improving working lives toolkit. Department of Health, Leeds

Department of Health 2001 Tackling health inequalities: consultation on a plan for delivery. HMSO, London

Department of Health and Social Security 1970 Standing Maternity and Midwifery Advisory Committee (Chairman J. Peel). Domiciliary midwifery and maternity bed needs. HMSO, London

Department of Health and Social Services Northern Ireland 1994 Delivering choice: the report of the Northern Ireland Maternity Unit Study Group. DHSS, Belfast

DeVries R 1993 A cross-national view of the status of midwives. In: Riska E, Wegar K (eds) Gender, work and medicine. Sage Publications, London

Dimond B 2002a Step 39: regulating health professionals. British Journal of Midwifery 10(3): 180

Dimond B 2002b Professional indemnity and the midwife. British Journal of Midwifery 10(8): 641–644

Donnison J 1988 Midwives and medical men. Historical Publications, London

Doyal L 1995 What makes women sick? Macmillan, London

Elston MA 1993 Women doctors in a changing profession: the case of Britain. In: Riska E, Wegar K (eds) Gender, work and medicine. Sage Publications, London

Ehrenreich B, English D 1979 For her own good. Pluto Press, London

English National Board 1999 Report of the audit of midwifery services and practice visits undertaken by the midwifery officers of the Board 1998/1999. English National Board, London

English National Board 2001 Report of the audit of midwifery services and practice visits undertaken by the midwifery officers of the Board 1999/2000. English National Board, London

Faludi S 1992 Backlash: the undeclared war against women. Chatto and Windus, London

Fenwick N 1998 Continuity of carer: the experiences of midwives. In: Clement S (ed) Psychological perspectives on pregnancy and childbirth. Churchill Livingstone, Edinburgh

Figes, K 1995 Because of her sex: the myth of equality for women in Britain. Pan Books, London

Firestone S 1979 The dialectic of sex: a case for feminist revolution. Women's Press, London

Flint C 1993a Midwifery teams and caseloads. Butterworth-Heinnemann, Oxford

Flint C 1993b Know your midwife. Continuity of care provided by a team of midwives. In: Robinson S, Thomson A (eds) Midwives research and childbirth, vol. II. Chapman and Hall, London

Flint C, Poulengeris P 1987 Know your midwife report (unpublished)

Gillen J 1995 Can midwives practise autonomously? British Journal of Midwifery 3(5): 245–246

Godfrey E 2002 Birth centres – a return to the natural way. Midwives 5(11): 368

Green JM, Curtis P, Price H, Renfrew MJ 1998 Continuing to care: the organization of midwifery services in the UK. A structured review of the evidence. Books for Midwives Press, Cheshire

Heagarty BV 1990 Gender and professionalization: the struggle for British midwifery 1900–1936. Unpublished thesis Michigan State University (copy in the RCM Library, 35 Portland Place, London)

Hearn J 1982 Notes on patriarchy, professionalization and the semi-professions. Sociology 16(4): 184–202

HMSO 1959 Cranbrook Report: Report of the Maternity Services Committee. HMSO London

HMSO 1980 Second Report from the Social Services Committee Session 1979–1980 (Chairman R. Short). Perinatal and Neonatal Mortality. HMSO, London

HMSO 1982 Maternity Care in Action, Part 1: antenatal care. A guide to good practice and a plan for action. First report of the Maternity Services Advisory Committee. HMSO, London

HMSO 1984 Maternity Care in Action Part II: care during childbirth (intrapartum care). A guide to good practice and a plan for action. Second report of the Maternity Services Advisory Committee. HMSO, London

HMSO 1985 Maternity Care in Action Part III: care of the mother and baby (postnatal and neonatal care). A guide to good practice and a plan for action. Third report of the Maternity Services Advisory Committee. HMSO, London

House of Commons Select Committee 1992 (Chairman Nicholas Winterton) Sessions 1991–1992 Second Report Maternity Service. HMSO, London

Hubbard R 1983 Social effects of same contemporary myths about women. In: Lowe M, Hubbard R (eds) Woman's nature. Pergamon Press, New York

Hunt SC 1996 Power, professionalization and midwifery. In: Symonds A, Hunt SC (eds) The midwife and society: perspectives, policies and practice. Macmillan, London

Hunter DJ 1994 From tribalism to corporatism: the managerial challenge to medical dominance. In: Gabe J, Kelleher D, Williams G (eds) Challenging medicine. Routledge, London, p 1–22

Janecek H 2002 Antenatal screening programme: information resource. RCOG Press, London

Kirkham M 1996 Professionalization past and present. In: Kroll D (ed) Midwifery care for the future: meeting the challenge. Baillière Tindall, London

Kirkham M 1999 The culture of midwifery in the National Health Service in England. Journal of Advanced Nursing 30(3): 732–739

Lewis P 2000 Daring to be different: future resolutions. British Journal of Midwifery 7(10): 4–6

Lowe M, Hubbard R (eds) 1983 Woman's nature. Pergamon Press, New York

MacArthur J, Lewis M, Knox EG 1991 Health after childbirth. HMSO, London

Martin E 1987 The woman in the body. Open University Press, Milton Keynes

McCourt C, Page L 1996 Report on the evaluation of one-to-one midwifery practice. Wolfson School of Health Sciences, Thames Valley University, London

Mitchell J, Oakley A 1976 The rights and wrongs of women. Pelican Books, London

National Health Service Litigation Authority (NHSLA) 2002 Clinical risk management standards for maternity services. NHSLA, London

Oakley A 1976 Wisewoman and medicine man. In: Mitchell J, Oakley A (eds) The rights and wrongs of women. Pelican Books, London

Oakley A 1980 Women confined. Martin Robertson, Oxford

Oakley A 1986 The captured womb: a history of the medical care of pregnant women. Basil Blackwood Ltd, Oxford

Oakley A 1987 The family in crisis 1. The woman's place. New Society 79(6): 14–16

Oakley A 1993 Essays on women, medicine and health. Edinburgh University Press, Edinburgh

Oakley A, Houd S 1990 Helpers in childbirth: midwifery today. Hemisphere on behalf of WHO Regional Office for Europe, London

Oakley A, Mitchell J (eds) 1997 Who's afraid of feminism? Seeing through the backlash. Hamish Hamilton, London

Parliamentary Office of Science and Technology 2002 Caesarean sections. The Stationery office, London

Pilcher R 1998 Hormones of hegemonic masculinity? Explaining gender and gender inequalities. Sociology Review February: 5–9

Pratten B 1990 Power politics and pregnancy. Health Rights, London

Raphael-Leff J 1991 Psychological processes of childbearing. Chapman and Hall, London

Rich A 1977 Of woman born: motherhood as experience and institution. Virago London

Robinson J 1995 Behavioural iatrogenesis. British Journal of Midwifery 3(6): 335

Rogers MF (ed) 1998 Contemporary feminist theory. McGraw Hill, New York

Royal College of Midwives, Royal College of General Practitioners 1995 'Responsibilities in intrapartum care' Working together: a joint statement by the Royal College of Midwives and the Royal College of General Practitioners. RCM/RCGP, London

Sandall J 1995 Burnout and midwifery: an occupational hazard? British Journal of Midwifery 3(5): 246–248

Sandall J 1996 Moving towards caseload practice: what evidence do we have? British Journal of Midwifery 4(12): 620–621

Sandall J 1999 Team midwifery and burnout in midwives in the UK: practical lessons from a national study. MIDIRS Midwifery Digest 9(2): 147–152

Scottish Office 1993 Provision of maternity services in Scotland: a policy review. HMSO, Edinburgh

Shorter E 1983 A history of women's bodies. Allen Lane, London

Spallone P 1989 Beyond conception: the new politics of reproduction. Macmillan Education, Basingstoke

Stevens T, McCourt C 2002 One-to-one midwifery practice part 4: sustaining the model. British Journal of Midwifery 10(3): 174–179

Tew M 1978 The case against hospital deliveries; the statistical evidence. In: Kitzinger S, Davis J (eds) The place of birth. Oxford University Press, Oxford

Tew M 1981 The effect of scientific obstetrics. Health and Social Services Journal 17th April: 444–446

Tew M 1990 Safer childbirth? A critical history of maternity care, 2nd edn. Chapman and Hall, London, p 55–65

Tong R 1989 Feminist thought: a comprehensive introduction. Routledge, London

Towler J, Bramall J 1986 Midwives in history and society. Croom Helm, London

United Kingdom Central Council for Nursing, Midwifery and Health Visiting 2000 Supporting women who intend to give birth at home. Registrar's letter 21/2000. UKCC, London

United Kingdom Central Council for Nursing, Midwifery and Health Visiting 2001 Supporting women who intend to give birth at home. Registrar's letter 21/2001. UKCC, London

Walby S 1990 Theorizing patriarchy. Basil Blackwood Ltd, Oxford

Walsh D 2002 Postmodernism and maternity care. British Journal of Midwifery 10(11): 662

Webb C 1993 Feminist research: definitions, methodology, methods and evaluation. Journal of Advanced Nursing 18(3): 416–423

Welsh Office 1991 Protocol for investment in health gain: maternal and early child health. Welsh Office, Cardiff

Witz A 1992 Professions and patriarchy. Routledge, London

World Health Organisation 1986 Having a baby in Europe: report on a study. WHO, Geneva

10

Feminist approach to midwifery education

Lorna Davies

INTRODUCTION

In this chapter I intend to consider whether it is possible to create changes within midwifery education using a feminist pedagogical approach.

As part of a Masters in Women's Studies, I originally set out to explore the significance of inquiry-based learning (IBL) as a vehicle for effecting such change within a midwifery education programme. During the process of the study it occurred to me that IBL enshrined many of the qualities espoused by feminist educational theorists. My focus therefore altered and centred more specifically on the value of IBL as a feminist pedagogical approach.

The chapter will include a brief history of midwifery education, an analysis of where we are now, an outline of problem-based learning, a summary of the study and the resulting analysis.

There is increasing evidence that midwifery in the UK is experiencing a crisis of identity and purpose (Downe 2001). Clarke (1999) suggests that within the obstetric medical model, midwifery has become virtually invisible. Many midwives are only able to identify their role in obstetric terms and this places birth as merely a physical event separated from the social, emotional, psychological and spiritual dimensions. Within this model childbirth is seen as normal only in retrospect. Additionally, the midwives' scope of practice is expected to embrace technocracy and the accompanying technical skills. Paradoxically, the midwife is simultaneously expected to provide a social model of birth characterised by freedom of choice, continuity of care, natural rhythms, support and encouragement. Women are seen as partners in the transition to motherhood, individuals who maintain their own identity.

The increase in emphasis on public health may be seen initially as a light at the end of the tunnel. By establishing a stronger community practice base, the public health role has the potential to provide midwifery with a key function to play in promoting women's and family health. However, conflicting demands have done much already to undermine the role of the midwife and this increased responsibility could create further dissonance by increasing the existing workload of the midwife, thus making further demands on the time and skills of those in practice.

It could be said that midwifery is in a state of confusion and apathy and education must recognise its part in this cycle of events and accept some responsibility for the onerous position that many midwives now find themselves in.

HISTORICAL PERSPECTIVE

For too many years midwifery education has subscribed to a patriarchal medical education archetype which adopts a rationalistic, scientific reductionist approach to the 'management' of pregnancy and childbirth.

In recent decades midwifery education has persistently implemented programmes of education which focus on the acquisition of knowledge as the procurement of factual, subject-based information. Midwifery education has allowed the experience of medicalisation to lead to the compartmentalism of midwifery subjects and definition of subject boundaries such as biology, psychology, sociology, medical sciences and so on. This approach does not facilitate the integration and synthesis which are characteristic of midwifery practice and has led to the acceptance of a body of knowledge that belongs to the medical model paradigm.

Throughout recorded history, midwives and the function that they serve have been grounded within a social model. In tribal culture this continues to be the case. It is only when a culture collides with Westernised allopathic medicine that childbirth becomes a pathological condition sited within a medical frame of reference (Oakley 1993). The terms used for the character of the midwife, both ancient and modern, reflect a role grounded in a social model. The word 'midwife' is derived from the Anglo-Saxon term 'with woman' (Aveling 1972).

Traditionally, midwifery was learned by apprenticeship. Knowledge and skills were passed down from generation to generation, by the oral tradition and hands-on experience. For centuries, the 'handywoman', as the village midwife was known, would provide her community with the knowledge and skills required to bring the next generation into the world (Sharp et al 1999).

However, by the end of the 19th century, the power of the emerging allopathic medical profession was finally successful in usurping the skills of the midwife in favour of obstetrics. Midwifery has subsequently undergone an evolutionary process that has left the profession as to all intents and purposes a branch of nursing, dominated by the medical discipline of obstetrics.

WHERE NOW?

The current age can be characterised by social and demographic shifts. Attitudes and value systems are volatile and the midwife needs to be dynamic, flexible and responsive to the ever-changing needs and demands of government and professional bodies, consumers and local service providers.

There are factors which suggest that change is necessary and long overdue. In a speech at the Royal College of Midwives Congress in May 2001, Alan Milburn, the Secretary of State for Health, emphasised his government's intention to increase choice for women and to provide £100 million to fund a much improved service (NHS NNLP 2001). The increase in the number of stand-alone birth units, and the value that users clearly place on them, give a clear message about the need for midwifery-led, woman-centred care. The home birth rate continues to rise, albeit slowly. However, arguably, in spite of these encouraging developments, without a clear understanding of the origin, nature and limits of midwifery knowledge (epistemology) the role of the midwife will remain ambiguous and a midwifery-led service will remain the privilege of a few women only. Midwifery education must play a key role in leading the midwife through this paradigm shift.

In order to re-establish a body of knowledge that is unique to its cultural embodiment, it may be necessary to create changes within midwifery education and with these changes, it may be possible to effect a shift from the existing hegemony towards a more pluralistic model within the current culture of childbirth.

FEMINISM AND MIDWIFERY

Feminism is not a concept which one immediately views as synonymous with midwifery. In spite of the fact that both disciplines are concerned with women and issues affecting women's lives, there has been little analysis or acknowledgement of relationships between the two.

Feminist theorists and midwives have to a large extent worked separately, rarely acknowledging in any formal sense the importance of the other. One would have imagined that the integration of midwifery into the academic sphere of the university in the early 1990s would have led to a mutually beneficial relationship between midwifery and women's studies departments. However, by and large this opportunity has not been grasped and the two have remained separate entities with little integration or collaboration in either the fields of research or learning and teaching. I know of not one university where midwifery sits within the women's studies field, although it appears within a range of other schools and faculties as far as accommodating the needs of midwifery education is concerned such as child health, medicine and nursing.

This current impasse is especially frustrating because it means that opportunities to forward feminist theories within a midwifery framework and vice versa are lost. These are opportunities that could be of fundamental importance in facilitating ideological and cultural shifts.

As a midwife teacher I believe that education is an essential catalyst if such paradigmatic shifts are to be fully realised. As a feminist I believe that feminist educational philosophy and methods could provide the vehicle to implement such change.

Using a feminist approach in midwifery education

In 1998 I was asked to take over the role of programme leader for the ENB A31 Enhanced Midwifery Practice Programme at Anglia Polytechnic University. This occurred during a period when considerable changes were being planned for the existing programme.

The programme had originally been designed in the early 1990s, when it was recognised that a framework for continuing professional development for midwives was essential to meet their advancing educational needs. At this time the A31 was intended to respond to this requirement and proved during its 6-year history to be highly valued by practitioners, educationalists and midwifery managers.

A curriculum development team was established in June 1998 to ascertain what changes were necessary and whether or how they could be implemented. During this development a conceptual analysis identified a concern that there was a heavy emphasis on the 'medical model' in the care of child-bearing women. This recognition suggested a need to identify and focus on the 'midwifery model', which emphasises the normality and physiology of the birth process.

The existing A31 of the time had sought to address this need also and midwives emerging from the programme were viewed in practice by colleagues and managers alike to be 'change agents', actively engaging in practice-based projects resulting from the programme. However, a study by Hillier & Sisto (1996), which examined the long-term value of such a programme for both practitioners and practice, demonstrated that although short-term gains were incontrovertible, the long-term changes were not so evident. These findings were also borne out in a paper published by the ENB which had similar findings. It was decided, therefore, by the curriculum development team that future development had to address how sustained changes could be achieved in practice as a result of exposure to the educational experience.

Effectively, we were being asked to create a programme of education for midwives that would effect change in their thinking in the long as well as the short term, in the belief that this would consequently change the way in which they addressed practice. What was needed was a fundamental change in our educational philosophy that would facilitate midwives to reclaim birth by challenging the existing paradigm and re-establishing a body of knowledge that is unique to the culture of midwifery.

The outgoing course had been built around a fairly traditional curriculum which did not appear to sufficiently foster thinking and critical analysis, to encourage the development of a lifelong learning approach. If we were to overcome this problem of long-term inertia then we needed to develop a more active way of learning which would initiate intellectual stimulation and motivation to go beyond factual knowledge to a deeper understanding. The comments within the review of the old programme seemed to indicate that the students had difficulty connecting basic principles and concepts to essential applications, i.e. there was a theory–practice divide which was not apparently being bridged.

Whilst studying for my Postgraduate Certificate in Education in 1997, I was introduced to the concept of problem-based learning (PBL). The discovery of this philosophy was a revelation, an approach to learning that could potentially meet the needs of adult learners. Problem-based learning is not a new concept. It was the dominant educational approach in the Classics; Plato and Socrates required their students to do the thinking, to retrieve information for themselves, search for new ideas and debate them in a scholarly environment, in contrast to the teacher-dominated approach evident in most educational establishments today. The approach was resurrected and developed at McMaster University Medical School in Ontario in 1969 (Chong et al 1984). It was developed in an attempt to overcome the apathy in the existing medical curriculum and the approach has since been adopted and adapted by many other professions and institutions and has been embraced significantly by healthcare disciplines (Barrows & Tamblyn 1980).

Problem-based learning is a facilitative educational method that challenges students to 'learn to learn', working co-operatively in groups to seek solutions to real-world problems. It prepares students to think critically and analytically and to acquire lifelong learning skills which include the ability to find and use appropriate learning resources (Boud 1997).

Problem-based learning transfers control of the learning process from the teacher to the student. The students formulate and pursue their own learning objectives and select those learning resources which are best suited to their current information needs. Teachers contribute to PBL by providing suggestions. In PBL, the traditional teacher and student roles change. The students assume increasing responsibility for their learning, giving them more motivation and more feelings of accomplishment, setting the pattern for them to become successful lifelong learners. Teachers do not prescribe or dominate. The classical model consists of 6–10 students who need to resolve a phenomenon or a set of events that require explanation (Sadlo 1994). There is a strong emphasis on the use of group dynamics to facilitate motivation and the elaboration of an issue.

From a philosophical perspective, it was felt that the commonly used term problem-based learning was inappropriate for midwifery where the practitioners are mostly engaged in situations that are not necessarily problematic or require resolving. The use of this method in medical education was founded very much on a hypothetic-deductive reasoning basis, which feels ill suited to midwifery, where I feel the concept of salutogenesis, which is the generation of well-being as opposed to the examination of illness (Antonovsky 1993), should be the guiding philosophical concept. The development team therefore chose to adopt the term inquiry-based learning (IBL).

It was agreed by the curriculum development team that IBL should be firmly placed at the heart of the curriculum, both philosophically and as the main learning and teaching methodology.

The modules were designed to reflect the three major curriculum themes which underpinned the curriculum philosophy: locus of control, paradigm shift and profession in transition. These themes were interwoven with the specific theoretical content of each module, thus allowing for the inclusion and integration of theory, philosophy and practice. It was felt that such an approach would result in a programme that encouraged the development of a more holistic practitioner, able to marry the theory and delivery of care in a flexible and responsive way. Therefore, the so-called 'divide' between theory and practice would be weakened and a seamless theory–practice continuum would replace the existing 'ideological hurdles' between theory and practice. It was anticipated that this would foster the development of practitioners who were 'change agents', able to provide the full spectrum of woman-centred, midwife-led care.

The use of IBL as a learning and teaching methodology was to facilitate the 'braiding' of the themes and the underlying philosophy by presenting lateral, real-life and practice-based perspectives.

The core modules were to be synchronised in terms of content and outcomes in a way which will encourage and support further exploration, consideration and possible resolution of issues.

FEMINIST PEDAGOGY – FEMAGOGY?

Whilst reviewing the literature on IBL, I recognised that the philosophy and method embraced many of the features that may constitute a feminist pedagogy, and one that as a result may have a particular value for midwifery education. The main principles of IBL, i.e. classroom as community, the value of personal experience, teacher as facilitator, are enshrined in the writings of feminist educational theorists.

… feminist pedagogy should engage students in a learning process that makes the world 'more real than less real' (Hooks 1989)

Whilst considering the possibility of placing IBL within a feminist pedagogical framework, I realised that I felt uncomfortable with the term 'pedagogy' in relation to women and learning. The word generally refers to the art and science of educating children and embodies teacher-focused

education. The word 'andragogy' is considered to be: 'the art and science of helping adults learn' (Knowles 1998), although it has taken on a broader meaning since it was introduced by Knowles (Jarvis 1985). The term currently defines an alternative to pedagogy and refers to learner-focused education for people of all ages. However, I feel that andragogy may be too inclusive and that by offering a generic home for all adult learners, it fails to identify the needs of specific groups, i.e. women. Perhaps it is time for feminist educators to consider the coining of a new term that would embrace the specific needs of women learners. The word 'femagogy', for example, could be adopted and this study would then be exploring the possibility of a 'femagogical' approach in midwifery education.

Within the IBL framework of the programme, the students are invited to analyse the unequal social relations embedded in the culture of birth and midwifery and to ask why these circumstances exist and what one can do about them. To achieve these goals, classroom process skills are utilised that are explicitly designed to empower students to apply their learning to social action and transformation, recognise their ability to act to create a more empowering service for women and become effective voices of change within maternity services.

Lewis (1992) suggests that the focus of feminist pedagogy must be the political struggle over meaning and the encouragement of students to: 'self consciously examine and question the conditions of our meaning-making and to use it as the place from which to begin to work toward change' (Lewis 1992).

Within the confines of what could be perceived as our patriarchal educational systems, the social values of females are emasculated. This process begins in primary education with a national curriculum which stresses intellectual competence, insists on a prescriptive and conservative intervention in the school syllabus, and ignores children's emotional needs. School-age children are often subjected to a learning environment which does not encourage student participation or involvement in learning (Caine & Caine 1995, Gardner 1993, Goodlad 1984).

Our current examination system leaves little room for an integrated approach within the curriculum. Caine & Caine (1995) stress the need for integration and the importance of challenging the theory that the brain does not easily learn things that are not logical and have no meaning. Girls naturally have a tendency to integrate information and resist learning isolated bits of information.

Hughes (1995) states that the current, Western educational system is based primarily on knowledge that has been generated and collected through the positivist approach to learning and meaning making. It is based on a reductionist approach and is largely aimed at delivering facts and information through cognitive lectures and content.

Most students view this educational setting as a passive way of learning. They are not actively engaged in the process. There is often little discussion, participation or engagement in the lecture by the student. Opportunities to challenge what the authority figure is saying and the freedom to propose alternative theories through personal experience are few and far between.

The pitcher metaphor is useful in relation to discussion of this didactic approach to teaching and learning (Samples 1987). The teacher acts as the pitcher that contains the knowledge. They pour knowledge into the empty vessel, which is the student. After the transaction, it is assumed that the glass is at least half full.

Hughes (1995, p 214–230), in a critical analysis of the education system, says that:

… men from a particular social group were in a position to construct and disseminate a world-view particular to themselves which, not surprisingly, helped to sustain a social order … (this) is the result of a deeply held value system which valorises that which is masculine, and denigrates that which is feminine. Consequently, it is objectivity, rationality, individuality, science, competitiveness, abstraction and things public which carry status, and their opposites (in a dichotomy) which are seen as feminine and therefore denigrated: subjectivity, emotion, co-operation, nature, collectivity, concreteness and things private.

The concept of IBL deconstructs many of the assumptions prevalent within traditional male-centred education.

Merriam & Heuaer (1996) suggest that there are three components to a woman-centred education programme, which I feel to be encapsulated within IBL.

1. First, they claim that students need to be introduced to a broad range of experiences and viewpoints.

Feminists have long recognised that women's experience is different (Weiner 1994). Traditional epistemology has tended to exclude women, by placing a boundary on knowledge, defining it through the means used to identify it, that is objective, empirical and scientific. Additionally, the object of inquiry is limited to issues pertaining to the public world, whilst the private domain usually associated with women has traditionally been excluded from scientific inquiry. Wickham (1999) argues that scientific evidence cannot supply all the answers when it comes to midwifery practice and that experiential knowledge and other concepts, equally difficult to evaluate and validate, play an important part in the process. Within midwifery education, although we are beginning to recognise and value the 'art' of midwifery as well as the science, there is a strong bias in favour of the scientific rationalistic perspective. Furthermore, the areas of reality that are considered worthy of scientific investigation generally pertain only to the external realities of life, matters that are quantifiable and measurable. They pertain much less to how people experience their reality.

The students draw upon a wide range of evidence, including research, anecdotal experience, the views of women, physiology and even intuition. In *Women's Intuition* (1989), Elizabeth Davis discusses the acquisition of information and suggests that Western society gives authoritative status only to the highly linear modes of inductive and deductive reasoning. She then adds that it is well established that there is no creativity in science, indeed, in any domain of creative activity, that does not entail intuition. Interestingly, midwives will often say things like 'I don't know why I did that, it just felt right at the time'. Yet because this 'evidence' cannot be quantitatively validated, it becomes lost knowledge.

A great deal of the discussion in the IBL tutorials and feedback sessions relates to the personal experiences of the students from their own areas of practice as midwives. Feminist educational theorists include personal experience as a basis for the production of knowledge, embracing the private sphere as a legitimate area of investigation (Kirby & McKenna 1989). Bel Hooks (1994) states that feminist pedagogy includes a goal of justice for all humans and allows students to be empowered through the recognition and validation of their own personal experience, and by encouraging them to draw on their personal experiences while learning about theory.

This is not to suggest that we should disregard scientific theory. Increased awareness of science is not necessarily in itself a negative development. However, it could be suggested that midwives need to face the challenge of becoming more 'scientific' without necessarily becoming more technological (Lewis 1997). One strategy to accomplish this is to distinguish 'physiological' (normal) birth from 'pathological' birth. Thus separated, midwives can use scientific methods to study normal pregnancy and birth and claim jurisdiction as experts in physiological birth. Science is used to assess technology itself, examining its appropriate and inappropriate uses. Carefully conducted, scientific studies can be used not only to enhance the image of a profession but to yield information useful to the promotion of the profession. As Downe (2001) states, midwives, as the so-called guardians of normal birth, should be grasping opportunities to undertake research about, for example, the physiology of normal birth.

2. Second, Merriam & Heuaer emphasise the significance of providing a safe environment for the learner.

As personal growth takes place in small steps, it is important that the learner feels safe enough to step into the unknown. In a threatening situation, people tend to hold closely to what is already familiar to them, thus inhibiting the learning process.

The IBL classroom offers an environment where the group can feel comfortable themselves and with each other. Women need space in order to develop a voice.

The basic structure of the IBL environment creates a space that feminists recognise to be a prerequisite for women's social and learning needs. The group gather in a circle, around a shared table, not in the traditional classroom format of rows.

There is something extraordinary about a circle. The circle creates a space with no beginning and no end – infinite connection. When women come together, for whatever reason, they create a circle. A sense of timelessness, safety, and strength permeates the space. No one enters without feeling it and no one leaves without feeling its loss. (Pinkola Estes 1992)

Pinkola Estes (1992), in her book *Women who Run with the Wolves*, suggests that women have always used storytelling circles to create a space of their own and to develop a voice. Circles offer an opportunity to discuss freely and in detail the issues that are most important to them. Such gatherings may also offer warm encouragement to develop ideas and aspirations.

The circle comes to represent shared power. Feminist pedagogy centralises women and the idea of a community within the classroom is important (Bogdan 1993). Community provides a foundation for trust within the group and trust is important because communication is difficult without it. The sense of community within the group is evident from the way in which the students relate and respond to one another. There is no sense of authority and the facilitator is part of the group: 'guide on the side' rather than 'sage on the stage'. Rather like a good midwife being 'with woman', the good facilitator is 'with student'.

3. Third, Merriam & Heuaer recommend that the educator should role model the kind of development they are seeking for the students.

This requires that educators share their views and perspectives with the learning group.

In their 1986 study, Belenky et al considered the idea of the teacher as midwife versus the teacher as banker, a metaphor which is particularly pertinent to the subject area of this study. The midwife-teacher helps a student to birth her own thoughts, while the teacher-banker deposits her own ideas in the heads of the students and then attempts to withdraw them for her own purposes.

Belenky et al (1986) suggest that women need to explore their own ideas to gain an understanding of the learning process and to view the teacher as an equal and understand that she goes through the same process as the students to acquire knowledge. The midwife-teacher creates an atmosphere where students can risk bringing out incomplete ideas and hunches. In a nurturing atmosphere, these ideas can be explored and expanded by input from the teacher and other students. Resources are made available for exploring what others have already discovered about these ideas. Students can personalise their learning, identify their position and apply the new information to their daily life, the place where learning and education make a difference.

In IBL through dialogue and reflection, the midwives in the cohort share knowledge and skills by talking about themselves, other women, their own lives and midwifery practice, spinning conversational threads and merging these into a structure of feminist theory in action.

ACTION RESEARCH

Between September 1999 and July 2001 I undertook an action research study, to explore the potential of IBL as a transformative educational philosophy and methodology for midwifery education, embedded within a feminist pedagogical framework.

A multimethod/multiperspective approach was used for data collection within the study which included feedback from students and educationalists. The majority of the data collection, however, was elicited from focus group discussions, with the remaining methods forming a scaffold, for purposes of triangulation.

In order to assist me in this endeavour, I used the work carried out by Belenky et al (1986). These researchers present the view that women learn differently from men and encourage us to think about what constitutes knowledge for women. The researchers identify five different perspectives from which women view reality and draw conclusions about truth, knowledge and authority: silence, received knowledge, subjective knowledge, procedural knowledge and constructed

Box 10.1 The five major epistemological categories identified by Belenky et al (1986)	
Silence	A position in which women experience themselves as mindless and voiceless and subject to the whims of external authority
Received knowledge	A perspective from which women conceive of themselves as capable of receiving and even reproducing knowledge from the all-knowing external authorities but not capable of creating knowledge of their own
Subjective knowledge	A perspective from which truth and knowledge are conceived of as personal, private and subjectively known or intuited
Procedural knowledge	A position in which women are invested in learning and applying objective procedures
Constructed knowledge	A position in which women view all knowledge as contextual, experience themselves as creators of knowledge and value both subjective and objective strategies for knowing

knowledge. They felt that these epistemological positions determined how women's self-concepts and ways of knowing are intertwined.

These epistemological perspectives can be seen to establish a continuum, with silence at one end of the spectrum and constructed knowledge at the other. Belenky et al speculate that it is possible to transcend the boundaries within the continuum.

The primary study cohort were the inaugural programme group, consisting of eight midwives from four different hospitals. Their age range was 32–49 and their ethnic background was Caucasian. Their time in practice and resulting experience and authority were varied. The most recently qualified group member had been in practice for 4 years and the most experienced for 25 years.

I was less concerned with what the students felt about IBL than the impact that it was having on them, because I felt that the resulting process was more important than the product. I did evaluate their impressions of IBL but I needed a way in which to evaluate the effect on attitude and behaviours as a result of the learning process.

The notes taken during interviews for the programme and the admission essays were used in the first instance to offer some insight into the attitudes, values and beliefs of the group members prior to the commencement of the course. These were useful landmarks in plotting the journey of the group from the onset.

Initially the group appeared to be firmly placed within a paradigm where the teacher delivers facts and anything that requires independent thought is viewed by most of the group members as an imposition.

S6: No disrespect to you but I've not enjoyed this. I've felt really threatened by this because it showed how little I do know, and how this must reflect when we do what we do.

However, by the end of the 6-month programme, the position of the group at large would appear to have markedly changed. During initial discussions, the group had demonstrated a leaning towards didactic learning as their 'comfort zone'.

S5: I always think that things like this are very woolly, and my grey matter doesn't stretch to this very well. I like things that are tangible, that you can touch, not things that you can't see.

As one of the facilitators observes:

F2: I know that several of you have struggled with the module as you went through the term. I know that and we expected that and we'd agreed that the triggers are very conceptual.

The students were focused much more on 'local' issues relating directly to the programme. By the end of the programme there is visibly a move to a self-directed stance and much more of a global perspective.

S7: ... it has really uplifted me, learning from other people.
S4: But it's obvious, just looking at each other as well since we first came together, each of us has kind of grown and adapted well to the learning.

There is barely reference to the modules or course structure and didacticism is no longer welcomed:

S1: I just felt that she was saying to us at the beginning there are no rights and no wrongs, then at the end of it she gave it to us ablast and she had a complete cut idea of what was one and what was the other and I thought why are you asking us then? There obviously was in her mind a right and wrong.
S2: Yes but she spoke very differently to everybody else.
S3: She was more of a lecturer.
S2: Yes she was the old-fashioned teacher, and we weren't used to it.
S1: Yes, she said, I've got here handouts and expected every one of us to sit here and go ...
F1: You wanted to be spoon-fed last semester.
S1: Yes
S4: That's right because I came out and said how frustrating it was.
F1: But you like lectures.
S1: Well we didn't know anything different, did we?
S2: And now we've all changed our minds.

From the position of received knowledge or even silence, the students can be seen to be moving towards a place where procedural reasoning is evident.

In relation to ownership of knowledge, the question of what forms evidence has particular significance. The admission essays for the group asked the students to discuss their understanding of evidence-informed practice and these essays also served to inform the researcher of the epistemological position of the participants at the outset of the programme. Although some of the students were able to recognise a range of evidence, this was limited and there was a heavy emphasis on research evidence and in particular, medical research evidence. Again this would suggest that the students were operating from a position of received knowledge, as yet unable to conceive of knowledge as anything other than that owned by others.

As they progressed, the students were seen to draw upon a wide range of evidence, including research, anecdotal experience, the views of women, physiology and even intuition, which suggested that the students were moving away from a positivist stance in relation to evidence and were recognising the value of other forms of evidence. They also appear to be grounding the theory within practice.

A turning point in the philosophical and epistemological bearing of the group would appear to lie in the field trip to The Farm Midwifery Center in Tennessee.

The trip was instigated at the request of some of the group about halfway through the programme. We were fortunate that one of our facilitators had an association with the midwives at The Farm, a midwifery centre with a philosophy firmly planted within the midwifery model. We were able to arrange a trip at relatively short notice and all but one of the eight midwives on the programme were able to make the visit. The Farm visit had a profound effect on all of us attending. This led me to question whether it was the programme or the visit to The Farm that had created change in the students. I have concluded that it would be impossible to separate the two as the trip was firmly embedded within the fabric of the programme. It was the programme that led the students to visit a practice which transcended the medical model and the visit reinforced the theory encountered during the programme.

One point that I have subsequently reflected upon is the epistemological grounding of The Farm midwives. The students recognised in those midwives a knowledge and a value system that facilitated an alternative paradigm for serving women during the child-bearing period. This knowledge could be construed to represent the constructed knowledge acknowledged by Belenky (1986) and her team as the: 'position in which women view all knowledge as contextual experience themselves as creators of knowledge and value both subjective and objective strategies for knowing'.

FACILITATING THE FACILITATORS

During the course of the study, a secondary cohort emerged in the form of the teaching team delivering the programme. The four midwifery teachers represented a broad range of experience and familiarity with the IBL process. It became apparent during the research that the process was having an impact on them as much as it was on the student group. It therefore became significant to include their voice as a subcohort.

Teachers who have worked in both traditional and PBL/IBL formats generally express a preference for PBL/IBL (Albanese & Mitchell 1993, Vernon 1995, Vernon & Blake 1993). The facilitators were emphatic about the benefits of IBL for the students and the issue of suitability for women learners emerged without prompting.

F1: I think that women are naturally great communicators. The emotional side of being a woman the IBL taps into that and feeds into that and given that opportunity that comes much more to life, than it does in that lecture theatre.

The PBL literature notes that as students pursue solutions to their classroom problem, they tend to assume increased responsibility for their learning and alter their view of teachers (Aspy et al 1993). The emergence of a far more autonomous group of students was at times difficult to accept and some of the facilitators found this process quite painful.

F3: They didn't want any direction whatsoever. No help. No mothering. It was very hard.

Another result of the exposure of the teachers to IBL was the realisation that they were able to clearly identify with the learning curve experienced by the student group and reported a parallel in their own practice.

F2: As they were learning things about the subject matter and their own philosophies, beliefs and comfort zones in relation to their practice as midwives, I also learned about my own in relation to my practice as a midwife teacher.

As previously stated, Merriam & Heuaer (1996) recommend that the educator should role model the kind of development they are seeking for the students. There was the recognition that they had to let go of their own long-held ideas and beliefs as much as the students did and the realisation that this was creating for them, at times, serious professional conflict.

F1: I must admit I find it really difficult to go back. I experience so much discord teaching big groups now. I don't like it, I hate it. The other thing I don't like as well is that I've built up very close relationships with the women on the course and I find it very hard to assume the assessor role. I'm not comfortable with that either.

In *Women's Ways of Knowing*, Belenky et al (1986) include a chapter analysing the concept of 'connected teaching'. The 'teacher as midwife' metaphor is particularly poignant and one of the facilitator group members spontaneously identified her role as teacher with students as being similar to that of midwife with woman.

F2: One of the really, really irritating things about IBL was that it does take over your life, which isn't irritating but the fact that you find yourself at 10 o'clock at night phoning up and going 'Just look at this on TV because it would make a great trigger'. And it does, your life becomes ruled by trigger opportunities. But that to me again parallels with what true midwifery is about. It becomes a lifestyle rather than something that you put away at 5 o'clock in the evening and go home.

By analysing the way in which they facilitated the group within the IBL process, the teachers were able to identify how in traditional lectures and other didactic approaches, they were taking away the experience of the learner in the same way that midwives could deny the mother the opportunity to grow and learn for herself.

The battlefield of objectivity versus subjectivity is apparent in both the realm of higher education and maternity services, where the 'professional' face of the role can discourage close personal relationships with the women they are 'caring' for or 'educating'. In midwifery we frequently use the term 'care' but the connotations of this word verge on the patriarchal. For instance, some of the ways in which we use this word include 'under the care of', 'care handed over to' and 'care taken over by'. This can be seen to render the woman a passive recipient of the process described as 'care', rather than being an autonomous person, making decisions about her body, her baby and her childbirth experience. Likewise, academics are discouraged from creating close relationships with their students for fear of breaching the professional–personal divide. There was a perceptible change in the boundaries between the students and the teachers within the study.

It seemed at times that the facilitators were struggling to find a voice in their attempt to make meaning from what at times was an extremely difficult process for them. One of the facilitators actually acknowledges that IBL has given her the means to step out of the realms of silence. It is almost as if the realisation that they are 'midwives of ideas' gives them a vehicle to express their feelings and frustrations.

In conclusion, it could be inferred from analysis of the dialogue that the facilitators have made almost exactly the same transition as the students.

It has been understood for some time that analysis of the language and discourse midwives use is essential to our development as an autonomous body. This has also been highlighted as being important in enabling us to understand issues of power and empowerment in professional interactions. As Walton (1995) notes, language has the ability to empower or disempower women through day-to-day clinical and social interactions.

The group came together for the final time in July 2001, one year after completing the programme. The language of the group at this meeting appeared to be far less medicalised than it had been previously. The group members never referred to women as patients or even clients, they were simply 'women'. The content is also markedly more empowering and facilitative in relation to women.

S3: We're hoping to get a low-risk area on the delivery suite where the doctors won't be allowed in and the women's names won't be put up on the board, the women won't be monitored, they won't have pethidine or epidural. A place for normal birthing women.

There is less claim to ownership on the part of the midwives. They do not refer to 'my women' or 'my delivery' but acknowledge an understanding that the experience belongs to the woman and not to them.

S1: You have to give them all of the information that you have, don't you? And enable them to find information for themselves. I have this great thing that women must be prepared to take on responsibility for themselves. It's a partnership, isn't it?

It emerged during the meeting that the perceived increase in confidence had arisen to some extent from the improved knowledge enjoyed by the group members as a result of the programme.

S2: I was really pleased with myself when I could turn around and say I can help you with this. I can tell you how to structure it, I can tell you where to get the information from, I can tell you what sort of things you need to know and I thought wow, listen to me. A year ago I couldn't even write a postcard. To see where I was and how I've moved on.

The group are very protective of 'normal' childbirth and recognise the role of protector that they are assuming. Their concerns do not, however, only relate to doctors but also to colleagues.

S2: You can pick up midwives who will have an abnormal case and you can see them come on and think, oh no, I have to be more vigilant with them than I would be with someone when I know that their philosophy is different. Sometimes they don't see what is normal, they don't understand what is normal. They go so far off the normal path that you can't bring them back and you end up with a section in the end that should never have happened.

A further interesting recognition during the final feedback session was that the sense of dissonance, which had been so apparent during the second focus group session, although still evident, had been reflected upon by all of those present. They appeared to have adopted a range of methods for managing any resulting conflict. One of my main worries at the end of the first run of the programme was that we may be 'setting the students up to fail'. I was concerned that we may be setting up change agents who would have the ideas and the motivation, but would not be able to match the might of the institution. However, the midwives by and large dispelled this fear with their self-awareness and coping strategies.

S1: I tend to be a bit more subversive than I was. Because the more times I've said about it, the more eyebrows went up and the sighs and I've said no I'm still going to do this my way and when you get results you can say look, it works.
S4: When you've done a course like this and you are becoming very different in your thinking to the people that you work with, you can only say it so many times to them before they stop listening.
F1: Do any of them ever take it on board and try it themselves?
S4: Yes they do.

This meeting was extremely heartening because for me it showed that the group did appear to have held onto the beliefs and values that they acquired or developed during the programme. The students also seemed to have developed strategies to manage the tension between conflicting

forces and elements in practice, which was enabling them to influence the thoughts and behaviour of colleagues.

During the course of the last year, most of the group members have been involved in some sort of project development. Three of the group have been promoted to senior midwife grades. One has left midwifery to commence a career in health visiting, but her reasons for leaving midwifery were related to problems with shift work.

To return to Belenky et al (1986), it may be useful at this juncture to revisit their study in relation to the 'educational dialectics' identified in *Women's Ways of Knowing*. This model presents the conflicting ideas that establish a continuum, with silence at one end of the spectrum and constructed knowledge at the other. Belenky et al speculate that it is possible to transcend the boundaries within the continuum. Throughout their journey on the programme and beyond, our group were closely monitored. This monitoring allowed me as researcher to explore their progress longitudinally and to gain insight into their experience and the effects of that experience. The educational dialectic model assisted me in mapping the transition, clarifying and making meaning out of what at times appeared to be chaos.

CONCLUSION

The study for me has demonstrated what happens when women come together in a dedicated temporal and physical space. The participating midwives' and the midwife-teachers' involvement in and recording of their experiences within this action research has revealed how long-held assumptions and institutionalised activities and practices are open to challenge, leading to enriched insights into and understandings of women's realities and needs, validation of their everyday knowledge and experiences, and increased audibility of their voices.

I recognise that the study was extremely small and that more research would be required to give further weight to the theory. However, in the light of the work carried out to date, I believe that inquiry-based learning does fit into the connected learning and teaching model identified by

Belenky et al (1986), which may 'help women toward community, power and integrity'.

I firmly believe that the only way in which midwives and women will reclaim birth is by challenging the existing paradigm and re-establishing a body of knowledge that is unique to the culture of midwifery. I consider that a 'femagogical' approach to midwifery education is a way of facilitating the educational needs of midwives and that inquiry-based learning is one way of helping to make this a reality.

Key points

- For too many years midwifery education has subscribed to a patriarchal medical education archetype which adopts a rationalistic, scientific reductionist approach to the 'management' of pregnancy and childbirth.

- Traditionally, midwifery was learned by apprenticeship. Knowledge and skills were passed down from generation to generation, by the oral tradition and hands-on experience.

- In order to re-establish a midwifery body of knowledge that is unique to its cultural essence, it may be necessary to create changes within midwifery education. Feminist educational philosophy and methods could provide the vehicle to implement such change.

- The philosophy and methods embraced by problem-based learning may be considered to constitute a feminist pedagogy and one that as a result may have a particular value for midwifery education.

REFERENCES

Albanese M, Mitchell S 1993 Problem-based learning: a review of the literature on its outcomes and implementation issues. Academic Medicine 68(1): 52–81

Antonovsky A 1993 The implications of salutogenesis: an outsider's view. In: Turnbull A, Patterson J, Behr S (eds) Cognitive coping, families and disability. Paul Brookes, Baltimore

Aspy DN, Aspy CB, Quimby PM 1993 What doctors can teach teachers about problem-based learning. Educational Leadership 50(7): 22–24

Aveling JH 1972 English midwives. AMS Press, New York

Barrows HS, Tamblyn R 1980 Problem-based learning: an approach to medical education. Springer, New York

Belenky M, McVickery Clinchy B, Rule Goldberger N, Mattock Tarule J 1986 Women's ways of knowing: the development of self, voice and mind. Basic Books, New York

Bogdan D 1993 When is a singing school not a chorus? The emancipated agenda in feminist pedagogy and literature education. http://srd.yahoo.com/srst/4290079/When+is+a+singing+school+not+a+chorus/1/2/*http://www.ed.uiuc.edu/EPS/PES-Yearbook/93_docs/Bogdan.HTML

Boud D 1997 The challenge of problem-based learning, 2nd edn. Kogan Page, London

Caine RN, Caine G 1995 The educated person. In: Beane JA (ed) Toward a coherent curriculum. Association for Supervision and Curriculum Development, Alexandria, VA, p 16–25

Chong JP, Neufeld V, Oates MJ, Secord M 1984. The selection of priority problems and conditions: an innovative approach to curriculum design in medical education. Procedure for the Annual Conference in the Research of Medical Education 23: 17–25

Clarke R 1999 Minding our own business. British Journal of Midwifery 4(4): 209–211

Davis E 1989 Women's intuition. Celestial Arts, Berkeley, CA

Downe S 2001 Is there a future for normal birth? Practising Midwife 4(6): 10–12

Gardner H 1993 Frames of mind: the theory of multiple intelligences. Basic Books, New York

Goodlad JI 1984 A place called school: prospects for the future. McGraw-Hill, New York

Hillier D, Sisto S 1996 Advanced midwifery practice: myth and reality. British Journal of Midwifery 4(4): 179–182

Hooks B 1989 Talking back: thinking feminist – thinking black. South End Press, Boston, MA

Hooks B 1994 Teaching to transgress. Education as the practice of freedom. Routledge, London

Hughes K 1995 Feminist pedagogy and feminist epistemology: an overview. International Journal of Lifelong Learning 14(3): 214–230

Jarvis P 1985 The sociology of adult and continuing education. Croom Helm, Beckenham

Kirby S, McKenna K 1989 Experience, research, social change: methods from the margin. Garamond, Toronto

Knowles M 1998. The adult learner: the definitive classic in adult education and human resource development. Gulf Publishing, Houston, TX

Lewis ?? 1992 Interrupting patriarchy: politics, resistance and transformation. In: Luke C, Gore J (eds) The feminist classroom. Feminisms and critical pedagogy. Routledge, London, p 167–191

Lewis P 1997 Frustration and fatigue. Modern Midwife 7(10): 4

Merriam SB, Heuaer B 1996 Meaning-making, adult learning and development: a model with implications for practice. International Journal of Lifelong Learning 15(4): 243–255

NHS NLLP: www.nursingleadership.co.uk/home.htm

Oakley A 1993 Essays on women, medicine and health. Edinburgh University Press, Edinburgh

Pinkola Estes C 1992 Women who run with the wolves. Rider, New York

Sadlo G 1994 Problem-based learning in the development of an occupational therapy curriculum: the process of problem based learning. British Journal of Occupational Therapy 57(2): 49–53

Samples B 1987 Open systems, open minds. Transforming Education Winter: 19

Sharp J, Hobby E, Woods S 1999 The midwives book: or the whole art of midwifery discovered (women writers in English, 1350–1850). Oxford University Press, Oxford

Vernon DT 1995. Attitudes and opinions of faculty tutors about problem-based learning. Academic Medicine 70(3): 216–223

Vernon DT, Blake RL 1993 Does problem-based learning work? A meta-analysis of evaluative research. Academic Medicine 68(7): 550–563

Walton I 1995 Words as symbols. Modern Midwife 5(2): 35–36

Weiner G 1994 Feminisms in education: an introduction. Open University Press, Buckingham

Wickham S 1999 Evidence based midwifery 1: what is evidence based midwifery? Midwifery Today Winter: 39–41

11

Feminism and ways of knowing

Sara Wickham

'The truth.' Dumbledore sighed. 'It is a beautiful and terrible thing, and should therefore be treated with great caution.' (Rowling 1997, p 298)

INTRODUCTION

This chapter sets out to explore issues surrounding the concepts of knowledge and evidence and how these relate to women, feminism and midwifery. Several aspects of this debate are explored, beginning with an exploration of ancient and modern history in this area, and analysis of how the situation we are faced with today is based on the ideas of those philosophers who have shaped our thinking over the last few hundred years. The responses of feminist theorists to both this situation and current theories of knowledge and evidence are considered, with a view to discussing the impact of all these issues on current and future midwifery practice.

GRANDMOTHER KNOWLEDGE

Although patriarchal ways of knowing and approaches to 'best' evidence have held sway for the last few hundred years of Western society, this is but a relative fraction of the time during which women's ways of knowing were those valued by cultures around the world.

While we can never be sure of exactly how ancient societies functioned, having to rely on our modern interpretations of the evidence, there are a few things of which we can be relatively certain. The first is that the study of history is subjective

(Carr 1985), rendering interpretations of any historical evidence relative to the prevailing social attitudes and values. Because the study of history itself was for many years a male-dominated discipline, we are only now seeing female and feminist interpretations of the evidence. Women have challenged the modern myths that men have always held a socially dominant position, citing archaeological evidence from around the world in support of their findings; instead, they suggest that women and men in ancient societies were equal and worked in partnership (Eisler 1995).

We can also make some inferences about ancient societies' ways of knowing. It is generally accepted that, before the written word, knowledge would have been passed on through oral traditions such as storytelling, song and myth, through art and possibly in other ways no longer used. The archaeological findings which place women at the centre of society and spirituality (Eisler 1995, Sjoo & Mor 1997) are supported by the fact that those ancient traditions which are still alive today have women placed firmly in the centre of learning and sharing knowledge. The menopausal woman who lived 30 000 years ago would not have been seen as 'past her prime'; she would have been revered and sought out for her great wisdom and experience. As in some societies today (Sargent & Bascope 1997), a woman would not have 'graduated' from her apprenticeship as a midwife until she was older, had seen many births and probably borne several babies herself. Experience was among the most valued and sought-after forms of knowledge.

Midwives would have learned their art alongside their mothers and grandmothers and directly from the experiences of the women they attended. Because midwifery would not have been seen as a distinct job or profession but as one aspect of a woman's life, there is no reason to presume that midwifery knowledge would have been viewed as a body of knowledge distinct from knowledge of other aspects of life.

PATRIARCHAL KNOWING

As cultures slowly changed from those described by Eisler (1995) as 'partnership societies' to those dominated by patriarchal thinking, men began to develop ideas about knowledge which differed from those they had learned from their grandmothers. The Greek philosophers Socrates, Plato and Aristotle built on each other's work to develop a tradition that rejected what they saw as the subjectivity of ancient wisdom in an attempt to think scientifically. Aristotle furthered his teachers' work in developing the process of reasoning, where existing knowledge is built upon in order to generate new knowledge (Aristotle 1928, Plato 1993). Even at this stage, knowledge was no longer seen as cyclic, circular and relative.

While Aristotle and Plato wrote about their ideas regarding logic and reasoning as far back as the fourth century BCE, the roots of modern approaches to scientific thinking and knowledge are generally attributed to philosophers such as Francis Bacon and Rene Descartes. The degree of sexism in their philosophy can be seen in Bacon's approach to the study of women: in inaugurating the hypothetical-deductive approach of modern science, he called for 'an aggressive male attack on women's secrets' (Sjoo & Mor 1997, p 323). For centuries, women have not been considered legitimate knowers; as recently as the mid-19th century, social Darwinists argued that women evolved from male fetuses whose development had been halted at an early stage. This theory was supported by doctors, who believed that development of the woman's brain could only occur at a cost to her ovaries (Schiebinger 1987).

Descartes, in an attempt to develop a science which would enable the physical world to be studied in order to generate knowledge (Magee 1987), initially held that we must begin by doubting all knowledge and throwing out every belief that we cannot prove (Descartes 1988). Once he took this argument to its logical conclusion, he then needed to begin by 'proving' his own existence, famously concluding with 'cogito ergo sum'; that he could know he existed because he could think. He also developed foundationalism, the desire to base any kind of knowledge on sound first principles which then anchored other evidence and knowledge (Urmson & Ree 1989).

Foundationalism remains a guiding principle of scientific thought today, where mathematics, as a theoretical discipline, is seen as a purer and more absolute form of science than the practical physical sciences. A distinction is made between a mathematical *proof* as an absolute and logical axiom and a scientific *theory*, which can only be supported or refuted but never proven (Singh 1997). The physical sciences in turn are deemed superior to the social and medical sciences, which involve the relatively messy concepts of social interaction and the influence of the mind of the person being studied, an issue that the scientist studying chemical compounds does not have to contend with. Yet Descartes also believed in dualism; that the mind and body were separate and that the physical could be studied without reference to the psychological, social or spiritual. While many people accept the fallacy of this belief today, its impact on current scientific thinking and practice – and thus scientific knowledge – is still evident.

By separating spirit and matter, patriarchal ideology has reduced physical existence to a mere observable mechanism, so-called 'practical reality', while spiritual existence is discarded or abstracted into 'the imagination' or 'the ideal'. (Sjoo & Mor 1997, p 72)

Is medical 'science' scientific?

While one debate in this area deals with the theoretical challenge to the knowledge produced by scientific means, it is equally important to consider to what degree the evidence that is considered scientific can actually lay claim to this label. Even where philosophers attempted to break down the world in order to produce scientific evidence, the methods of those at the forefront of 'scientific' medical thinking led to conclusions which we would view differently today. During the Renaissance period:

The most practised and scientific methodologies of the day included astrology, incantations, alchemy, mercury ingestion treatments, bleeding, purging, leeches, lancets and fumigations. (Southern 1998, p 37)

The practice of 'bleeding' people to cure them appears to originate from the Greeks' observation of a hippopotamus who cut itself on rocks as it thrashed against them (Brown 1998). After several of these animals were seen to exhibit this behaviour, the assumption was made that this was a 'good' thing to do. In reality, this may have been accidental behaviour, where the hippos did not intend to cut themselves. It might have been an extremely stupid form of behaviour, in that they did not learn from their previous mistakes. It could be true that, for hippos, bleeding is a beneficial activity; this does not, however, mean that this is the same for humans.

Despite these possibilities, bleeding became a common medical treatment and remained so for several centuries. Some of those who were bled managed to survive the procedure. Proponents of bleeding then saw this as providing evidence of the success of this intervention. As Brown (1998) notes, because the body has the ability to heal itself, undue credit was often given to baseless methods and this 'scientific' process.

Empiricism as a method, especially when pressed into service of Greek philosophy, is no more immune to unfounded conclusions than medicine based on magic. (Brown 1998, p 18)

During the same period, midwives and other healers still practised their arts, even in the context of a society which had become wholly patriarchal. Their methods of developing knowledge could also be described as empirical, building as they did upon their experience of trial and error, cause and effect. Whether or not they enjoyed better results than their medical counterparts is difficult to ascertain; however, they were clearly not in alignment with those who held power. Consequently, they were sought out and killed in their thousands (Sjoo & Mor 1997).

One might argue that the methods (of knowledge generation) of midwives at this point were just as scientific in their way as those of the newly developing medical profession. Yet, because of the prevailing political structures, the dominant group was able to suppress and discredit the work of the less dominant group, both to gain power for themselves and to cause their own theories and knowledge to become normative. Doubt is still thrown on the degree to which medicine can be described as a science (Taylor 2001); some feminists see Western medicine as a fundamentally political structure which sets out to control society.

Although medicine touts itself as rational and objective, it is in reality deeply influenced by the prevailing ideology and power structure of the society in which it operates. (Coney 1995, p 45)

Sadly, this effect can still be seen today, where those groups who hold power in the field of childbirth manage to retain their 'norms', even against the weight of scientific evidence which does not support these. To see this in practice, one only has to look at the large numbers of clinical trials which show that routine electronic fetal monitoring in labour is not useful (NICE 2001, Wagner 1994) and contrast this with the situation in many hospitals, where women still experience this as a routine intervention.

It is also important to note that, in Western culture, safety has become the dominant rationality in childbirth (as in other areas of life) and that this impacts on professional interpretation of knowledge and evidence in practice. This is clearly illustrated where women who are seeking an experience which may be considered 'alternative' to the norm, such as home birth or physiological third stage, are often overtly or subtly berated for putting their own spiritual or psychological well-being above the physical well-being of their baby. Whether or not the scientific evidence supports the woman's choice – and often it does – the emphasis is placed on the physical above and beyond any other aspect of the woman's or baby's experience.

As Mernissi (1988, p 20) notes: 'The weapon of knowledge seems to be the most formidable weapon of all'. Knowledge is always open to interpretation and subject to politics.

Challenging scientific knowledge

Initially, the most widely cited challenges to scientific knowledge came from men, notably Thomas Kuhn and Karl Popper. In the latter half of the 20th century, Kuhn (1996, p 5) criticised the practice of science for attempting to 'force nature into conceptual boxes', a position which may appeal to many midwives. He also suggested that 'normal science ultimately leads only to the recognition of anomalies and to crises' (Kuhn 1996, p 122). In his analysis of the history of science,

he considers the concept of 'paradigm shifts', which render previously cherished 'facts' as ridiculous fallacies. With a wider perspective on knowledge over time, it is easy to see how knowledge is relative, existing as it does as 'fact' only in a given context.

Karl Popper (1959) also challenged the existence of absolute fact, although he took a different perspective, focusing on the principles and procedures of verification. He suggested that, for a scientific theory to hold any weight at all, it had to be potentially falsifiable. For instance, one might develop a theory that a 'normal' physiological labour could not last for more than 30 hours without there being some negative impact on the woman or baby. This theory is potentially falsifiable. As soon as a woman experiences physiological labour lasting 31 hours, with no ill effects to her or her child, this theory is shown to be false. But, as long as the theory is not shown to be false, it is also not 'proven'; evidence may come along which supports the theory but there is always the possibility that one case might disprove the theory. Because of this possibility, Popper asserts that nothing can be considered absolute fact.

Midwives might agree with this approach, surmising that there are very few objective facts in midwifery; there will almost always be the exceptional experience which falsifies the 'rule'. The woman who waited 8 hours for her placenta at home with no ill effects, the baby born at 32 weeks gestation at home who survived in a basket on the oven door; for every exceptional story there is a theory waiting to be disproved. Midwives' reluctance to use the words 'always' and 'never' may stem from their own knowledge and understanding about this issue.

Despite the prevalence of criticism regarding the scientific method, this is still held in high regard in Western society. Equally, despite the failure of scientific evidence to support many of the practices employed by proponents of Western medicine, this is still held to be a useful science by many people. In fact, medicine may be better viewed as a pseudo-science, a set of ideas that claim scientific weight but which are based on theories rather than 'proven' scientific evidence. As can be seen in this section, the weight that our society places on scientific and patriarchal approaches to knowledge has been challenged on a number of different theoretical grounds. The feminist approach, while sharing some common ground with other critics of science, looks at the problem from the perspective of politics and gender as well as from a theoretical philosophical standpoint.

FEMINIST THINKING

In her critique of what we consider to be 'knowledge' and 'fact', Simone de Beauvoir (1952, p 161) suggested that:

Representation of the world, like the world itself, is the work of men; they describe it from their own point of view, which they confuse with absolute truth.

The field that has grown out of feminist challenges to knowledge and knowing has been termed 'feminist epistemology'. Theory in this area is as political an issue as in many other areas of interest to feminists. Here, feminist thinking has led to challenges to current and past epistemological positions and theories – which have usually been proposed by men in the context of patriarchal societies – and to reflection by feminists about the extent to which we can ever be really sure we 'know' anything. This is particularly the case when it comes to knowledge of how it is to 'be' another person or in another situation from our own. Feminists are more likely to embrace the subjectivity of each person's individual experience than to see value in seeking the elusive 'objective facts'.

A number of women have challenged existing knowledge in their particular field by returning to earlier work and reappraising its value in relation to our knowledge about women. Carol Gilligan (1993) showed clearly how models of psychological thinking and knowledge could be seen as gender based in her work on ethical dilemmas. Previously, the (male) psychologist Kohlberg had interviewed children to study their level of ability to reason through moral dilemmas. Following their responses to the question of whether a man whose wife was terminally ill should steal the drug that would cure her,

Kohlberg suggested that girls were less adept at moral reasoning than boys.

In her turn, Gilligan (1993) suggested that, while the boys had tended to demonstrate the ability to debate whether the man 'should' or 'should not' steal the drug, many of the girls had responded in a different way. They approached the question by thinking about whether he should 'steal' the drug or whether he could find a way around the issue of theft, through communication, negotiation or via relationship with the people involved. Gilligan argues that their approach to the question was simply different – and arguably more creative – but because Kohlberg's researchers were looking for the answers they expected from male respondents, the girls were perceived as less able.

This illustrates one of the key issues in this area; that, following the patriarchal domination in the fields of learning, knowledge and knowing during the last few hundred years, women are now having to discover and establish ways of knowing which are more appropriate to the feminine and feminist.

Categories of knowledge are human constructions … Recognition of the relativity of judgement infuses our understanding … when we begin to notice how accustomed we have become to seeing life through men's eyes. Gilligan (1993, p 6)

As part of the feminist backlash against the received view of science and knowledge, Gilligan does not see the dominant 'male' forms of knowledge as better but as a symbol of the incompleteness of our understanding of knowledge.

The failure of women to fit existing models of human growth may point to a problem in the representation, a limitation in the conception of human condition, an omission of certain truths about life. (Gilligan 1993, p 2)

Three feminist theories on science

Feminist criticisms of received and traditional scientific thinking have, as above, built upon some of Kuhn's and Popper's arguments. Sandra Harding (1986) discusses the three main feminist epistemologies which deal with questions concerning the links between women, science and knowledge.

Feminist empiricists stand by the main principles of scientific inquiry; that the world can be known objectively as it exists outside the person knowing it and that all knowledge is gathered via experience which is itself gathered through our senses. Feminist empiricists believe that the androcentric approach which characterises science is correctable by stricter adherence to the rules of science.

In a midwifery context, proponents of this approach might suggest that quantitative research should remain the gold standard for evidence and focus on improving the approach to that research. These people may not see the value in exploring alternative forms of evidence, believing that, if this cannot be done from within an objective scientific framework, the lack of objectivity renders this a pointless exercise.

On the other hand, critics of this theory would use similar arguments to Kuhn and Popper in suggesting that foundationalism and empiricism themselves do not lead to any kind of absolute knowledge and that the fact that women rather than men are carrying out scientific research does not cause this to be more objective or further removed from human experience and bias.

From within the *feminist standpoint*, there is more of an emphasis on the political domination of women and a belief that women, as the subjugated members of society, can have a clearer understanding of what is happening than the men who are in a dominant position. This perspective, which has links with the work of Karl Marx, can be seen in those groups of women who seek to gain knowledge of what it is like to be a particular woman having a particular experience. They are primarily concerned with our need to understand what it is like to be in the position of the individual woman.

The work generated from such a position can have a tremendously positive impact in enabling professionals to think about what they are doing and reflect on practice. However, a problem arises when this theoretical position is used as a basis for trying to gather evidence and build knowledge. Qualitative research based on this approach may be tremendously useful in enabling us to understand the viewpoint and experience of a small number of women but when we consider the massive differences between women around the world, it is difficult to see how we could reconcile all of these viewpoints into a coherent 'women's standpoint theory'.

The *feminist postmodernist* position challenges both of these views. As far as empiricism is concerned, feminist postmodernists believe that objectivity and universal truth are completely unattainable goals. They are therefore unlikely to see scientific research as any kind of gold standard, although some may see it as one potentially valuable form of evidence when used with other forms, perhaps those which are more in line with women's ways of knowing. Feminist postmodernists may also be interested in deconstructing aspects of knowledge and evidence, along with those midwives who are attempting to deconstruct terms such as 'normal birth' and challenging the language used in midwifery and obstetrics. Ultimately, the feminist postmodernist would assert that knowledge is wholly relative and can only be held by the 'knower': in this case, the pregnant woman.

As Harding (1986) shows, one of the problems faced by feminists using the strategy developed by Kuhn (1996) in arguing that science is value laden and relative only to the cultural context is that these critics (including Kuhn himself) fail to present their own work as culture laden. In arguing that the received view is dependent on cultural context, we must acknowledge that the argument against this is also dependent on its own cultural context. If it were not for the work of the earlier feminists who gave their time and sometimes their lives to secure voting and other rights for women, it is unlikely that we would be able to write and publish chapters such as this. Equally, the thinking and priorities of those women (and men) who have come before us have influenced the stance we take.

The greatest criticism of the feminist postmodernist stance is that, while it is all very well to hold a position of relativism in theory, this again does not necessarily take us any further forward in developing knowledge or theories in practice. It does not seem particularly helpful or productive to decide that we simply cannot 'know' anything absolute. We may as well all give up and go home! In fact, taking the position that we cannot know anything absolutely is a Godelian paradox: an undecidable statement of position which may be true but which cannot be proved. Either we do know something absolutely (which is that we cannot know anything absolutely) or we do not know anything absolutely, in which case we cannot know absolutely that we cannot know anything absolutely!

Does this mean we have reached scientific stalemate? While the scientific method might not hold the key, taking a position where we decide that everything is subjective and individual is not useful either. In order for any kind of theory of knowledge to be useful in the real world – which is, after all, where we practise midwifery – it needs to be guided by some kind of objective standpoint and standard. Within this context, objective does not have to mean scientific or reductionist; we need to explore this issue further, particularly in relation to midwifery. While we can clearly show the failures of existing models of knowledge and evidence, I would argue that this is not a useful exercise in itself if we do not attempt to build models of our own.

MIDWIFERY KNOWLEDGE – RECLAIMING WOMEN'S WAYS OF KNOWING

Having briefly explored the history of this area and looked at some of the key theoretical positions taken by those who have come before, we can now look at these issues in relation to midwifery practice. From its roots as an ancient art learned through storytelling, experience and reflection on practice, Western midwifery now sits in a cultural – and medical – context where scientific research is valued above all other forms of evidence.

It is certainly true that a small number of scientific research studies carried out by midwives in the 1970s and 1980s had a major positive impact on changing midwifery practice and enabling the removal of some of the routine interventions which were shown to be unnecessary (Page 2000). However, the emphasis placed on scientific and quantitative evidence in the current culture of the maternity services leads to a reluctance to consider other forms of evidence.

> … It appears we have problems discussing anything related to things that are not tangible, that cannot be demonstrated through research. (Hall 2001, p vii)

Yet it is also clear that scientific research evidence can provide us with only a small amount of the knowledge we need for practice (Page 2000, Wickham 1999) and that there are fundamental problems with the tenets on which normal science is based. Furthermore, we have established that medical 'science' is no more scientific or based on the outcomes of sound research studies than midwifery or any other related discipline. There is no more scientific back-up for the truth of the medical model over that of the midwifery model; in fact, it might be argued that the latter has more support in the form of both quantitative and qualitative evidence.

Many midwives also struggle with the idea that scientific research evidence alone could provide us with all the answers we need. While science attempts to look for certainty, midwives understand that doubt and inconsistency remain at the very heart of birth and life. While people often express distress and amazement that 'in this day and age' women and babies still die in childbirth, midwives 'know' that, however hard we try, we simply cannot offer guarantees.

The realisation that evidence may come about by means other than the scientific method and the acceptance that we may not find 'absolutes' in our search for midwifery knowledge lead us to the possibility that it is both useful and productive for midwives to seek and explore other forms of knowledge and evidence on which to base their practice. Indeed, a number of midwives have reached this point and begun to explore the alternatives.

Reclaiming narrative and experiential learning

Midwives commonly use stories of their own and birthing women's experiences as evidence in practice. Midwives tell stories as a fundamental part of their 'being with' women, often to help the woman to gain trust in her own body and her ability to birth. Ina May Gaskin (personal correspondence, 1999) describes the way in which she and the midwives she works with tell women experiencing long labours the story of Pamela, one of their colleagues, who was herself in labour for 3 days. On occasion they ask Pamela to come and see the labouring woman so that she can see for herself that Pamela survived the experience.

Some midwives have described their feeling that learning and knowledge derived through experience is greater than that which can be gained through books. In an interview by Gaskin (1989, p 6), midwife Candice Whitridge says:

When I went to school, I became knowledgeable about fundamentals. I learned, as midwives initially learned, how to measure everything: uteruses, pelvises, blood, urine, blood pressures, everything. I began to gather skills, I began to gather knowledge, but I don't think I began to learn midwifery until I began to care for women. The art, the craft, that came later. The women themselves became my teachers. I learned my midwifery from pregnant women. That's when I began to gain some wisdom.

Midwives also teach students and each other by explaining how they learned about midwifery by watching women and noting what helped them in labour and what did not appear to be useful. While this process may not be as rigorous as a controlled trial in assessing the benefit of a single intervention, it may be a useful way of learning from the complex and multilayered reality of practice, especially where the knowledge generated is tested by sharing it with other midwives and modifying the theory as appropriate.

In my own research, I have observed a number of groups of midwives where one will begin a dialogue by asking a question, perhaps about the use of a particular technique. Commonly, one midwife will take the lead in responding with details and stories about her experience in the area. Other midwives will then join in the conversation, both to support the aspects of this midwife's understanding which have also been their own experience but also to share stories of their own where their experience has differed. Often, this appears to be a good way of finding

the case where the general maxim does not fit the general rule which has been proposed. Not only does this lead to a degree of theory modification, it also tends to generate reflection as to 'why' this exception occurred. This, in turn, often causes midwives to think laterally and look for other types of knowledge (such as that gained from the study of women's physiology) to help develop their ideas.

The use of stories as evidence may also be midwives' way of claiming the need for the individual experience or story in a context where, following the basic tenets of science, the generalised average is the focus. As Page (2000, p 35) notes: 'In practice, an individual is not a statistic'. It is all very well for women to be told that if they follow a certain course of action, there is a 99% chance their baby will survive. This gives the woman in question a clearer idea of the probabilities of a certain outcome and she will know from this statement that her baby's chances of survival are better than if the odds were 50-50, but it does not enable her to know whether her baby will be in the 99% who survive or in the 1% who do not. In the absence of that kind of concrete information (which is almost always an impossibility in the uncertain world in which we live), exploring the experiences of other women may help her work through her own feelings and make a choice in the face of relative uncertainty.

Intuition and body wisdom

Another area which has recently begun to be explored by feminists and midwives is that knowledge which is gained through intuition. Again, this is an ancient and primal way of learning (Sjoo & Mor 1997) which does not fit into the parameters of normal science and is, as a result, derided by scientists. Yet, while the medical profession are seeking to remove the use of intuitive knowledge from decision making in evidence-based obstetric practice (Olatunbosun et al 1998), some midwives and social scientists are arguing that this is a potentially useful form of evidence which can be added to other kinds of knowledge in order to advance practice (Davis-Floyd & Davis 1997, Wickham 1999).

Briefly, there are two types of knowledge generation which are commonly described as intuition. The first of these has also been termed 'pattern recognition' or 'tacit knowledge' (Benner 1984) and comes about as a result of an expert 'knowing' what to do as a result of great experience in an area. In Benner's view, the expert has internalised her knowledge and experience to such a degree that she is unable to explain how she came to her decision or generated her knowledge.

An example of this would be a midwife attending a woman in labour who has a gut feeling that although everything appears to be going well externally, something is 'not quite right'. Although there is always the danger that our feelings about the outcome of a woman's labour may actually influence the woman's experience and render this a self-fulfilling prophecy, the midwife in this position who can manage to keep her fears and feelings to herself may discover that she was right. This does not necessarily mean she gathered the knowledge from the ether; she may have seen other women experiencing the same situation or problem in the past and while her rational brain did not consciously see the same signs or pattern, her subconscious may have recognised the situation and caused her discomfort.

The exploration of this kind of intuition does not tend to upset too many people. Although it is incredibly problematic to discover through research exactly how people 'know what they know', as a society we do not find it difficult to accept the existence of pattern recognition. On the other hand, the other kind of intuition – that mystical knowledge which does not appear to be based on any rational knowledge or experience – is more difficult for some people to accept. This kind of evidence sits firmly outside the realms of normal science and so-called rational thinking. Yet, by ascribing all examples of intuition to pattern recognition, we may be missing an opportunity to explore the kind of intuition which is found to be more uncomfortable – and thus derided – within a rationalist framework. Feminists have suggested that we need to deconstruct issues of gender and knowledge in order to explore these issues fully.

We as women have all taken a profound devaluing of the feminine into our bodies like mother's milk ...

Unless and until we examine this unconscious distrust of the feminine, we will never inhabit our bodies fully and never trust our intuitive wisdom. (Reeves 1999, p 124)

Another form of knowledge which may be linked with intuition may work within the physical body as well as on a psychological or spiritual level. Shelton (1995) discusses the concept of 'primal wisdom' – a genetic quality passed through generations of people, irrespective of experience – and suggests that some of our knowledge comes about at a cellular level. Certainly we know that most babies come with reflexes which assist their survival; is it reasonable to assume that this kind of knowledge exists only in the neonate?

Ackerman (1990, p 149), in contemplating the relationship between the woman who experiences food cravings in pregnancy and her body's need for particular nutrients, also suggests that: 'At least for certain nutrients, some gustatory yen or body wisdom takes over'. While many midwives would support the suggestion that some women experience a craving for the kinds of foods they need, it is unlikely in current practice that a woman who craved a bag of chips during the transitional phase of labour would be given this as a priority. It is more likely, especially in the context of a hospital birth, that the woman would either be counselled against eating in labour or would be offered something lighter to eat. Again, knowledge is subject to the social context of that knowledge.

Women's ways of knowing

During the 1980s, four women set out to research 'women's ways of knowing', ultimately writing a book of the same title (Belenky et al 1997). Having interviewed 135 women of varying ages and backgrounds, they proposed a fluid model which described the differing types of knowledge held by the women they talked with. While women continually highlighted the importance of their first-hand experiences and gut reactions in knowing, they were seen to fall into a number of different categories depending on their personal philosophy and approach to knowledge. (Further details of this research are discussed in Chapter 10.)

Some of the women were termed as 'silent', having not found their voice (in the context of patriarchal society). Some accepted the 'received view', having not yet discovered the possibility of challenging their socialisation. Then there were the women who had discovered liberation through subjective knowledge. Finally, a small group of women had moved through all of these stages and had become what the researchers termed 'constructed knowers'. These women gathered evidence from a variety of sources and used this to formulate a more holistic understanding of the place of knowledge in their lives and in the fields in which they worked. Critics of this research point out that these categories may be based as much on social class and other demographic factors as gender; we have no data from male 'knowers' to compare this with. Despite this, Belenky et al's study is often given a key place in discussions of feminist epistemology and it may also be useful in informing the development of midwifery knowledge.

WHERE DO WE GO FROM HERE?

Midwifery is faced with a situation where the culture of the current maternity care services and society as a whole values patriarchal, pseudo-scientific, medical knowledge above that held by women and midwives. Many midwives working with this system are governed by policies and guidelines which attempt to use reductionist thinking to define the normal and set general parameters for practice, often with little consideration of the needs of the individual woman. How can an understanding of feminist theory in this area help us to advance midwifery practice and knowledge within this context?

We have seen that normal science – even when this is woman centred – cannot realistically play a large part in further increasing our knowledge of midwifery and childbirth. While the randomised controlled trial may be useful for evaluating single interventions, it is extremely limited in its ability to help us make sense of the complex reality of women's experiences and midwifery practice. We have also suggested that, while it is useful to use qualitative approaches to explore the experiences of small numbers of women, taking a feminist standpoint may also not be wholly useful in enabling us to develop wider theories and knowledge. The stance of the feminist postmodernist, in pulling apart much of what has gone before, may help us to see where the problems lie. However, this may not be useful if this does not lead to alternative forms of knowledge generation.

Even the term 'evidence', which I have used in this chapter in line with current discussion of midwifery knowledge, may be problematic. It is most commonly used as a legal word and, in many of its meanings, relates to the concept of 'proof' (Kirkham, personal correspondence 2002). Having established that there is little we can prove or disprove with certainty, perhaps we should reconsider our use of this word in relation to midwifery knowledge.

One solution may exist in the development of a 'constructed midwifery knowledge', using multiple sources of knowledge to build and test theories. Another possibility lies where feminists are joining with theorists from other, related, standpoints in an attempt to build theories of knowledge which have meaning and relevance to women, are inclusive of women's ways of knowing and which can take this debate forward. One of the current debates in this area considers whether it is helpful to generate theories of knowledge which are specifically based on women's (as opposed to men's) ways of knowing. Would it be helpful to consider how women know or to build a specifically feminist epistemology or would this, by its very inclusivity, be less than helpful in the wider world of epistemological debate? How do we know that women are any less biased and that their knowledge is less based on social constructs than men? The answer is that we cannot remove our personal bias any more than can another theorist, and that we are equally situated within our own social constructs.

While midwifery itself is primarily about women, there are many other related fields which are not; it may be that, by joining with thinkers from other areas, we can build a more holistic model through which we can generate, explore and evaluate knowledge. Sjoo & Mor (1997) talk about the possibility of developing a 'holistic epistemology' – where the subject and object are in sympathetic resonance with each other. Even scientists such as the physicist Capra (1982) have begun to talk about the need for a holistic view in contrast to the current approach involving hierarchies, compartmentalisation and mechanistic thinking. Modern philosophers Riane Eisler (1995) and Ken Wilber (2000) both discuss the development of a 'new science', which integrates new thinking with a spiritually based perspective.

However we move forward in our search for midwifery knowledge, two fundamental problems remain to be solved in practice. First, in an age where some degree of objective evaluation of knowledge is seen as essential, how can we develop tools for evaluating the women-centred knowledge which midwives use? Second, should we also be working on a political level – even if this is within a partnership framework – to encourage our culture to see those forms of knowledge favoured by women as valid, just as science is seen by many as the most valid form of knowledge generation today? Just as it did in the time of the early feminists, knowledge equals power. This power can either be used against women or in a way which empowers them and their midwives towards a holistic approach to knowledge and the range of choices which are open to them.

Questions for Reflection ?????

To what degree do you feel your own thinking is based on traditional (male) or feminist approaches to knowledge?

With which of the feminist positions (if any) do you feel the most sympathy? How does this manifest in your life and work and in your attitudes towards the different types of evidence which are available to women?

To what degree do you feel the type of education or training you experienced has influenced your current viewpoint in this area?

What types of evidence are valued by the women you most respect? How does this impact on your personal philosophy in this area?

In practice, how much value do you place on women's knowledge and intuition? How much value do you place on your own?

Would the best way forward in this area be to continue to explore forms of knowledge which are particularly used by women or to join with other groups of thinkers who are challenging the current situation in order to develop a more inclusive epistemology?

In what ways do you and your colleagues already evaluate 'alternative' forms of knowledge?

How can we work towards a situation where women's and midwifery knowledge – particularly those forms which would be considered 'alternative' – is validated and valued in our culture?

Key points

- 'Ways of knowing' have, historically, tended to be based around male ideas, with few women contributing to philosophical and epistemological debate until relatively recent times.

- Taking a historical perspective on the development of knowledge highlights that there are many things we once thought we 'knew' which we now label as 'myth'; this raises questions about how certain we can ever be.

- Knowledge is not simply about 'what we know'; it is a personal, political, social and economic issue.

- There are vast questions surrounding the issue of whether midwifery and/or medicine are sciences and whether scientific methods are able to increase our knowledge in these fields.

- Midwives and other women have suggested that there are more 'ways of knowing' than through scientific method alone and we are beginning to unpack some of these in relation to women's lives and midwifery practice.

REFERENCES

Ackerman D 1990 A natural history of the senses. Random House, New York

Aristotle 1928 The Oxford translation of Aristotle (trans. Ross WD). Oxford University Press, Oxford

de Beavoir S 1952 The second sex (trans. Parsley HM). Vintage, New York

Belenky MF, Clinchy BM, Goldberger NR, Tarule JM 1997 Women's ways of knowing. The development of self, voice and mind, 2nd edn. Basic Books, New York

Benner P 1984 From novice to expert. Addison Wesley, New York

Brown C 1998 Afterwards, you're a genius. Faith, medicine and the meta-physics of healing. Riverhead Books, New York

Capra F 1982 The turning point: science, society and the rising culture. Simon and Schuster, New York

Carr EH 1985 What is history? Text of the George Macaulay Trevelyan lectures delivered in the University of Cambridge. January–March 1961. Penguin, London

Coney S 1995 The menopause industry, 2nd edn. The Women's Press, London

Davis-Floyd RE, Davis E 1997 Intuition as authoritative knowledge in midwifery and home birth. In: Davis-Floyd RE, Sargent CF (eds) Childbirth and authoritative knowledge. Cross-cultural perspectives. University of California Press, Berkeley, CA

Descartes R 1988 Descartes: selected philosophical writings (trans. Cottingham J, Stoothoff R, Murdoch D). Cambridge University Press, Cambridge

Eisler R 1995 The chalice and the blade, 2nd edn. HarperCollins, New York

Gaskin IM 1989 Interview with Candice Whitridge. Birth Gazette 5 (3): 6–12

Gilligan C 1993 In a different voice. Psychological theory and women's development. Harvard University Press, Cambridge, MA

Hall J 2001 Midwifery, mind and spirit. Books for Midwives, Oxford

Harding S 1986 The science question in feminism. Open University Press, Milton Keynes

Kuhn TS 1996 The structure of scientific revolutions, 3rd edn. University of Chicago Press, Chicago, IL

Magee B 1987 The great philosophers. Oxford University Press, Oxford

Mernissi F 1988 Doing daily battle. Interviews with Moroccan women (trans. Lakeland MJ). The Women's Press, London

National Institute for Clinical Excellence (NICE) 2001 The use of electronic fetal monitoring: the use and interpretation of cardiotocography in intrapartum fetal surveillance. National Institute for Clinical Excellence, London

Olatunbosun OA, Edouard L, Pierson RA 1998 Physicians' attitudes toward evidence-based obstetric practice: a questionnaire survey. British Medical Journal 316: 365–366

Page L 2000 The new midwifery: science and sensitivity in practice. Churchill Livingstone, London

Plato 1993 Republic (trans. Waterfield R). Oxford University Press, Oxford

Popper KR 1959 The logic of scientific discovery. Harper Torchbooks, New York

Reeves PM 1999 Women's intuition: unlocking the wisdom of the body. Conari Press, Berkeley, CA

Rowling JK 1997 Harry Potter and the philosopher's stone. Bloomsbury, London

Sargent CF, Bascope G 1997 Ways of knowing about birth in three cultures. In: Davis-Floyd RE, Sargent CF (eds) Childbirth and authoritative knowledge. Cross-cultural perspectives. University of California Press, Berkeley, CA

Schiebinger L 1987 History and philosophy. In: Harding S, O'Barr JF (eds) Sex and scientific inquiry. University of Chicago Press, Chicago, IL

Shelton HM 1995 The myth of medicine. Cool Hand Communications, Boca Raton, FL

Singh S 1997 Fermat's last theorum. Fourth Estate, London

Sjoo M, Mor B 1997 The great cosmic mother: rediscovering the religion of the earth. Harper and Row, San Francisco, CA

Southern J 1998 On trial: women healers. Midwifery Today 46: 35–39

Taylor M 2001 Thoughts on science, RCTs and midwifery knowledge. Midwifery Matters 91: 3–8

Urmson JO, Ree J (eds) 1989 The concise encyclopaedia of Western philosophy and philosophers. Unwin Hyman, Boston, MA

Wagner M 1994 Pursuing the birth machine: the search for appropriate birth technology. ACE Graphics, Sydney

Wickham S 1999 Evidence-based midwifery 1: What is evidence-based midwifery? Midwifery Today 51: 42–43

Wilber K 2000 A theory of everything. An integral vision for business, politics, science and spirituality. Shambhala, Boston, MA

12

Midwifery partnership with women in Aotearoa/New Zealand: a post-structuralist feminist perspective on the use of epidurals in 'normal' birth

Ruth Surtees

Finally, the ideology of technology shapes motherhood. No longer an event shaped by religion and family, having a baby has become part of the high-tech medical world. But as an ideology, a way of thinking, technology is harder to pin down, so pervasive has it become in Western society. The ideology of technology encourages us to see ourselves as objects, to see people as made up of machines and part of larger machines. (Rothman 1989, p 28)

INTRODUCTION

In 1996 Barbara Katz Rothman was a keynote speaker at a New Zealand College of Midwives (NZCOM) conference held in Christchurch, Aotearoa/New Zealand. As the conference was drawing to a close, she called upon the midwives in the audience to be mindful of the ways in which epidural analgesia serves to separate the mind from the body, saying '…don't make the same mistake with epidurals in normal birth as we have in America…back there we have two whole generations of women now who simply don't know how it feels to give birth'. As someone who is convinced that home is the preferable place for both birth and death, and that these transitions are spiritual, rather than medical events, I was deeply concerned about this image of epidurals as standard practice in normal birth in the USA. This use of technology was inconsistent with my participation in the home births of one of my nieces and various friends' babies, and with most of my experiences as a pakeha* midwifery student. Since 1996, however, my engagement with feminist post-structuralist analysis and my research with midwives in Aotearoa/New Zealand have pushed me to think in different ways about medical technology, epidurals and the practice of partnership between midwives and birthing women.

My contribution to this book offers a particular perspective from a discourse analytic methodological approach to some of the issues surrounding women's choice of epidural pain relief in normal labour and what this may mean for midwives' scope of practice. It is based on the ethnographic fieldwork undertaken for my doctoral research into the practice of midwifery in one city in Aotearoa/New Zealand.** This involved interviews and participant observation in a variety of different contexts: a base obstetric hospital, a birthing centre, two small semi-rural hospitals and several differing self-employed midwifery practices, some of which included home birthing as an option. I begin by outlining some issues specific to midwifery in Aotearoa/New Zealand. This is followed by a discussion of discourse theory and analysis based on feminist post-structuralism in the context of its relevance for midwifery. Finally, I discuss some of the data from my fieldwork, highlighting the importance of language and desire in the (re)production of contestable meanings around childbirth. My focus is on how midwives committed to partnership and joint decision making with birthing women may find themselves using epidural analgesia, despite their concerns about its use in normal labour.

CONTEMPORARY MIDWIFERY PARTNERSHIP IN AOTEAROA/ NEW ZEALAND

Midwives in Aotearoa/New Zealand have relatively recently re-emerged as autonomous practitioners whose professionalisation processes are now articulated through a prevailing discourse of partnership. The complex history and medicalisation of birthing and midwifery in Aotearoa/New Zealand from colonial times until 1990 cannot be adequately discussed here and is well documented elsewhere (see Banks 2000a, Daellenbach 1999, Donley 1998, Guilliland & Pairman 1995, Mein Smith 1986, Papps & Olssen 1997, Smythe 1998, Tully 1999). After the political struggles these authors document between groups of birthing women, doctors, midwives and nurses, public and private hospitals, health reforms and the state, the Nurses' Amendment Act of 1990 finally restored midwives' professional autonomy. This secured their position as specialists in normal birth and as a profession that is now distinctly separate from medicine and nursing (Pairman 2002). At the core of the discourse articulating their status as birthing professionals has been midwives' commitment to work in partnership with women.

This concept of partnership with birthing women has emerged as a distinctly feminist form of professional practice, explored by Tully (1999).

---

*The term 'pakeha' refers to a non-Maori person of European descent, born in Aotearoa/New Zealand. The term 'Maori' refers to the indigenous people of Aotearoa/New Zealand (and see 'tangata whenua', footnote on p 171). These names signify '... the colonial relationship between "Maori" and "Pakeha", the non-indigenous settler population' (Tuhiwai Smith 1999, p 6). The self-identification by some researchers with the term 'pakeha' may signify a politicised positioning within discourses of biculturalism. At the same time, these politics remain troubled by an engagement with postcolonial and post-structural texts (Glamuzina 1992, Gunew & Yeatman 1993, Tuhiwai Smith 1999). Banks (2000b) suggests that pakeha midwives address the power of pakeha in terms of numbers, resources, and leadership in midwifery, by 'accepting and understanding' the need for separateness in the voice(s) of the Maori midwives' collective Nga Maia o Aotearoa me te Waipounamu, while holding 'tight to the common threads we share as we walk the with-woman path' (Banks 2000b, p 5). The NZCOM, in its commitment to biculturalism, maintains a role in supporting Maori midwives and communities in the pursuit of Maori-identified interests (Tully et al 1998).
**My academic background is in feminist/gender studies and education, where I have focused on feminist discourse analytic research in health/education, and it is this critical perspective, rather than a midwifery practice base, that I bring to the field.

Tully details the ways in which partnership '... developed out of mutually supportive relations between domiciliary midwives and homebirth consumers in the 1970s/80s, [and] was formalised in the philosophy of the NZCOM which was formed in 1989' (Tully 1999, p 17). Daellenbach notes that in the decade prior to the establishment of the College of Midwives in 1989, home birth activists and domiciliary midwives forged understandings of partnership '... out of a shared sense of marginalisation in relation to the dominant medical profession' (Daellenbach 1999, p 204). During this time the Direct Entry Taskforce was formed specifically to re-establish direct entry midwifery education (Save the Midwives Direct Entry Taskforce 1990). This arose from a pressure group called 'Save The Midwives', to which a number of home birth and consumer activist organisations belonged (Daellenbach 1999, Donley 1986, Guilliland & Pairman 1995).

Also important during this decade of feminist activism in health was the inquiry into the treatment of women for cervical cancer at the National Women's Hospital, which investigated the denial of women's right to informed consent (Cartwright 1988). The report arising from this inquiry recommended practices of accountability, patient-centred care, self-determination and cultural sensitivity in the health service. The implementation of these practices included patient advocates in hospitals and consumer representation on medical committees (and see Bunkle 1992, 1994, Cartwright 1988, Coney 1993, Guilliland & Pairman 1995 for critical analyses of these issues).

Guilliland & Pairman also describe the establishment of ideals of partnership as arising from a commitment to biculturalism. They note that the constitutional and legislative structures of society in Aotearoa/New Zealand are based on the Treaty of Waitangi, signed in 1840 between tangata whenua* and the Crown. Principles inherent to the Treaty and which are intended to govern this relationship are partnership, participation,

protection and equity (Ramsden 1995, p 3). These are also important contributing contextual factors in the development of and continued shaping of differing and complex ideas of partnership.

The defining attributes of this midwifery model arising from these understandings of partnership are that midwives are autonomous practitioners, recognise pregnancy and birth as normal life events and deliver continuity of care that is woman centred (Guilliland & Pairman 1995, Tully et al 1998). These attributes are central to midwifery's claims to feminist professional practice and function as counterclaims to the medical model of birthing (Tully et al 1998, p 249). In relation to this, the introduction of *The Midwifery Partnership – a Model for Practice* states: 'It is because of this political and personal involvement with women that midwifery accepts its responsibilities as an emancipatory change agent' (Guilliland & Pairman 1995, p 1). The midwifery model of care encourages pregnant and birthing women to retain decision making and control over their own bodies and experiences (Tully & Mortlock 1999). Guilliland & Pairman state (1995, p 2): '... the midwifery profession identifies, acknowledges and requires partnership as part of practice, and provides guidelines for the practice of partnership within its Code of Ethics ...'. This midwifery model of partnership has had a significant effect on the articulation of professional discourse within midwifery in Aotearoa/New Zealand.

The commitment to partnership between individual women and midwives is extended to organisational partnership between midwives and consumer members of the NZCOM. This includes the incorporation of consumers on national and regional committees of the College and consumer involvement in the evaluation of professional practice through the 'Standards Review' process for practising midwives, as well as significant consumer input into the Direct Entry Bachelor of Midwifery degree programmes.* This both reflects and reinforces the midwifery model of partnership where the

---

*'Tangata whenua' means the indigenous people of Aotearoa; literally, people who stand on the land in which the placentas that sustained their life in the womb have been buried (Banks 2000a, Donley 1998).

*For historical analyses of the development of Direct Entry midwifery education in Aotearoa, see Donley 1986, Papps & Olssen 1997, Pairman 2002, STM DE Taskforce 1990.

woman/consumer is at the centre of care. After some conflict with the International Confederation of Midwives (ICM) over the issue of consumer membership in the NZCOM, the confederation adopted the policy statement submitted by the NZCOM in 1993 which articulates midwifery as a profession founded on its partnership with women (Guilliland & Pairman 1995, Tully 1999). The New Zealand midwifery model of partnership is now hailed internationally as an innovative model of consumer-centred care (Bryar 1995, Young 1996).

From July 1996, and within the context of continuing complex health reforms, significant changes were made to the funding of maternity provision (see Abel 1997, Cumming & Salmond 1998, Guilliland 2002, Larner 1997). Women are now required to nominate a lead maternity caregiver (LMC), who may be a midwife, obstetrician or general practitioner. That provider holds a budget, which is claimed for under modules of care. This budget is the same regardless of professional discipline. Continuity of care is recognised as being vital to the well-being of the woman under the LMC system (Guilliland 1999), the costs of which are met by the state.** By 2001, 70% of women chose a midwife as their LMC, while 15% chose a general practitioner. Most of the remaining women have a private obstetrician. A small minority present straight to hospitals for care (Guilliland 2002, p 7) and 6–10% of women choose home birth with a midwife who may either offer this as one option in her practice or who may maintain a specifically home birth-centred practice. Midwifery is now clearly a well-established profession in Aotearoa/New Zealand. Midwives acting as LMCs may consult with an obstetrician for specialist advice and allocate money from the budget for this but they remain lead caregivers. This provides the continuity valued by women and reduces the need to transfer to another professional group (Guilliland 1999, p 12).

**The LMC system is now provided for and funded under section 88 of the New Zealand Public Health and Disability Act 2000, which sets out terms and conditions for payment to the provider of maternity services. (See Guilliland 1999, 2000, 2002, for details of LMC funding and related policy issues.)

In her thesis examining the ways in which midwives in Aotearoa/New Zealand 'do professionalism differently' from doctors and nurses, Tully (1999) discusses the ways in which the language of 'empowerment' and 'choice' in childbirth, drawn from radical feminist critiques of medicalisation, shaped midwifery's definition of itself as a distinctly feminist profession. This conception of empowerment through choice also informed home birth activism in the 1980s. Daellenbach argues that this activism was more successful in prompting women to question which maternity services they wanted, rather than to actually birth at home in large numbers, and popularised '... the rhetoric of "choices for childbirth"' (Daellenbach 1999, p 192). Tully et al note that rather than the college involving two philosophically aligned and mutually dependent groups, as it appeared to during its inception over a decade ago, '... it now embraces a range of differently positioned practitioners and consumers with potentially different understandings of what partnership involves' (Tully et al 1998, p 251). Partnership in any arena remains a contested and slippery concept and, in relation to biculturalism, has been critiqued by Maori activists involved in ongoing disputes over Treaty negotiations with the Crown and, in relation to birth, by some home birth activists engaged in negotiations with the NZCOM. Daellenbach (1999, p 202–207) argues that these negotiations over partnership (which merge and intersect in the NZCOM between Maori/pakeha and consumer/midwife) highlight complex differences as well as some similarities between sets of actors who have been defined as 'partners'.

FEMINIST DISCOURSE PRACTICES AND MIDWIFERY

An analysis of discourses *within* midwifery partnerships as well as those between midwifery and obstetrics is useful in exploring some of the differences in positioning between midwives and consumers, and the effects of these differences. While advocating post-structuralist theorising here I am not concerned with feminist debates about its ir/relevance for feminism or feminist action (Ahmed 1998, Fraser & Nicholson 1990,

Miller 2000, Zalewski 2000). Instead, I want to suggest that feminisms that strategically appropriate Foucault's theories about discourse, power and knowledge may make a real contribution to midwifery praxis. The task is to explore differences between women and midwives without fragmenting midwifery's emancipatory goals. While there are many different types of discourse analysis, Miller describes a common premise.

The fundamental premise of discourse analysis … is that language constitutes rather than reflects reality, and that speakers use talk strategically to accomplish their purposes in particular settings. In the parlance of social constructionists, language is a 'claims-making' enterprise … Here I use 'claim' in the specific sense of an account or story which is designed to further some practical goal. (Miller 2000, p 317)

Miller suggests that it has been Foucault's great contribution '… to have shifted the discussion of power away from properties of classes and individuals to ways of saying and knowing' (Miller 2000, p 316). Particularly helpful to any analysis of institutions involved in the practical goals of the regulation and monitoring of bodies, such as in childbirth, is the idea of power as a capillary network. The 'microphysics' of power involves the subtle, multiply directional relations between specific individuals. This provides scope for a much broader feminist analysis of power as something that is widely distributed, rather than the property of a few people, and generated within fields of knowledge, including midwifery as a field of professional practice. Power in this sense, then, is seen as productive and diffuse, rather than repressive and exclusionary (Burman 1996, de Ras & Grace 1997, McNay 1994, Ussher 1997).

Marion McLaughlan is one midwife who has used discourse analytic methodology in Aotearoa/New Zealand in this way. She has noted that there are two predominantly available discourses of birthing, either the 'medical' or the 'natural'. While the medical discourse prevails during the pregnancy and birth of the first baby for women, this also provides a potential point of resistance for subsequent births. She notes that where women receive continuity of care, the '… docile body is replaced with a more self-determining possibility' (McLaughlan 1997, p 134).

McLaughlan suggests that midwives may be positioned in either discourse or may also be 'straddling the two' at different times and different places of work (McLaughlan 1997).

Social discourses available to women in a given culture at a given time, such as those identified by McLaughlan above, provide subject positions, constitute our subjectivities and reproduce or challenge existing gendered relations (and see Gavey 1989, Jaworski & Coupland 1999, Wetherell et al 2001). The discourse of partnership developed during the inception of the NZCOM assumed that midwives and women share common interests. My research shows how these shared interests may be deployed strategically, and shift and change at different times for different practical purposes, and to make different claims about certain forms of partnership. Two questions I brought to the transcripts of the interview texts for analysis were: 'What actions, in which situations, constitute partnership? What are the effects of these actions?'.

THE SEDUCTION OF SEDATION

I think that the technology is very seductive in that epidurals, for example, they have appeal … a lot of women are very seduced by the thought of something, anything that would take the pain away … in labour at a critical point – I think that women are vulnerable in labour to the suggestion that there is something that can remove the pain. They believe that it's completely safe … and yeah, I can see that it would be very seductive. So I think that a lot more women do really make uninformed choice about things like epidurals because they're not aware of the possible risks or dangers or implications of what might happen next … it's sometimes referred to as a cascade of interventions. (Mandy*, birthing centre midwife)

In the UK the *Changing Childbirth* Department of Health report of 1993 identified the concepts of 'choice, continuity and control' as vitally important in empowering women in childbirth (Sandall 1995). In Aotearoa/New Zealand these concepts are echoed in ideals about partnership between midwives and women that involve '… trust, shared control and responsibility and shared

---

*All midwives' names here are pseudonyms.

meaning through mutual understanding' (Guilliland & Pairman 1995, p 1). The midwives who participated in my project and who talked about the provision of pain relief describe their actions as a response to the desires of the women who chose them as caregivers. Women's choice to use epidurals as pain relief poses particular challenges for midwives committed to minimising medical intervention in normal birth. Below I examine discourses of partnership and choice in the context of epidural analgesia in normal birthing, chosen as a focus here because many midwives in my study were concerned about the effects of what they sometimes called an epidural 'epidemic'. The effect this has on what is seen as normal birth is briefly explored, as are the results of these networked intersections of knowledge/power in constructing midwifery professional identity and subsequently shaping individual scope(s) of practice.

Embracing 'empowerment' through women's choice

... but it's also the whole culture of childbirth that seems to have become so ... there's been such an embracing of medicalisation. You know, a frightening embracing of it really. Last week I had a woman arrive in saying oh, I don't like pain, I'd like an epidural cos all my friends had said, you know, have an epidural cos you don't have pain and ... it could easily be the type of client that I have ... . People go straight for epidurals, often it seems to be where they take their antenatal classes, all their education things. But the thing is epidurals have their own complications really ... the fact that you're more likely to get interventions as a result. (Gillian, self-employed midwife)

How can midwives value choice for women, yet also provide professional advice about alternative options in birthing? Some midwives suggested that, while choices in childbirth are important, some women may feel overwhelmed at times with choices or that the very availability of the choice of an epidural itself impacts on women who would prefer to resist it, such that:

I think it's a lot harder for women to birth these days with that choice because they know that choice is there ... I mean, you know yourself if you're in a lot

of pain, and you think you can get out of it then you'll get out of it ... and I just admire women so much that they do have the choice and they don't go for it ... I think it's a lot harder for them than it was for us, when epidurals weren't available. (Eva, self-employed midwife)

Choosing or resisting an epidural as analgesia is a historically specific action; when and where it was not available, it was not an issue and midwives focused on constant support and care during labour (Rooks 2000). The possibility of this specific type of pain relief intensifies its demand.

We were talking about this at work this morning and it's just not that simple, to tell women they can have a normal birth is not that simple. They have gone the other way, they have not embraced the normal, they have embraced the medical and technological model. So it's all very well for consumers to tell us as midwives how to do our job, but it's not easy if women for a whole lot of cultural, social and political reasons have embraced the medical model. I have an epidural certificate so I can stay with a woman if her care becomes less than normal, women feel betrayed if suddenly things are a bit off the track or not normal, and what do you say? See you later, I'm out of here, you're not normal any more? I want to be able to stay right through with all my women; that is something that is important to me. (Natalie, self-employed midwife)

In the excerpt above, Natalie distinguishes between 'consumers', as politicised birthing activists who are critical of midwives involved in using epidurals in normal births, and individual women. This is central to feminist debates around 'women' as a singular category of identity and embodied subjectivities of difference and desire (Butler 1990). Midwives identify their partnership with individual women as something that results from the women feeling in control of their experience, whether that involves embracing or rejecting the medical technological model. Women who choose epidurals may see themselves as birthing normally and positively as long as they feel in control of the situation. Some midwives are also more interested in partnership with individual birthing women than with women who 'represent' birthing women collectively. In Natalie's narrative, professional identity as a midwife comes from continuity of care and facilitating choice. This is enhanced by the ability to follow the woman into the field of secondary care provision. Both home birth and secondary care are sites at which knowledge and power intersect in childbirth. Both are sites in which midwives may practise continuity of care and facilitate the empowerment of birthing women (Annandale & Clarke 1996, Kent 2000, Sawicki 1991).

Often midwives' talk about choice and control was linked to the evidence that choosing an epidural as analgesia in an otherwise normal labour would very often lead to a cascade of intervention, sometimes thwarting midwives' goals of normal birth and significantly directing their scope of practice. Some midwives felt that women are demanding epidurals because they are fully informed about the choices for pain relief available to them. On the other hand, women are also seen to demand epidurals despite being informed (of the probable cascade of intervention).

So I think the intervention rate is about the culture of our facilities … that whole expectation, women are demanding epidurals all around the country and they're fully informed and there's no problem, women's choice, and that's what they want but I still question that; is it really an informed choice in all cases but it's still – that's just like the woman who's demanding obstetrics … you know, the obstetrician as her primary carer and they'll pay for it … and they do. (NZCOM midwifery advisor)

Being informed is seen as a positive and empowering experience for women. However, some women's access to the possibility of pain relief intensifies demand for technological intervention in birth, at a time when midwives rather than doctors are the predominant professionals working with birthing women. There is a parallel between the use of twilight sleep by middle-class (usually non-Maori) women in the 1930s and the suggestion by some midwives in my study that there are sometimes links between social class, ethnicity and 'choices' for pain relief. The relationship of resources (financial, social, cultural) to the desire to avoid pain is borne out by the large Australian study by Roberts et al which indicated that amongst all low-risk birthing women, private patients were '… significantly more likely to have interventions before birth (epidural, induction or augmentation)' (Roberts et al 2000, p 137).

The complex relationships between choice, control, social class and pain relief in labour are further addressed by Lazarus (1997) and by Donley (1998).

Woman-centred and continuity of care discourses – negotiating ideas of 'normal'

While most midwives supported low technological intervention in normal births, the majority I interviewed had their epidural certificates or were working towards them. Holding an epidural certificate meant that they could support and respect women's choices by providing this service to women who choose epidural pain relief. Giving women choices with respect to epidurals was seen as a way to empower women and part of a woman-centred practice that prioritised continuity of care.

The challenges for midwives of responding to women's choices were illustrated by a conversation I had with a midwife in a small rural unit. Susan had worked for a long time in the base hospital as a core midwife doing rostered shifts on the labour ward, then for a spell on the base hospital community/domiciliary teams providing continuity of care, and was now working in a small semi-rural hospital. In the extract below, Susan talks about rates of intervention when she practised as a core midwife at the base hospital.

Susan: I think you try harder here because of the very fact that you're away from town and … you know, I mean there it's quite easy to pop along and get the anaesthetist … just pop along round the corner and he'll come and put an epidural in and it's great. I mean my epidural rate was very high. Well, it was in keeping with the hospital, but it was very high … I mean I did standards review and I was quite surprised.
RS: What sort of rate are we talking about … what percentage of births?
Susan: Oh, about 60%, 70% … my Caesar rate was 22% which was obviously the same as the hospital's. My ecbolic rate was 100% …

The context of our discussion was her enjoyment of her new worksite, which necessarily involved lower rates of interventions. Susan is able to position herself as working in a woman-centred way if she adapts her practice to the choices women make about birthing.

There is a lot to weigh up ... but you can't deny somebody an epidural. Who are we to say you cannot have an epidural ... your pain isn't as great as you think it is. Pain's really subjective. I try not to judge women ... if they don't have an epidural and they have a nice normal birth it's absolutely fantastic. But I don't judge them and think they're weak because they wanted an epidural, you know, each to their own ... and that's being woman centred. I think to deny them an epidural when they really want one is not being woman centred and that happens, cos the midwife doesn't like epidurals or she doesn't want to give pethidine cos it would ruin her record that she's set for the last 2 years. But that's not being woman centred, is it?

Susan's talk highlights the way in which the provision of effective pain relief constitutes her as providing woman-centred care and working in partnership with women. Providing what women choose, regardless of who they are or where they come from, is to empower women in their choices for (pain relief in) childbirth. If women are made aware of the risks involved, then they are exercising informed consent. They are making choices. In other words, in the conversation above, supporting, rather than 'judging' their choices, is seen as the appropriate action to empower women.

Supporting/empowering some women in their desire to have an epidural can simultaneously be seen as disillusioning for some midwives if they feel at times that there is a discrepancy between what women want and what midwifery might offer.

And I had this woman saying oh she'd like an epidural and I was trying not to frighten her but saying I don't think it's a brilliant idea for you to go in there thinking of having one. But you can't help them ... that's what's coming through. So the whole option of natural midwifery seems to be going and a lot of the women don't actually seem to care ... they all want it. (Yvonne, community midwife)

Angela, a midwife in a rural unit, talks about the various influences on women's choice of epidural for pain relief.

Yeah ... they want epidurals because that's what the medical practitioners tell them they need and because they've been told by people that nobody should endure pain and because people tend not to sit down and explain to them that pain is normal in birth and in most cases with assistance can be coped with. Many women don't have the implications of an epidural explained to them. Things like the increased risk of instrumental delivery, caesarean section or the risks of other intervention being needed, or the risks to the baby. Frequently the husband influences the woman, as he can't cope with her pain. (Angela, midwife, rural unit)

Medical practitioners, other people, both lay and medical, and 'frequently the husband' often tell the woman what she needs or influence her decision in other ways. Yvonne says, '... but you can't help them ... they all want it'. And Natalie, in the excerpt below, reinforces this conclusion by drawing on a consumer survey undertaken by the base hospital.

... and they did this wee consumer sort of thing last year to see what women wanted ... women wanted to make sure they could get epidurals, you know ... there was no consumer response at a political level to work at reclaiming normality and getting pools into the rooms and getting, you know, things that would potentially make it a more personable kind of experience to be in there ... that just ... it wasn't there. (Natalie, self-employed midwife)

It may be that for many women/consumers now, 'normality' is about choosing pain relief in the form of epidural analgesia, simply because it is so common and so readily available (Rooks 2000, Weston 2001). The resultant freedom from pain itself is seen as empowering, despite the increased likelihood of further medical intervention. It is chosen over and above what different midwives and women may consider the ideal normal birthing experience. This is similar to MacDonald's (1999) analysis of contemporary meanings of 'normal' and 'natural' in midwifery discourse in Ontario. For the women in MacDonald's study, just as midwives report in mine, prioritising choice, control and continuity of care with a known midwife may be the most important issue for birthing women now. This may be so regardless of the woman's individual relationship to medical technologies, whether embracing, rejecting or otherwise strategically deploying them. What may now constitute 'normal' birth may be the presence of a midwife who offers 'variety of choice' for birthing, as Bess, a new graduate midwife, explained.

This last year has been about learning to be a technician – that's just part of the process, we're almost having to become mini-obstetricians. I've just done a reiki massage course and want to offer that as well – I can offer the full smorgasbord of medical stuff, now I want to balance it all up again. (Bess, self-employed midwife)

Some midwives spoke to me about their philosophical reasons for resisting the acquisition of an epidural certificate. Rosalie's talk positions her in partnership with a birthing woman as they together resist hegemonic hospital discourses around pain relief during a situation of transfer from birthing unit to labour ward.

… and I said she does not want an epidural … do not push her into it, she will know if she needs one … now within an hour the woman did want an epidural, but the one thing for her out of that whole birth experience was that I had said to them that she didn't want one. And I mean it takes … it takes a long time to feel able to do that with them. (Rosalie, birthing centre midwife)

Rosalie's story suggests that it is possible to negotiate issues around hospital protocols and timetabling. Bargaining together over procedures and protocols constitutes aspects of the partnership between the birthing woman and her LMC midwife during the time in the hospital. As Rosalie highlights above, the LMC midwife also has simultaneous professional and collegial relationships to negotiate. Learning to constructively resist powerful hospital discourses 'takes a long time', something many new practitioners also mentioned. Pressure is exerted at different times by some midwives who do have their epidural certificates on those who do not for different reasons, such as to provide back-up or to relieve pressure on core midwives in a busy labour ward. Of central importance here is the effect of intertwined discourses of 'normality', 'continuity of care', 'choice' and 'empowerment'. Midwives are constructed as the guardians of a conceptually mobile ideal and midwifery is constantly reconstructed around shifting ideals of 'normal' birth. The midwives I spoke to who did not yet have or did not want their epidural certificates

for a variety of reasons often saw themselves as occupying a position frequently interpreted as resistant or transgressive.

Midwifery scope of practice – in which direction now?

In one group interview with newly graduated practitioners, the concept of 'normal' is linked to birthing practices that would not include the use of an epidural simply for pain relief.

Ange: But it's not something that … if a woman comes in here saying, I'm pregnant … I want a midwife and I want an epidural then you know, it makes us question really whether …
Beth: Whether they're coming to the right place.
Ange: And we actually now … I don't make any excuses for saying to women well, you know, this is the way we work, and this is how we view epidurals. If you need an epidural after going through and trying all these things and it's really appropriate and we just thank God that epidurals have been invented at those times because they really are appropriate, but to use them inappropriately for me, as a midwife, is not good practice. So we don't do that.

In these instances, having an epidural is not seen as part of normal birth. The provision of epidural care in an otherwise low-risk labour would be seen as outside the individual midwife's scope of practice and not part of the group practice philosophy. Since an epidural can only be provided in a base hospital and requires the (initial) presence of an anaesthetist, followed by the continual presence of a midwife with an epidural certificate, it constitutes secondary care. In other instances, midwives said that because epidurals can be considered part of normal birth now, they should all work towards gaining the epidural certificate which enables midwives to top up the anaesthetic dosage after the delivery catheter has been initially inserted into the woman's epidural space.

This position was particularly evident in the talk of midwives where continuity of care was of primary importance in constituting their partnership with women. As one midwife said to me: '… what do I say, see you later, you're not normal any more?'. This particular repertoire parallels midwives' administration of chloroform from

Murphy's inhalers in the 1930s at the St Helen's hospitals.* As soon as some midwives become trained in what is essentially seen as doctors' work (Donley 2000, Strid 2000), pressure can be brought to bear on other midwives to provide the same service. If midwives do not wish to provide the service or are not trained to do so, women may choose another practitioner so the midwife risks 'losing business' as an LMC. Some self-employed midwives talked about the ways in which the woman's choice of epidural for pain relief has an effect on their (scope of) practice and relationships with core labour ward staff.

I don't have an epidural certificate ... which isn't against the law ... and I should be able to take a woman over and say I'm handing my client over because she wants an epidural and I can't do epidural care ... that bit's really clear. I'd say to them, but she wants an epidural and that's her choice and that's her right ... and so to provide her with an epidural I have to hand her over to you, because you're the guys that do the epidurals. Even if I got my certificate ... which is very unlikely cos you have to have X number of women, I wouldn't be skilled at it. It isn't in my field of expertise ... and I think there are midwives who work in base hospitals who have epidural certificates and do it every day ... look after women with epidurals every day ... and of course there shouldn't be such a high epidural rate ... that's a different story ... and so those women deserve to be looked after by people who are good at it. And that's their field of expertise. (Frida, self-employed midwife)

Frida's talk in this account constructs her 'field of expertise' in which the provision of epidural care is not included; instead, when the limits of this field are reached, her desire is to hand over care to secondary (core) midwives who have a broader scope of practice (in the medical sense).

What is missing from this and other accounts where claims are staked to a different ideal of normality is the space/time/energy to talk about

*The Midwives Act 1904 established state control of midwives and provided for the establishment of the 'St. Helens Hospitals' managed by the then Department of Health. These hospitals were to provide training facilities for midwives and subsidised care for 'married working class women' and were initially run by midwives until the access of medical students in the 1930s led to eventual control by the medical profession, a process continually contested and negotiated by various groups of women and midwives (see Donley 1986, Mein Smith 1986, Papps & Olssen 1997).

forms of pain relief other than epidurals (Leap 1997). The very existence of epidurals in normal birth has set the terms of the debate; midwives/women are drawn into the discourse in some way regardless of their position on it; it can be resisted but not ignored (and see Rooks 2000). DeVries (1993) argues that the availability of medical technologies may act to diminish traditional midwifery skills, as well as changing patterns of midwife recruitment and significantly altering the sources of knowledge that surround birth. The midwives in my study were acutely aware of these issues in their consideration of the various meanings around childbirth and midwifery in their working lives.

DISCUSSION

Despite midwives' re-emergence as specialists in, and guardians of, 'normal' birth, there is rising concern that medical intervention in childbirth is increasing both within Aotearoa/New Zealand and internationally (Banks 2000a, Donley 1998, 2000, Lazarus 1997, Pollock 1999, Rothman 1991, Tew 1995, Wagner 1994). While the intervention rate in Aotearoa/New Zealand '... has been at a much slower rate than the rest of the western world ...' (Guilliland & Campbell 2002, p 5), it is still of concern to many midwives and women (Banks 2000b, Calvert 2002, Guilliland & Campbell 2002, Strid 2000). At the 2002 NZCOM conference it became obvious that increasing intervention rates are cause for (inter)national alarm (Bree 2002, Guilliland 2002, Guilliland & Campbell 2002, McAra-Couper 2002, Savage 2002).

The articulation of internal debates between the participating midwives in my study about the provision of epidural pain relief in an otherwise low-risk, healthy or 'nice normal' pregnancy/labour reflects some issues that are beginning to emerge from the international literature. Some midwives in my study were concerned that normal birth appears to be a diminishing goal for women (and see Downe 2001, Hartley 1997, Lazarus 1997, MacDonald 1999, Rooks 2000). Their concern is based on evidence that the use of epidurals for normal birth results in a cascade of intervention (Banks 2000a, Guilliland 2000,

Guilliland & Campbell 2002, Roberts et al 2000, Savage 2002). This impacts on the meaning of normal birth when this is used to define midwifery's scope of practice. It also has implications for midwifery as a profession, if a central tenet of midwifery philosophy is that midwives are to remain the 'guardians of normal birth' (Strid 2000). Normal birth may mean different things to different women, however, as it does to different midwives (Davies 1996, Downe 2001, Hartley 1997).

Whether or not the attainment of an epidural certificate and the provision of epidural care is part of contemporary normal birth or part of something else (neo-medicalisation?), the knowledge that care is likely to become secondary rather than primary if an epidural procedure is used provides significant points of tension for a midwife. This is especially pertinent if the provision of primary care is what constitutes her professional identity as a midwife. Interpreting the individual woman's choice as 'empowering' for her, despite the risks of interventions thereafter, constitutes the midwife as having provided woman-centred care that has been appropriate for a particular woman and her specific circumstances.

Deliberately maintaining ambiguity about the demarcatory boundaries of 'normal' could be interpreted as colluding in the woman's desire for what some might call medicalisation. On the other hand, if the woman sees this as allowing her to maintain a measure of control over her birthing situation, the same midwifery actions are undertaken within a discourse of empowerment (and see DeVries et al 2001, Lazarus 1997). Midwives are able to make important claims in their strategic utilisation of, and positioning within, these discourses around choice and normality. These claims further different practical goals for individual midwives in diverse sites of work.

A number of feminist theorists using aspects of post-structuralist theory have evaluated the critique of medicalisation offered by radical feminisms (Grace 1991, Lupton 1997, Sawicki 1991, Wajcman 1991). Differences in feminist thought about medicalisation hinge on an array of approaches to theorising about biomedical technology as well as about gender. These points of tension between differing feminist viewpoints are highlighted in the data drawn from my interviews with midwives who talk about the relationships between women and technology. The freedom from pain that some women demanded as every woman's 'right' during the twilight sleep years has contemporary parallels (Donley 1998). Contemporary discourses around the obstetrical promise of freedom from pain in childbirth appear just as seductive as they did 70 years ago, but women's responses to it are framed within and organised around discourses of desire and consumer 'choice', rather than those of women's 'rights' to pain-free birthing. This medicalised focus appeared to lessen with the reintroduction of midwifery based on partnership with women, but it seems that women's desires for pain relief may disrupt earlier notions of 'normal' birth. Normal birth is redefined as much by women as by midwives.

How are analysts to interpret the argument that women 'choose' epidurals? Are midwives and birthing women merely docile bodies subjected to the hegemonic regimes of medical dominance? Or can we see women, with midwives, as those who appropriate 'elements of the technology in order to gain a measure of control' over their lives? (Hunt & Symonds 1996, p 87). Is this one example of partnership in action, just as resisting this same technology is another partnership action? As Davies suggests: 'Until we address the question of who decides what constitutes "normality", we will only be paying lip service to the ideal of being "woman-centred"' (Davies 1996, p 286). And as Bordo notes: 'While it is true that we may experience the illusion of "power" while actually performing as docile bodies, it is also true that our very "docility" can have consequences that are personally liberating and/or culturally transforming' (Bordo 1993, p 192). Midwives in my study, in their analysis of the 'epidural epidemic' and women's choices, appear to rupture the dualism between 'active consumer' and 'passive recipient'. Their articulation of the power of desire is discussed by Sawicki.

If patriarchal power operated primarily through violence, objectification and repression, why would women subject themselves to it willingly? On the other hand, if it also operates by inciting desire, attaching individuals to specific identities, and addressing real needs, then it is easier to understand how it has been so effective at getting a grip on us. (Sawicki 1991, p 85)

The desire for painless childbirth *is* a real desire. Epidural analgesia, provided in an otherwise normal birth, even if that birth may then become obstetrically interventionist, is a perceived source of control for some women. This disrupts the notion that some people, such as doctors, have/hold power and others, such as women, do not. The value of continuity of care is especially important to midwives in mobilising a discourse of empowerment here, as it is influential in some midwives' decisions to maintain an epidural certificate. This means in effect that they have a broader scope of practice in one sense, encompassing secondary as well as primary care, and can carry on the provision of care while utilising the base hospital facilities but without having to officially hand over care to the hospital staff.

The valuing of individual women's choices, and the desire to stay with the woman throughout her child-bearing experience by gaining (and, significantly, maintaining) the skills required for an epidural certificate, will be interpreted as part of a rationale for a type of woman-centred partnership. The skills that are developed and crafted, however, are necessarily based on medical technology. For other midwives, revaluing and developing different forms of midwifery knowledges and practices related to pain are important in their rejection of epidural certification in their positioning as the guardians of normal birth.*

CONCLUSION

I have identified some of the ways in which differently positioned midwives negotiate and

contest different modes of knowledge production in the field. This highlights the actions they take in constructing themselves in those networks as contemporary subjects of knowledge/power in childbirth. This has resulted in complicating some previous feminist criticisms of medicalisation and empowerment. Choosing or rejecting an epidural as pain relief in normal labour provides subject positions for women in discourses which arise from different feminist analyses of embodiment, choice and empowerment. On the one hand, empowerment is seen to rest in women's emancipation *from* bodily processes, by avoiding the (potential) pain of childbirth. On the other, and as part of a different claim, empowerment is constructed through and *in* the birthing body and is manifest in the refusal of the epidural, even if this refusal is temporary. This may be seen to further a practical goal of experiencing normal/non-interventionist birth and, for midwives, acting as guardians of the same.

This feminist analysis of discourses within midwifery stresses the importance of attending to the ways in which midwives-being-with-women is constituted within discourses and practices that utilise liberal-humanist notions of choice that may be in tension with the ideal of 'natural' childbirth (and see Bogdan-Lovis 1996). These choices have significant impact for a profession purporting to specialise in normal birth. We can see that partnership discourse involves articulating a relationship between mutually empowered and equal actors but practising partnership is not easy (whether between Maori/pakeha or birthing women/midwives). Setting up these emancipatory goals and articulating the ideals are often followed by negotiations about what this means in practice. Utilising post-structural theories of power and discourse in research analysis such as this means that midwives, feminists and researchers who are 'interested' (MacDonald & Bourgeault 2000) in the politics of childbirth can strategically attend to some of the differences, as well as the similarities, between and among differing groups of women/consumers and midwives. Most importantly, such analyses should attend to the effects of these differences.

---

*Homeopathy, hot water, massage, acupuncture/pressure, responsiveness, love, etc. and see Nicky Leap (1997) who has noted the remarkable difference in birth outcomes when midwives talk with pregnant women about 'working *with* pain', rather than 'pain *relief*' (whereby a 'menu' of different analgesia is offered to the woman for her to choose from). The midwives who adopted the former approach '... represented an overall philosophy of reflecting on practice, embracing uncertainty, recognising that nothing is absolute ...' (Leap 1997, p 263).

Questions for Reflection ?????

Are the issues raised here similar to those in your own place of work?

How might an understanding of feminist discourse analysis help you to think about these issues?

What discourses and practices underpin the Changing Childbirth (1993) report in the UK?

What sorts of assumptions do we make about the role of technology in normal childbirth? Why?

What is your response to the statements made by Barbara Katz Rothman at the start of this chapter?

How can midwives and women work strategically together to maintain women's choice, continuity and control in childbirth, whilst acknowledging the diversity within and between us?

Key points

■ Midwives committed to partnership and joint decision making with birthing women may find

themselves using epidural analgesia, even though they prefer to minimise intervention in normal birth.

■ Midwives identify their partnership with individual women as something that results from the women feeling *in control* of their experience. The woman's wish to be in control may involve embracing, or rejecting, the medical technological model.

■ Normal birth may mean different things to different women, as it does to different midwives.

Acknowledgments

Enormous thanks as always to my thesis supervisors, Elody Rathgen, Rosemary Du Plessis and Daphne Manderson, for their critical feedback on earlier drafts of this chapter. Rosemary's specific knowledge of the field in particular has been of invaluable help to me. Many thanks also to Liz Smythe for her insightful comments, enthusiasm and friendship along the thesis journey. I am indebted to Valerie McClain IBCLC for her extensive research into patients on products and methods exploiting human milk constitutents.

REFERENCES

Abel S 1997 Midwifery and maternity services in transition: an examination of change following the Nurses' Amendment Act 1990. Unpublished PhD thesis, University of Auckland, Auckland, New Zealand

Ahmed S 1998 Differences that matter: feminist theory and postmodernism. University of Cambridge Press, Cambridge

Annandale E, Clarke J 1996 What is gender? Feminist theory and the sociology of human reproduction. Sociology of Health and Illness 18(1): 17–44

Banks M 2000a Home birth bound: mending the broken weave. Birthspirit Books, Dunedin, New Zealand

Banks M 2000b Nurturing our strengths. Paper presented at the Seasons of Renewal NZCOM Conference, Cambridge, New Zealand

Bogdan-Lovis EA 1996 Misreading the power structure: liberal feminists' inability to influence childbirth. Michigan Feminist Studies 11: 59–79

Bordo S 1993 Feminism, Foucault and the politics of the body. In: Ramazanoglu C (ed) Up against Foucault: explorations of some tensions between Foucault and feminism. Routledge, London

Bree S 2002 Plenary session: keeping birth normal. Paper presented at the Diversity Within Unity NZCOM National Conference, Dunedin, New Zealand

Bryar R 1995 Theory for midwifery practice. Macmillan, London

Bunkle P 1992 Becoming knowers: feminism, science and medicine. In: Du Plessis R, Bunkle P, Irwin K, Laurie A, Middleton S (eds) Feminist voices: women's studies texts for Aotearoa/New Zealand. Oxford University Press, Auckland, New Zealand, p 59–73

Bunkle P 1994 Women's constructions of health. In: Spicer J, Trlin A, Walton JA (eds) Social dimensions of health and disease: New Zealand perspectives. Dunmore Press, Palmerston North, New Zealand, p 219–239

Burman E (ed) 1996 Psychology discourse practice: from regulation to resistance. Taylor and Francis, London

Butler J 1990 Gender trouble: feminism and the subversion of identity. Routledge, New York

Calvert S 2002 Being with women: the midwife–woman relationship. In: Mander R, Fleming V (eds) Failure to progress: the contraction of the midwifery profession. Routledge, London

Cartwright S 1988 The Report of the Committee of Inquiry into Allegations Concerning the Treatment of Cervical Cancer at National Women's Hospital and into Other Related Matters. Government Printing office, Auckland, New Zealand

Coney S (ed) 1993 Unfinished business: what happened to the Cartwright Report? Women's Health Action with the Federation of Women's Health Councils, Auckland, New Zealand

Cumming J, Salmond G 1998 Reforming New Zealand health care. In: Ranade W (ed) Markets and health care: a comparative analysis. Addison Wesley Longman, New York, p 122–146

Daellenbach R 1999 The paradox of success and the challenge of change: home birth associations of Aotearoa/New Zealand. Unpublished PhD thesis, University of Canterbury, Christchurch, New Zealand

Davies S 1996 Divided loyalties: the problem of normality. British Journal of Midwifery 4(6): 285–286

de Ras M, Grace V (eds) 1997 Bodily boundaries, sexualised genders, and medical discourses. Dunmore Press, Palmerston North, New Zealand

DeVries R, 1993 A cross-national view of the status of midwives. In: Wegar K (ed) Gender, work and medicine: women and the medical division of labour. Sage, London

DeVries R Salvesen HB, Wiegers TA, Williams AS 2001 What (and why) do women want? In: DeVries R, Benoit C, Teijlingen ERV, Wrede S (eds) Birth by design: pregnancy, maternity care, and midwifery in North America and Europe. Routledge, London, p 243–266

Donley J 1986 Save the midwife. New Women's Press, Auckland, New Zealand

Donley J 1998 Birthrites – natural vs. unnatural childbirth in New Zealand. Full Court Press, Auckland, New Zealand

Donley J 2000 The culture of home birth in New Zealand. Paper presented at the Seasons of Renewal Midwifery Conference, Cambridge, New Zealand

Downe S 2001 Is there a future for normal birth? Practising Midwife 4(6): 10–12

Fraser N, Nicholson L 1990 Social criticism without philosophy: an encounter between feminism and postmodernism. In: Nicholson L (ed) Feminism/postmodernism. Routledge, London

Gavey N 1989 Feminist poststructuralism and discourse analysis. Psychology of Women Quarterly 13: 459–475

Glamuzina J 1992 A lesbian-feminist approach to the histories of Aotearoa: a Pakeha perspective. In: Du Plessis R, Bunkle P, Irwin K, Laurie A, Middleton S (eds) Feminist voices: women's studies texts for Aotearoa/New Zealand. Oxford University Press, Auckland, New Zealand

Grace V 1991 The marketing of empowerment and the construction of the health consumer: a critique of health promotion. International Journal of Health Services 21(2): 329–343

Guilliland K 1999 Managing change in midwifery practice: the New Zealand experience. Birth International

www.acegraphics.com.au/resource/papers/guilliland01.html4/10/2001]

Guilliland K, 2000 Midwifery autonomy in New Zealand: how has it influenced the birth outcomes of New Zealand women? Paper presented at the NZCOM Seasons of Renewal Conference, Cambridge, New Zealand

Guilliland K 2002 CEO's forum: submission on maternity services notice – December 2001. Midwifery News 24: 7–11

Guilliland K, Campbell N 2002 College viewpoint. Midwifery News 24: 5

Guilliland K, Pairman S 1995 The midwifery partnership – a model for practice. Department of Nursing and Midwifery, Victoria University, Wellington, New Zealand

Gunew S, Yeatman A (eds) 1993 Feminism and the politics of difference. Allen and Unwin, St Leonards, NSW, Australia

Hartley J 1997 Normal pregnancy and labour: is it limiting midwifery practice? British Journal of Midwifery 5(12): 773–776

Hunt S, Symonds A 1996 The midwife in society: perspectives, policies and practice. Macmillan, London

Jaworski A, Coupland N (eds) 1999 The discourse reader. Routledge, London

Kent J 2000 Social perspectives on pregnancy and childbirth for midwives, nurses and the caring professions. Open University Press, Buckingham

Larner W 1997 'A means to an end': neoliberalism and state processes in New Zealand. Studies in Political Economy 52(Spring): 7–38

Lazarus E 1997 What do women want? Issues of choice, control, and class in American pregnancy and childbirth. In: Davis-Floyd RE, Sargent CF (eds) Childbirth and authoritative knowledge: cross-cultural perspectives. University of California Press, Berkeley, CA, p 132–158

Leap N 1997 Birthwrite: being with women in pain – do midwives need to rethink their role? British Journal of Midwifery 3(5): 263

Lupton D 1997 Foucault and the medicalisation critique. In: Peterson A, Bunton R (eds) Foucault, health and medicine. Routledge, London

MacDonald M 1999 Expectations: the cultural construction of nature in midwifery discourse in Ontario. Unpublished PhD dissertation, Department of Anthropology, York University

MacDonald M, Bourgeault IL 2000 The politics of representation: doing and writing 'interested' research on midwifery. Resources for Feminist Research 28(1/2): 151–168

McAra-Couper J 2002 What is shaping midwifery and obstetric practice in relation to intervention in childbirth? Paper presented at the Diversity Within Unity NZCOM National Conference, Dunedin, New Zealand

McLaughlan M 1997 Women's place: an exploration of current discourses of childbirth. Unpublished MA thesis, Victoria University, Wellington, New Zealand

McNay L 1994 Foucault: a critical introduction. Polity Press, Cambridge

Mein Smith P 1986 Maternity in dispute, V.R. Ward. Government Printer, New Zealand

Miller L J 2000 The poverty of truth-seeking: postmodernism, discourse analysis and critical feminism. Theory and Psychology 10(3): 313–352

Pairman S 2002 Towards self-determination: the separation of the midwifery and nursing professions in

New Zealand. In: Papps E (ed) Nursing in New Zealand: critical issues, different perspectives. Pearson Education New Zealand, Auckland, New Zealand, p 14–27

Papps E, Olssen M 1997 Doctoring childbirth and regulating midwifery in New Zealand: a Foucauldian perspective. Dunmore Press, Palmerston North, New Zealand

Pollock D 1999 Telling bodies, performing birth. Columbia University Press, New York

Ramsden I 1995 Cultural safety: implementing the concept. Paper presented at the Social Force of Nursing Conference, Wellington, New Zealand

Roberts CL, Tracy S, Peat B 2000 Rates for obstetric intervention among private and public patients in Australia: a population based descriptive study. bmj.com/cgi/content/abstract/321/7254/137

Rooks JP 2000 Topic: epidurals during labour and birth. MidwifeInfo.com. www.midwifeinfo.com/topic-epidurals.php

Rothman BK 1989 Recreating motherhood: ideology and technology in a patriarchal society. WW Norton, New York

Rothman BK 1991 In labour: women and power in the birthplace. Norton Books, New York

Sandall J 1995 Choice, continuity and control: changing midwifery, towards a sociological perspective. Midwifery 11: 201–209

Savage W 2002 The caesarean section epidemic. Paper presented at the Diversity Within Unity NZCOM National Conference, Dunedin, New Zealand

Save the Midwives Direct Entry Taskforce 1990 Direct entry to midwifery. Save the Midwives Newsletter 23 May: 12–20

Sawicki J 1991 Disciplining Foucault: feminism, power and the body. Routledge, London

Smythe L 1998 'Being safe' in childbirth: a hermeneutic interpretation of the narratives of women and practitioners. Unpublished PhD thesis, Massey, New Zealand

Strid J 2000 Revitalising partnership. Paper presented at the Seasons of Renewal NZCOM Conference, Cambridge, New Zealand

Tew M 1995 Safer childbirth? A critical history of maternity care. Chapman and Hall, London

Tuhiwai Smith L 1999 Decolonizing methodologies: research and indigenous peoples. Zed Books, London

Tully L 1999 Doing professionalism 'differently': negotiating midwifery autonomy in Aotearoa/New Zealand. Unpublished PhD thesis, University of Canterbury, Christchurch, New Zealand

Tully L Mortlock B 1999 Professionals and practices. In: Davis P, Dew K (eds), Health and society in Aotearoa/New Zealand. Oxford University Press, Auckland, New Zealand, p 165–180

Tully L, Daellenbach R, Guilliland K 1998 Feminism, partnership, and midwifery. In: Du Plessis R, Alice L (eds) Feminist thought in Aotearoa/New Zealand. Oxford University Press, Auckland, New Zealand, p 245–253

Ussher JM (ed) 1997 Body talk: the material and discursive regulation of sexuality, madness and reproduction. Routledge, London

Wagner M 1994 Pursuing the birth machine: the search for appropriate birth technology. ACE Graphics, Sydney, Australia

Wajcman J 1991 Feminism confronts technology. Polity Press, Cambridge

Weston R 2001 What is normal childbirth? The midwife practitioner's view. Practising Midwife 4(6): 13

Wetherell M, Taylor S, Yates SJ (eds) 2001 Discourse theory and practice: a reader. Sage, London

Young D 1996 The midwifery revolution in New Zealand: what can we learn? Birth 23(3): 125–127

Zalewski M 2000 Feminism after postmodernism: theorising through practice. Routledge, London

13

Journey to midwifery through feminism: a personal account

Nicky Leap

INTRODUCTION

Each version of a story has its own truth. And our myths, whether of the universal, numinous kind or of the more prosaic, family variety, are used by us to tell and retell truths in ways that mean we can make sense of our world. (O'Neill 1990, p 145)

When asked to contribute a chapter to this book, I balked. I realised that I could not write about feminism and midwifery as theory in the abstract. For over 20 years there has been an embodied entwining of these concepts that is played out in my life and in every aspect of my engagement in midwifery practice, education and research. To write about this would require examples and a personalised account. It would necessitate 'real-life' explanations of my motivation and the ways in which I believe feminist principles are woven through midwifery practice and philosophy. Would people think such reflection was self-indulgent? Would anyone be interested in the subjective point of view and experience of one midwife?

One tentative email later, I was encouraged by editor Mary Stewart to write about feminism and midwifery by drawing on my own experiences in the feminist tradition of seeing the personal as political and placing individual experience in the context of a gendered world. I accept that to do so limits any portrayal of the complexity of midwifery practice and the multiple lived experiences of midwives. However, I hope that aspects of my story and perceptions will resonate for others in the ongoing process of making changes in midwifery practice that put women at the centre of care; changes that enable women to take the power that potentially transforms lives.

I came to midwifery via the women's liberation movement of the 1970s. Midwifery was for me the ultimate political arena in which to work 'with women' and strive to 'make a difference' to women's lives. In the Association of Radical Midwives (ARM), the support group that nurtured me throughout my perilous training and thereafter, I found many other midwives who were similarly motivated by feminist politics and a fierce sense of altruism. Many of today's midwifery leaders emerged from the ARM of the 1980s – Belinda Ackerman, Tricia Anderson, Mary Cronk, Soo Downe, Caroline Flint, Jane Grant, Deborah Hughes, Billy Hunter, Kate Jackson, Ishbel Kargar, Mavis Kirkham, Judy Rogers, Jilly Rosser, Meg Taylor and Holliday Tyson, to name a few.

Many of us did not come to midwifery through nursing. We struggled our way through the dwindling 'direct entry' courses of the 1970s and 1980s, gritting our teeth and tempering our fury at the atrocities we saw perpetuated on women and their bodies. We had to work within hospital systems with rigid and often brutal hierarchical structures, 'designed for the army and adapted for nurses' (Flint 1988, p 25). As women with political consciousness and a commitment to social justice, we came together to interpret and explore the gendered nature of the oppression around us. Long before any of us had heard of 'Foucault' or 'postmodernism', we defined our experiences and the society around us in terms of the dynamics of power relationships within the 'the patriarchy', which was personified within maternity services. The oppression of women in society was mirrored by the oppression of women in their experience of maternity care, which in turn was mirrored by the way midwives, as a predominantly female profession, experienced their working lives.

The rhetoric of our midwifery training offered us the opportunity to be a 'practitioner in your own right', capable of 'hanging up your shingle on Day 1 of qualification'. For us, this meant that if we could survive the wretched lot of the student midwife, we could qualify and provide a service that would aim to enable women to feel powerful through their experience of childbirth. Implicit was the understanding that we would talk, write and campaign about the 'why' and 'how' of every aspect of creating changes for child-bearing women. We referred to this process as 'the Cause'* since this was the colloquial term we employed (with tongue-in-cheek irony) to describe the embodied concept of feminist midwifery activism that became the focus of our lives. The Cause motivated us to write and speak out at every opportunity in the interest of creating changes that would benefit child-bearing women. In this chapter, I shall outline some of the rhetorical means of persuasion* that were employed by myself and others and will identify where this might fit in an understanding of feminist midwifery practice.

MY JOURNEY TO MIDWIFERY
Social politics and gender

… Women's liberation has given expression to a new consciousness among women and it came out of a social reality which is peculiar to the kind of life possible in advanced capitalism. (Rowbotham 1973**, p ix)

My understanding of how feminism influenced me as a midwife is steeped in my subjectivity as a white, middle-class woman involved in the politics of the women's liberation movement in the 1970s and 1980s in London. It therefore does not allow for an exploration of the revolutions that were taking place in the 20th century in terms of the diverse politics of economic and cultural oppression, in particular black politics and what was then described as 'Third World struggles'. I am also aware that the ideological revolution that enabled the promotion of 'feelings' and the 'politics of experience' has its limitations in a society that has continued to see emotionality as a female characteristic and resisted socio-economic change that would address gender inequalities. Bearing such limitations in mind, I shall attempt to paint a backdrop of the social politics that influenced me and that eventually would affect the way I practise as a midwife.

---

*Cause: what produces an effect: person or thing that occasions something; reason or motive; justification; side in a struggle, principle etc. to further which people strive; united efforts for a purpose (Australian Pocket Oxford Dictionary, 1985).
**A concept borrowed from Aristotle who spoke of 'the faculty of observing in any given case the available means of persuasion' (Bizzell & Herzberg 1990).

I was born in 1948. My mother was of a generation of British women who were encouraged back into the home to enable the jobs that they had undertaken for the war effort to be made available to men. Overt and covert ideology underpinned this move, with an emphasis on women's fulfilment and duties in the role of wife, homemaker and mother. My mother suffered the increasing isolation of women in nuclear families and the dissatisfaction and yearning that Betty Friedan (1963) first described in her groundbreaking text as 'the problem that has no name'.

I was the eldest of five children, born in the South London Hospital for Women and Children. As an adult, I was part of the occupancy of this hospital by women campaigning (unsuccessfully) to prevent the last major women's hospital in London from closure. My mother visited during the occupation and showed me the corridor where she had laboured alone with a classic stop/start posterior labour – beds were at a premium following the war – and then the room where she gave birth to me. She noted that the light fitting that had been the focus of her lonely experience had not changed. My brother was born at home a couple of years later, followed 15 months later by a sister, also born at home. I have vivid memories of being taken to see 'the new baby' in my mother's bedroom and of rolling cotton wool into balls and baking these in cake tins in preparation for the births. I received clear, positive messages about babies being born at home for which I am grateful. After an 8-year gap, my mother gave birth at home to (undiagnosed) twin girls. She tells me that each time she gave birth to a daughter, she apologised to my domineering father that the baby was not a boy.

In the early 1990s I was interviewed by Caroline Kelly and Sara Breinlinger for their study on 'Women's participation in a range of activities aiming to bring about social change in the context of gender relations'*. This study identified the

importance of personal experiences of inequality in motivating women to engage in collective action. Like some other women in this study, I identified gender relations in my family as a major source of a sense of injustice.

I know that even when I was a little girl, I went around saying, 'It's not fair'. I was forever seeing things that weren't fair. I was the eldest and I had a brother, and my mother absolutely adored my brother. And because he was a boy he used to get lots of privileges – he was allowed endless slices of the white bread we were brought up on – with butter – but I was only allowed two slices with butter and then I had to have margarine, which was pretty diabolical in those days! Little things like that – he didn't have to do the washing up and I did. I grew up really grumbly because of this brother, who got all these privileges that I didn't get and I think I got an anger about things that aren't 'fair' and that is quite a motivation I think for me. If I see an injustice, I want to do something about it. Who knows if it's about having that brother and the slices of bread and margarine. (Kelly & Breinlinger 1996, p 87)

In the late 1960s, it was my turn to grapple with the inequalities that came with motherhood and female roles in a patriarchal society. However, it was not until I read Germaine Greer's *The Female Eunuch* (1970) that I discovered a way of seeing my world that made sense of my experience, my feelings and an embryonic, but pressing, awareness of social justice issues. As for many women, this book politicised me and gave me the courage to make profound choices as to how I would interact with the world. The women's liberation movement and the 'consciousness-raising groups' of the 1970s provided some of us with the opportunity to meet regularly, to support each other and to explore the gendered experiences of how our individual lives had been governed by sexism and patriarchal societies. The personal became political and for many of us this included collective action in the form of active campaigning, in particular for women's refuges, contraception, abortion on demand and the right to define our sexuality.

Childbirth activism

… the exercise of personal agency is a political struggle for each woman against a dominant institutional voice which argues that her compliance with its norms must frame the outer limit of her actions during pregnancy

---

*Published as: Kelly C, Breinlinger S 1996 *The social psychology of collective action*. Taylor and Francis, London. The authors identify six distinct themes that emerged as reasons why women became involved in women's groups: personal background and personal characteristics, social beliefs, life events, services offered by the group and an element of chance.

... continuing efforts by activists and midwives, feminists and non-feminists alike, to resist and contest that image of incapacity over the last four decades have not dislodged obstetric medicine from its position as the principal authority on the birth process. (Murphy-Lawless 1998, p 4)

A series of publications were significant for those of us who became involved in the women's health movement and childbirth activism. *Our Bodies, Ourselves* by the Boston Women's Health Collective in 1971 was a landmark in terms of women coming together to share information and demystify all processes to do with our health, including childbirth. Alongside the women's health movement, a small but significant alternative birth movement was gaining momentum in the USA where midwifery had faded almost into oblivion. Birth had become a highly medicalised event with women in hospitals being rendered passive to the point of being handcuffed to beds (Arms 1975). Birth at home with lay midwives was seen as a way of reclaiming birth for women, a social and spiritual event with profound potential for learning and empowerment. Publications from this movement had a significant effect on midwives throughout the Western world, notably Ina May Gaskin's (1980) *Spiritual Midwifery*, Raven Lang's (1972) *Birth Book* and Suzanne Arms' (1975) *Immaculate Deception.*

The 1970s also saw the increase of support groups and organisations associated with campaigns to change maternity services. Organisations such as the National Childbirth Trust (NCT) and the Association for Improvements in Maternity Services (AIMS) in the United Kingdom (UK) and the National Association of Parents and Professionals for Safe Alternatives in Childbirth (NAPPSAC) in the USA gathered momentum. Campaigners for reform in childbirth, such as Doris Haire in the USA and Sheila Kitzinger in the UK, emerged from these organisations. Their early publications – *The Cultural Warping of Childbirth* (Haire 1972) and *The Experience of Childbirth* (Kitzinger 1962) – heralded a stream of activity and writing from childbirth activists that influences governments as well as individual women to this day.

Midwives were also beginning to organise themselves into groups and campaign for improvements in maternity services. In the USA, the Midwives Alliance of North America began to publish journals and bring together midwives, mainly those who were attending births at home and teaching each other through apprenticeships. In the UK in the late 1970s, a small group of student midwives were so appalled by what they saw happening to women in childbirth in hospital that they placed an advertisement in a national newspaper calling for others to contact them if they felt equally outraged. Thus, the Association of Radical Midwives (ARM) was born, an organisation that would eventually enable the notion of 'woman-centred care' to become enshrined in government documents.

I shall explain later how being a member of the ARM enabled me to explore the connections between feminism and midwifery. First, though, I shall return to explaining the personal events that led to me becoming a midwife.

BECOMING A MIDWIFE
The motivation of giving birth

She dries you, bundles you up and removes you to the other side of the room. My arms ache to hold you but she is busy: busy with you, bathing you, measuring you, weighing you. I watch from the other side of the room, desperate to hold you, my body and mind suffused with relief bordering on ecstasy. What could be more wonderful than this? I have survived something huge. I am triumphant! I am capable of doing anything ...

Eventually she brings you to me, all wrapped up, exquisite little doll face peeping out, blinking at me. I am overwhelmed with tenderness, with joy. I think you are the most beautiful thing I have ever laid eyes on. Immediately I am so in love with you. A ferocious all-consuming mother love that will always be there. And in this moment I know that such unconditional love will render me forever vulnerable to losing you. My life will never be the same. I feel so clever for having grown you, for having been through that extraordinary pain and survived, both of us, survivors of something indescribable. (from: 'For Lucy, born 7th October 1968, Musgrove Park Hospital, Taunton, Somerset, England')

I knew I wanted to be a midwife when I gave birth to my first child in 1968. At this time I did not know that I was a feminist although I might have had an inkling; news of the women's liberation movement gaining momentum in major cities throughout the world had barely reached my home in rural England. The above account of the moments following the birth of my first child reflects powerful feelings that I was to experience with equal intensity in two subsequent births. I had read no literature to prepare me for the fact that giving birth could leave me feeling so powerful that I would feel I could achieve anything in life. I had been very scared of labour during pregnancy and did not see myself as brave or particularly accomplished at physical activity such as sport. After giving birth, the feeling of having been pushed to the limits of my endurance to a place where I had to deal with an overwhelming sense of uncertainty, aloneness and selfhood transformed my view of myself. To have grown a little person in my body; to have dealt with such overwhelming pain in labour; to have given birth and then produced the perfect food with which to continue to nurture this vulnerable, exquisite baby – all of this seemed so intensely *clever*. This was my first insight into the potential of birth as empowerment that can act as an insurance policy for the challenges of new motherhood.

In later years, time and again I saw and heard of women experiencing this sense of discovery of their strength through giving birth. Informally, midwives have described themselves as 'birth junkies' when discussing the exhilaration of being alongside women at such a powerful time. The sensation of returning home from a birth, often physically and mentally exhausted but totally 'high', is one that many midwives can relate to, particularly where birth has taken place in the intimacy of a woman's own home. This potential for women to be transformed by their experience of giving birth can be conceptualised as the 'notion of triumph' that is linked to the pain and uncertainty of labour (Leap 1996, 2000a).

Enabling safe situations where women can experience the full potential of birth as transformation and empowerment is a central tenet of midwifery practice. This notion is directly related to feminism and activism since there are often complex obstacles that get in the way of enabling situations where women feel powerful around birth. Systems involving power and control and the essentially gendered struggles that surround childbirth often lead to situations where women are rendered powerless and traumatised. An understanding of the difference between 'giving birth' and 'being delivered by others' and the potential long-term consequences motivates many of us who become childbirth activists. I shall return to exploring these issues in more detail but in the interest of chronological order, I shall return to my own story of becoming a midwife.

Inspiration

I don't know whether you go into midwifery because you're a bit of a square peg in a round hole or whether you get like it. Maybe it's a bit of both, but midwifery has always attracted individualists … because it offers independence. (Mollie T, retired midwifery tutor, in Leap & Hunter 1993, p 190)

My role models for midwifery were not the bustling women in nurses' uniforms in the hospital where I was persuaded, against my better judgement, to go to give birth to my first child. These women with their strict regimes did little to gain my attention other than through intimidation. Midwifery care was metered to a strict timetable that involved a lot of 'allowing' during the 7 days enforced stay for 'first time' mothers. This was my first understanding of the implications of the word 'confinement'. In between performing regular perineal washes on the bedpan, the midwives 'allowed' us 'patients' various activities in sequence as we struggled through that first week of new motherhood – getting out of bed, making the bed, the demonstration baby bath culminating in the nerve-wracking 'test' bath where these 'guardians of the newborn' towered over us to correct our fumbled attempts to get things right. Those of us who were breastfeeding had to line up at the sink at 4-hourly intervals to scrub our nipples and breasts in 'preparation' for breastfeeding our babies when they were marched to the bedside from the nursery, where they had spent most of the time in lines of cribs being cared for by nursery nurses. The system was so obviously *wrong*. This early indignation was the first of many that would motivate me to find ways of joining with others to change maternity care systems.

By contrast, the local community midwives were inspirational. Sister Jones and Sister Sykes shared a home and engaged in a triple role as the village midwives, community nurses and health visitors. I thought that they probably knew everything about every family in the area but never did they betray confidences. They were kind, discreet and non-judgemental. They exuded wisdom during my contact with them for antenatal care, during their daily postnatal visits to my home and later during the baby clinic visits. Less than 2 years later, they attended me for the birth of my second baby at home and during the postnatal visits I quizzed them about how to become a midwife.

A traumatic custody battle and a chance meeting were to change my life further. Gwen Rankin, a founder member of the National Childbirth Trust (NCT), found me weeping and walking my goats in a Somerset lane. 'My dear, what on earth is the matter?' She invited me to her home for a cup of tea and in spite of our differences over 'women's liberation politics', she became my mentor. Since the 1960s, the NCT has trained teachers to prepare women and their partners for childbirth and becoming parents. I sat in on the antenatal classes Gwen ran in her home and knew that this was important work that made a difference to people's lives. As an NCT teacher in the following years in both Somerset and then in London, I often sat alongside women in labour who had no-one else for support. Increasingly I knew that I had to find a way to become a midwife. Meanwhile, with others, I set up and worked voluntarily in Women's Aid refuges, in girls' groups and young mothers' groups and hostels. I became a trainer in sex education with the Family Planning Association and talked to schools, women's groups, youth clubs and voluntary organisations about a range of subjects from relationships and sexuality to domestic violence and women's liberation. I continued to be actively involved in feminist campaign groups.

It was at this stage in my life that I started exploring the concept of facilitating antenatal groups instead of teaching antenatal classes. This developed into a model that became the lynch pin of the midwifery group practices that I would be part of once I became a midwife. The basic idea is that women can come to an antenatal group at any

stage of their pregnancy. Each week, women come back to the group with their new baby and tell the other women about their experiences of giving birth and being a new mother. The friendships that develop are continued in postnatal groups and through informal networks and play a significant role in reducing the isolation of new motherhood.

The strategy of putting women in touch with other women so that they can learn from each other and develop support structures is an important midwifery skill. It is based in fundamental feminist principles, in particular the notion of minimising dependency on health professionals. Women who made a video about their experiences of attending an antenatal group in South East London (Leap 1991) described this shifting of power dynamics.

I think it's the only place I go where people don't try to *tell* you how you're supposed to feel… It sort of makes me feel like I'm the one that's got the power and I used to think that everyone else had the power over me. … It wasn't about 'experts/novices, women/us'… we were all seen as having a valuable contribution to make; we were seen as having our own expertise.

The 'training'

…It is ARM's vision that midwifery education, through its content and processes, will be individually and collectively liberating in terms of gender, class, race, sexuality and creed … Visionary midwifery is enabled by non-hierarchical relationships and this needs to be reflected in the way we educate future midwives. (ARM 1999)

In 1979 after the birth of my son, I finally had the opportunity to enroll in a 'direct entry' midwifery programme. My partner and I engaged in a role swap – he gave up his job to be at home with the baby – a decision that was to challenge both of us almost beyond endurance. It took me 2 hours on public transport to cross London, 1½ hours on the motorbike. In between 'early' and 'late' shifts I breastfed the baby. I nearly gave up my training on almost a daily basis as the ideals that had inspired me to become a midwife floundered in a hierarchical system that I would later describe in terms of 'horizontal violence' (Leap 1997).

Unlike current programmes, my own 'training' left a lot to be desired and I hesitate to call it 'midwifery education' except in the context of the mentors who inspired me along the way. There were six of us and we were a motley crew from various countries and with very different backgrounds. All we had in common was that we wanted to be midwives.

We were told at the beginning of the course that this was the last direct entry course and that if we wanted to 'go anywhere in midwifery' we would have to undertake nursing training immediately after our midwifery course. This was my first introduction to the politics of direct entry midwifery education. Later, campaigns that I would be involved in led to a situation where the majority of midwives in the UK are now educated through 3-year direct entry programmes. At this stage, though, the climate was such that some of the midwives I encountered in the hospital who had trained through this route hid the fact that they were not nurses.

At the beginning of our midwifery course, we were 'sent across to the general side' for the first 6 months and did not see a midwifery teacher during that time. We joined in with the new student nurses in an intensive course in bed making, laying patients' food trays, bedpan, bathing and sluice skills, 'taking the basic obs' and anatomy, physiology and pathology in that seeming order of importance. We were then hurtled into placements working full-time 'shifts' on a women's medical ward, followed – with some relief – by the gynaecology and paediatric wards. The staff and patients 'on the general side' tolerated us midwifery students with various degrees of lack of interest and amusement. There were lots of jokes, particularly when we were assigned to elderly patients – 'Mr Smith, you've got the midwife looking after you today'. It was a sobering induction into hospital culture but I was an avid learner and picked up a lot of useful practical skills – in particular, basic assessment, aseptic techniques, surgical and recovery nursing skills – as well as an understanding of how to survive the hierarchies of a regimented system in a struggling National Health Service that even then was severely resource depleted.

Having 'done time on the general', we were relieved to go back to the maternity unit where we rotated round the wards, working 'shifts'

with one day a week in school. We were called by our surnames – no first names – unless we were married, in which case 'Mrs' was added as a prefix. First names were forbidden in all situations for staff and for the women. I learnt that uniforms were the outward manifestations of status, starting with the number and colour of bands on those dreadful, slippery cardboard waitress hats. We had to cope with qualified midwives' dismay that the 'direct entrants' no longer wore yellow epaulets or yellow belts to denote their 'inferior' position. Worse, we certainly had done nothing to earn our white uniforms, which were the pride and status symbol of those who had graduated from the NHS blue check of the student nurse. How were they to tell how ignorant we were?

At the bottom of the pecking order, on a rung just below the student nurses who rotated into the maternity unit, we often clung to each other in tears in the sluice room and developed strong solidarity. I soon learnt that it was unwise to let on that I had been a childbirth educator for some years and 'worse' still, given birth to three children, two of them at home. The safest thing to do was to bite my lip, knuckle under and get through. We all exerted untold energy trying to be accepted and liked because the alternative was too debilitating. This was the era representing the height of intervention, with 70% of women having their labours induced, where shaves and enemas, routine episiotomies and birth in lithotomy were the order of the day. Most days I cried on the journey home across London – tears of indignation and powerless fury at how women were being treated, at how I was being treated.

The mentors

... to have someone more experienced and who cares about the midwifery profession and mothers, who can advise, encourage, teach and reminisce, who can be a role model, and who can be the older and wiser friend ... (Flint 1986, p 192)

In class we sat in rows and were drilled in Maggie Myles rote learning. There was little room for discussion. The saving grace was Molly Turner, the delightfully eccentric retired midwifery 'tutor' who was brought in to work with us in the classroom and who changed for ever my experience of public transport.

Student Midwives – on your way to work on the Tube [London Underground] observe the head shape of all the bald men in the carriage. Today I observed a breech, a persistent occipitoposterior, a caesarean section and a variety of deflexed occipitoanteriors!

She told us riveting stories about being 'on the district' during the war – stories about sweet coffee enemas and acacia gum intravenous infusions for postpartum haemorrhages in air raid shelters. Stories about student midwives cycling home from births to find the placenta was no longer in the basket on the back of the bike: 'Student Midwives – you have a statutory duty to ensure that the placenta does not become a public nuisance'. She continuously reinforced the message that we were to be 'practitioners in our own right', that midwifery was a separate profession from nursing and that we were to learn to be responsible for the total care of 'mother and baby', referring to 'doctor' only where there was a problem.

The other saving grace in my fraught midwifery 'training' was the system of having 3-month placements with a community midwife interspersed throughout the course. Olive Jones, 'my' community midwife, was an inspirational mentor who, years later, was to set up the famous free-standing Edgware Birth Centre. She reinforced my belief in the safety of home birth for the majority of women, she taught me how to do kind 'Guthrie' tests with the baby breastfeeding, and role modelled how to listen to women and give them the message that you trust them to be the baby's expert, drawing on their instincts and common sense. We had great conversations in the car as we travelled from one postnatal visit to the next and if she tired of all my questions, she never showed it.

Other midwives who inspired me were some of the night duty staff, who were able to practise unhampered by the constant presence of doctors. In particular, I remember an African midwife who showed me that a baby could emerge without the midwife's hands fiddling around and pressing on the baby's head with the pronged fork action that we had been taught was essential 'to keep the baby's head flexed'. Towards the end of my 'training' I noticed a very quiet midwife,

newly back from living and working in a developing country, who gently encouraged women and seemed to do little else. For the first time I saw women giving birth kneeling and on all fours and it made sense. This midwife was Jane Sandall who later became a friend and continued to be a mentor for me, as she became a well-known researcher of midwifery models of care.

It was not only midwives who inspired me. Perhaps the biggest eye-opener of the whole course was my day out with the district nurse. We went from home to home, dressing leg ulcers, moving stranded elderly and disabled people on and off the commode and providing a lifeline for carers and those who faced isolation in the community. I was humbled and forced to consider where midwifery politics sits in the wider picture of public health service provision.

THE ASSOCIATION OF RADICAL MIDWIVES: SUPPORT AND VISION

Emergence is the surprising capacity we discover only when we join together. (Wheatley & Kellnor-Rogers 1996, p 67)

I would not have finished my midwifery training if it had not been for the Association of Radical Midwives (ARM). The ARM was formed in 1976 by a small group of student midwives from different training schools who were alarmed by the apparent trend towards maternity nurse status and the way women were treated in the maternity system. Many of the early members of ARM were drawn to midwifery through feminist politics and had been shattered to find a system that we saw as brutalising and disempowering for child-bearing women and midwives alike. We mirrored the feminist processes of consciousness-raising groups and political action in carrying out the objectives of the organisation:

1. To re-establish the confidence of the midwife in her own skills.
2. To share ideals, skills and information.
3. To encourage midwives in their support of women's active participation in birth.
4. To reaffirm the need for midwives to provide continuity of care.

5. To explore alternative patterns of care.
6. To encourage evaluation of development of our field.

The ARM became a lifeline for me during my training and continued to be a major source of support until I moved to Australia in 1997. Once a month I knew that I would come together with midwives – representing every level of the hierarchy of maternity services – who shared the same politics about changing the culture of childbirth and supporting each other. Managers, teachers, students, new midwives and midwives who had been around for a long time shared a common aim to enable women to be powerful in their experiences of pregnancy, giving birth and during the time of new motherhood. Several times a year we would also come together from across the UK to national meetings. ARM members continue to meet in this way to share ideas, stories and skills and to strategise around how to make changes happen. The dual role of support and collective action offered by ARM provides a powerful vehicle for engendering solidarity and for working together on changes to the ways in which we practise and the conditions for birthing women.

In the last two decades, the influence of the ARM on the development of maternity service policy throughout the Western world has been substantial. In 1985, a group of ARM members spent a weekend together in order to formulate a 'vision' for the maternity services of the future. The ensuing document, *The Vision: Proposals for the Future of the Maternity Services* (ARM 1986), proposed a system that would now be recognised as caseload practice within midwifery group practices, based in the community, where midwifery care follows the woman (Leap 1996). We were aware that articulating a vision is a political strategy to promote change in policy, particularly where individual and collective efforts work at strengthening beliefs that it can be achieved (Plant 1987, p 58). As members of the ARM, we ensured that the small booklet was widely disseminated and 'talked it up' at every opportunity. *The Vision* became a blueprint for the development of midwifery services and its ideology and practical recommendations continue to be incorporated into policy documents in

---

> **Box 13.1**   Principles outlined in *The Vision* (ARM 1986)
>
> - That the relationship between mother and midwife is fundamental to good midwifery care
> - That the mother is the central person in the process of care
> - Informed choice in childbirth for women
> - Full utilisation of midwives' skills
> - Continuity of care for all child-bearing women
> - Community-based care
> - Accountability of services to those receiving them
> - Care should do no harm to mother and baby

---

the UK. *The Vision* identified clearly for the first time the inherently feminist principles that should underpin policy in maternity service provision (Box 13.1). Each of these principles was referenced to literature explaining the concept – an early example of identifying evidence-based practice as a rhetorical means of persuasion.

Midwives in other Western countries also used *The Vision* as the basis of their recommendations for change in maternity service provision. Documents produced in the late 1980s by midwifery professional bodies negotiating public funding for midwifery services in New Zealand and Canada reflect the framework suggested by *The Vision*. Although there was little international collaboration at this point, the models proposed in each country were strikingly alike. They evolved through a similar process of negotiation by feminist midwifery activists with a common vision to implement woman-centred continuity of midwifery care within state-funded health services. Comparisons of our experiences of these processes reveal that we shared similar informal strategies for negotiation and creating change in policy. These strategies are similar to those used by feminist activists in other organisations and are identified in Box 13.2.

CONTEMPLATING THE LANGUAGE OF MIDWIFERY AND POWER

This baby must be a boy, he's giving you so much trouble … Now then dear, we're just going to put a little tube in here … Let's put Baby in here and Dad can keep an eye on him while Mum hops up onto the bed after having popped into the loo to do a little wee. (Leap 1992, p 60)

Box 13.2   Strategies for negotiation and creating change in maternity service provision

- Strong alliances with women in campaigning and influencing people
- Understanding the politics and strategies of the new market economy in health services
- 'Seizing the moment' in terms of strategies that capitalise on the neoliberalist policy of promoting individual choice, control and continuity
- Promoting midwifery as a public health initiative
- Identifying friends, enemies and those who might be convinced
- Developing meeting and negotiation skills
- Developing skills in proposal writing and polished presentations
- Highlighting cost-effectiveness issues and the evidence for change
- Ensuring good publicity and a high media profile
- 'Talking it up' at conferences, workshops and in teaching sessions
- Publishing in midwifery, medical and health services journals
- Sharing our ideas and building support networks

It was in ARM gatherings that I first started to question language that potentially disempowers women. Long before any of us engaged in any formal study of 'discourse', in ARM meetings we would discuss how the words we use both reflect and construct who has the power in any given situation. We identified the dynamics of 'allowing' and 'managing' words, of sexist innuendo, 'jolly talk', 'baby talk' and phrases that belittle and trivialise women. We identified the flawed notion of 'informed choice' in terms of the power of the person who gives the information and encouraged each other to talk about 'women' and not 'girls' or 'ladies'. Always we encouraged each other to write articles about such issues as a deliberate strategy to disseminate ideas and change culture.

BEING A MIDWIFE

Woman-centred practice

Midwives need key skills in order to sustain relationships that help women to feel safe and able. One central example is midwives' belief in women, which enhances women's belief in themselves and is the key issue in trust, with all its positive benefits. (Kirkham 2000, p 243)

After I finished my training, I went to work for 6 months in the Day Care Abortion Unit (DCAU) at Mile End in East London, which was headed up by feminist obstetrician Wendy Savage. There was a curious tradition of newly qualified direct entry trained midwives going straight to the DCAU at Mile End to work for a while 'to heal the soul'. This was a place with a reputation for employing a feminist approach to women's health. Here we were able to work in a non-hierarchical, woman-friendly environment that was at the cutting edge of putting feminist principles into practice in terms of enabling women to make choices that would give them more control over their lives.

At this time, I also began working alongside independent midwives who guided me through my first year of practice providing continuity of care for women who chose to book with us to have their babies at home. Along with other midwives in the Western world, I began to articulate a philosophy of practice that places women at the centre of care. The notion of 'woman-centred' care is often challenged by those who say, 'What about fathers? What about the baby?'. In such circumstances I have found it helpful to explain this is a 'concept' that can be understood in terms of the recognised global notion of the ripple effect of enabling women to become more powerful – if women are empowered, they enable their families and communities to become more powerful. It is up to individual women (rather than health professionals) to identify and negotiate those relationships.

My definition of woman-centred care (Box 13.3) arises from feminist notions of midwifery practice. In putting this together recently for a regulatory board in Australia, the intention was to describe the notion of woman-centred midwifery care, as requested, for the purposes of setting standards. Such definitions are also deliberate strategies to shape and change midwifery practice in order to shift the locus of control to women.

Practising as an independent midwife and being alongside women giving birth at home taught me to quell my fear and believe in women's ability to give birth. I learnt to be acutely aware of my own power as a professional with expertise and to recognise the expertise of women. I learnt that the messages a woman receives from

---

> **Box 13.3** Woman-centred midwifery care – a definition
>
> • Focuses on the woman's individual needs, expectation and aspirations rather than the needs of the institution or professionals
> • Recognises the need for choice, control and continuity of care from a known caregiver or caregivers
> • Encompasses the needs of the baby, the woman's family and other people important to the woman as defined and negotiated by the woman herself
> • Follows the woman across the interface of community and acute settings
> • Addresses social, emotional, physical, psychological, spiritual and cultural needs and expectations
> • Recognises the woman's expertise in decision making

her midwife throughout pregnancy, labour and the early postnatal period must enable her to build and reinforce her own belief in her capabilities. In particular, when a woman is disadvantaged by psychosocial dynamics, she needs to hear that the midwife is confident that she (the woman) has the potential to monitor her baby's well-being and respond appropriately according to her instinct and common sense.

Midwifery as a public health strategy

Public health is a natural territory for midwives … Midwifery sees each woman holistically, taking into account her social, psychological and emotional needs as well as her physiological state. Midwifery understands that a woman's confidence and sense of control, her relationships with those who are important to her, and her home situation are as important as the clinical interventions provided to her in determining her overall well-being throughout pregnancy and early motherhood. (Kaufmann 2002, p 524–525)

Once I understood the concept of 'the personal is political' for myself, I was able to view women's lives in a wider social context than the parameters of their individual situations. This has motivated me to join with women and other midwives and to continue to work towards changing the 'big picture' of policy making in relation to maternity services. If we recognise the social context of all women, we cannot avoid our responsibility to work towards social change. As identified by Karen Guilliland and Sally Pairman (1995, p 8) in their feminist analysis of the midwifery partnership,

'It is because of this political and personal involvement with women that midwifery accepts its responsibilities as an emancipatory agent'. In New Zealand and Canada the enabling of publicly funded midwifery practices presents living proof of what can be achieved where midwives and women come together to campaign for change.

An understanding of the ideological framework underpinning policy and process has played an important role in my work as a midwifery activist. Such understandings continue to contribute to my experience as a midwife committed to making changes that improve women's experiences of childbirth. An exploration of the values and power dynamics that underlie policy decisions can contribute to strategic planning in developing woman-centred maternity services. This is particularly relevant with regards to opportunistic 'seizing the moment' and an understanding of social justice, community development and the primary healthcare principles listed below:

• equity and access
• services based on need
• community participation
• collaboration
• community-based care
• affordable care
• sustainability.

These principles underpin the rhetoric that is used in our efforts to persuade others to engage in systems change, in particular around the notion of midwifery as a public health strategy (Box 13.4).

As a feminist, while working as an independent midwife, I had difficulty with the ethics of working outside the NHS, providing a privileged service to women who could afford to pay. A small group of like-minded independent midwives in South East London felt the same way. We were drawn together by a common philosophy and the practical need to provide support and midwifery cover for each other. Increasingly we were offering our services to local women who could not afford to pay but asked us to book them. We rationalised this in terms of providing a 'Robin Hood' service – the wealthy subsidising the poor – but we began to work intensively towards contracting our services to the NHS. Underpinning our negotiations

---

Box 13.4   Midwifery as a public health strategy

- Midwives based in the community are ideally placed to provide locally responsive, woman-centred services.
- Where continuity of midwifery care 'follows the woman', midwives work across the interface of community and acute services.
- The opportunity to tackle health inequalities and social exclusion/isolation.
- Midwives can network and activate social support for women.
- Women with pressing needs may benefit from establishing a trusting relationship with midwives.
- The importance of 'dovetailing' and liaising with child health services and community-based organisations.

Box 13.5   Access policy: South East London Midwifery Group Practice 1994

- Women who have previously had low birthweight babies
- Women from Vietnam and other minority groups
- Women from specific housing estates
- Women with housing difficulties
- Women on income support
- Women who are unsupported
- Women with disabilities
- Women with mental health difficulties
- Women who are under 18 or over 38
- Women who are lesbians (and at risk of homophobia)
- Women with a previous childbirth or pregnancy bereavement
- Women who are referred by their GPs or health visitors as being in particular need
- Women who are HIV positive
- Women with a history of substance abuse

---

were principles associated with social justice and an awareness of how some women are more disadvantaged than others in society. In particular, we had a common vision that the type of care we were offering should be implemented throughout the NHS and therefore be free at the point of service. We developed skills in writing proposals that would 'sell' a quality, cost-effective service that was evidence based and aimed at long-term health gain. This involved a conscious effort to understand the management-dominated culture and marketplace economy of the new NHS.

In the early 1990s this group of midwives formalised its partnership and, as the South East London Midwifery Group Practice (SELMGP), we negotiated the first NHS contract between a local health authority and self-employed midwives. We strategically argued for funding that would address inequalities in health and promote long-term health gain. We proposed accessing community-based, continuity of midwifery carer to women who have poor health outcomes and who tend to be the most disadvantaged in society and in their experience of maternity care. Thus our contract was to work with women in the groups outlined in Box 13.5.

In 1997, I moved to Australia and started a new chapter in my life. Simultaneously, midwives in the SELMGP formed the Albany Midwifery Practice and moved from Deptford to Peckham, having negotiated a new NHS contract, this time with King's College Hospital. The success of this midwifery group practice in terms of a public

health strategy has been widely acclaimed (Sandall et al 2001, Warwick 2000) and continues to inspire me. The Albany midwives care for women in an area with particularly high socio-economic disadvantage. With a 43% home birth rate, the Albany practice has significantly different outcomes when compared to other midwifery group practices at King's.

- Lower induction rate
- Higher vaginal birth rate
- Lower elective caesarean section rate
- Higher intact perineum rate
- Lower episiotomy rate
- More use of the birthing pool
- Less use of pethidine and epidurals
- Higher breastfeeding rates at birth (Sandall et al 2001)

LIVING FEMINIST CONCEPTS: PROCESS AND REFLECTION

In a group committed to feminist process, differences ultimately strengthen the integrity of the group, because the group members value and acknowledge their differences openly and work towards reaching mutual understandings of these differences. (Eldridge Wheeler & Chinn 1991, p 20)

In my experience, there is a particular style of interaction that arises from involvement in the

> **Box 13.6** Feminist group processes in midwifery
>
> - Starting and finishing with a round
> - Striving for non-hierarchical structures
> - Encouraging story telling as a vehicle for reflection
> - Interpreting individual situations through a sociopolitical framework
> - Identifying a vision and strategies for change
> - Valuing female friendships
> - Consensus decision making

women's movement. Feminist group processes are incorporated into the way many of us interact in midwifery group practices. These processes are also played out in meetings, training programmes, workshops or when running antenatal groups (Box 13.6).

For many of us who were active in the early days of the ARM, our experience of being in women's groups – consciousness-raising groups, campaign groups and ARM meetings – means that we engage in feminist analysis and critique, not just of our practice and the systems and cultures within which we work, but also our relationships with each other and our personal lives. Story telling and reflection on the dynamics of power relationships became a process subconsciously incorporated into our lives and interactions. Such an approach engenders a sense of control and efficacy (Andrews (1991, p 32). Identity, belonging, solidarity, support and having a 'safe place' to say what you want are important aspects of group participation (Kelly & Breinlinger 1996). These factors encourage us to disclose our uncertainties and insecurities and to take risks with our explorations of self.

Some years ago I conducted a small (unpublished) observational study in a midwifery group practice of which I was a member. I noted every time that I saw midwives engaging in processes of formal and informal reflection. In our structured midwifery group practice meetings, we spent a lot of time reflecting on how to change our systems and practice to better meet the needs of women but it seemed that whenever we came together, we told each other stories and asked questions such as: 'I'm not sure about how I handled that … What would you have done? … Have you ever been in a situation like that? … Do you know if there's any

evidence about this? … How does the evidence fit with this woman's situation?'. Stories of everyday interactions were explored in situations where midwives were travelling together, making tea and coffee, washing up, in the toilet and particularly through laughing at ourselves and our foibles – we hardly stopped reflecting on our practice and our lives. This aspect of working in a midwifery group practice is akin to what is identified as 'solidarity' in feminist polemic. It therefore does not surprise me that research on avoiding 'burnout' in midwifery group practices (Sandall 1997, Stevens & McCourt 2002) consistently identifies the following factors for success:

- the ability for midwives to develop meaningful relationships with women
- occupational autonomy
- regular meetings with colleagues
- support at home and at work.

I would add that the single most important recipe for midwives working together in partnerships providing continuity of care is 'generosity of spirit'. Most midwives are women and therefore there is the potential for double disadvantage in any given situation at home and at work. Recognising the pressures colleagues may be exposed to, particularly around family commitments and crises, and going on call for each other at times of stress, knowing that this will be reciprocated at some stage in a 'swings and roundabouts' continuum, is the essence of solidarity in action.

With other midwives who have experience of providing continuity of care, I have identified some of the important factors in the way successful midwifery group practices operate that reflect feminist ways of working (Box 13.7).

FEMINISM AND THE RHETORIC OF EMPOWERMENT THROUGH MIDWIFERY

Midwifery begins with a critique of professional powers, and extends into a critique of media depictions of midwifery, patriarchal elements of law enforcement, and critiques of state allocation of health resources. At its core, midwifery is a celebration of diversity and new possibilities. It not only restores ancient elements of community and

Box 13.7 Midwifery group practices: feminist ways of working

- Each woman has a primary midwife as her first point of contact who provides a 'safety net' and ensures that the woman has access to all appropriate services
- Building and activating community support for women
- Facilitating antenatal groups where women can learn from each other's stories, support each other and build friendships, minimising women's dependency on midwives
- Midwives networking across community and acute services, putting women in touch with each other and organisations
- Addressing conditioning, 're-socialisation' through groups, word of mouth and a home visit at 36 weeks with the woman's supporters
- Midwives having their own premises in the community – being visible and accessible
- Non-hierarchical self-management and choosing who we work with encourages pulling together and autonomous practice
- All midwives are paid the same – equal pay for equal work
- Flexible negotiations about time off call and recognition of domestic pressures
- Midwives meeting together often to reflect – room to explore uncertainty
- Midwives learning from each other through working in different pairs

female familiarity, but argues for an honouring of these elements. (Burtch 1994, p 53)

In recent years in Australia, I have continued to come together with other midwives and women to engage in midwifery activism: campaigning, writing and speaking out in activities that aim for a 'vision' that is not dissimilar to that articulated in the ARM *Vision* of 1986. The rhetoric emerging from my teaching and research activities addresses the same gendered issues of inequality and power relationships.

Engaging with students, I frequently discuss their enthusiastic tendency to talk in terms of 'midwives empowering women'. Such a notion is contradictory to feminist thinking, I explain. Power cannot be given; it has to be taken. As midwives it is possible that we can enable situations where women are able to take up power through an approach that:

- minimises disturbance, direction, authority and intervention

- maximises the potential for physiology, common sense and instinctive behaviour to prevail
- places trust in the expertise of the woman
- engages with women around uncertainty (Leap 2000b).

Reflecting with other midwives continues to offer me the opportunity to explore how, as midwives, we can enable situations that shift the locus of power to women.

CONCLUSION

To be a midwife is to be 'with woman' (the meaning of the Anglo-Saxon word) – sharing their travail, their joys and their delights. To be a midwife is to engage in a close and intimate relationship, which often lasts only as long as the pregnancy, birth and puerperium, but the effect of which travels down through the centuries in the image women have of themselves and their abilities and worth … Midwives and women are intertwined, whatever affects women affects midwives and vice versa – we are interrelated and interwoven. (Flint 1986, p viii)

I was a student midwife in an era when feminism was easily identified as integral to midwifery practice by those of us who were active in the early days of the ARM. In the 1980s in England, particularly in London in the heady political days of the GLC*, words like 'sexism' and 'racism' were prevalent in tabloids and on billboards. Support groups and campaign groups proliferated and were funded. By contrast, today in Western countries, we are living in an era of individualism, in a culture that (ironically) privileges the me-culture of 'choice, control and continuity'. It would seem that for many people, indeed many midwives, feminism is either taken for granted or not identified as being central to the multiple issues facing women in a postmodern world. I am reminded of seeing a group of young women lifesavers on an Australian beach being interviewed about their engagement in a holiday job that is traditionally done by men. When

---

*The Greater London Council, led by Ken Livingstone and later disbanded by the Thatcher government, made a commitment to funding initiatives that would raise awareness about antidiscrimination issues.

asked whether they thought this was a 'feminist statement', they replied, 'We haven't studied that in history at school yet'!

It would be easy to write off feminism in relation to midwifery as a 'dinosaur' approach but my understanding of feminism in a postmodern world that privileges diversity and difference is that there are multiple 'feminisms' under the umbrella of 'equal opportunity' and that complex analyses of power dynamics still form the central tenet of these discourses. Key life experiences led me to midwifery and these experiences and understandings continue to resonate in the values and motivation that I bring to all areas of my working life.

Key points

- Life experiences have a significant effect on who we are as midwives and how we are 'with women'.

- The women's liberation movement of the 1970s and 1980s was a major catalyst for consciousness raising and midwifery activism through the Association of Radical Midwives in the UK.

- The notion of 'woman-centred' practice has its roots in feminist ideology and the principles of social justice and primary healthcare.

- Mentors play a significant role in motivating and inspiring midwives.

- The language we use both describes and constructs the culture of midwifery and has the potential to trivialise or disempower women.

- Collective action is an important strategy for change, support and reflection in midwifery.

Questions for Reflection ?????

What issues in my background motivate me as a midwife to change things: my identity/character, social beliefs, politics, life events...?

How do I employ 'rhetorical means of persuasion' in my midwifery life?

How are power dynamics played out in my working life and at home? Are there similarities?

What relevance do books like The Female Eunuch *(Germaine Greer) have for women's lives today?*

Who are the role models/mentors who have inspired me as a midwife?

REFERENCES

Andrews M 1991 Lifetimes of commitment: ageing, politics, psychology. Cambridge University Press, Cambridge, UK

ARM 1986 The vision: proposals for the future of the maternity services. Association of Radical Midwives, Ormskirk, Lancashire

ARM 1999. A vision for midwifery education. Association of Radical Midwives, Ormskirk, Lancashire

Arms S 1975 Immaculate deception: a new look at women and childbirth in America. Houghton Mifflin, Boston

Bizzell P, Herzberg B (eds) 1990 Aristotle. Rhetoric, Book 1. The rhetorical tradition: readings from classical times to the present. Bedford Books, Boston

Boston Women's Health Collective 1971. Our bodies, ourselves. Simon and Schuster, New York

Burtch B 1994. Trials of labour: the re-emergence of midwifery. McGill-Queen's University Press, Montreal

Eldridge Wheeler C, Chinn PI 1991 Peace and power: a handbook of feminist process. National League for Nursing, New York

Flint C 1986 Sensitive midwifery. Heinemann Midwifery, London

Flint C 1988 On the brink: midwifery in Britain. In: Kitzinger S (ed) The midwife challenge. Pandora, London

Freidan B 1963 The feminine mystique. Dell, New York

Gaskin IM 1980 Spiritual midwifery. The Book Publishing Company, Summertown, Tennessee.

Greer G 1970 The female eunuch. MacGibbon and Kee, London

Guilliland K, Pairman S 1995 The midwifery partnership: a model for practice. Victoria University of Wellington, New Zealand

Haire D 1972 The cultural warping of childbirth. International Childbirth Education Association, Minneapolis

Kaufmann T 2002 Midwifery and public health. MIDIRS Midwifery Digest 12 (suppl 1): S23–26

Kelly C, Breinlinger S 1996. The social psychology of collective action: identity, injustice and gender. Taylor and Francis, London

Kirkham M (ed) 2000 The midwife–mother relationship. Macmillan, London

Kitzinger S 1962 The experience of childbirth. Victor Gollancz, London

Kitzinger S 1988 The midwife challenge. Pandora, London

Lang R 1972 Birth book. Genesis Press, Felton, CA

Leap N 1991 Helping you to make your own decisions: antenatal and postnatal groups in Deptford, South East London. VHS video available from Birth International: info@birthinternational.com

Leap N 1992 The power of words and the confinement of women – how language affects midwives' practice. Nursing Times 88(21): 60–61

Leap N 1996 Midwifery perspectives on pain in labour. Unpublished Masters thesis. South Bank University, London

Leap N 1997 Making sense of horizontal violence in midwifery. British Journal of Midwifery 5(11): 689

Leap N 2000a Being with women in pain in labour: towards a midwifery perspective. MIDIRS Digest 10(1): 49–53

Leap N 2000b The less we do, the more we give. In: Kirkham M (ed) The midwife–mother relationship. Macmillan, London

Leap N, Hunter B 1993 The midwife's tale: from handywoman to professional midwife. Scarlet Press, London

Murphy-Lawless J 1998 Reading birth and death: a history of obstetric thinking. Cork University Press, Cork, Eire

O'Neill G 1990 Pull no more bines. The Women's Press, London

Plant R 1987 Managing change: and making it stick. Fontana/Collins, London

Rowbotham S 1973 Woman's consciousness, man's world. Penguin, Harmondsworth

Sandall J 1997 Midwives' burnout and continuity of care. British Journal of Midwifery 4(12): 620–621

Sandall J, Davies J, Warwick C 2001 Evaluation of the Albany Midwifery Practice: final report, March 2001. Florence Nightingale School of Nursing and Midwifery, King's College, London

Stevens T, McCourt C 2002 One-to-one midwifery practice: sustaining the model. British Journal of Midwifery 10(3): 174–179

Warwick C 2000 Address to the launch of the All Party Parliamentary Group on Maternity. House of Commons, 29th November

Wheatley MJ, Kellnor-Rogers M 1996 A simpler way. Berret-Koehler, San Francisco, CA

Index

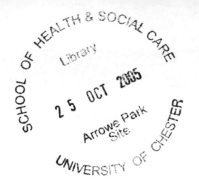

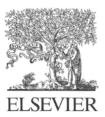
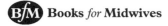
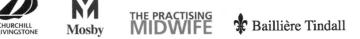
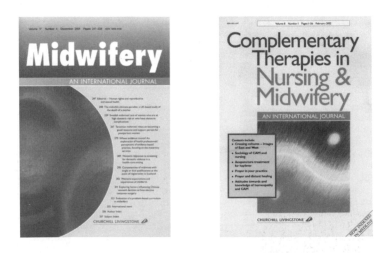
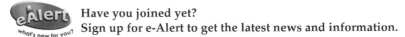